Other Books by Dr. Ronald Hoffman

Seven Weeks to a Settled Stomach
Tired All the Time: How to Regain Your Lost Energy
Natural Approaches to Attention Deficit Disorder
Natural Approaches to Lyme Disease
Natural Approaches to Mitral Valve Prolapse
Intelligent Medicine
How to Talk with Your Doctor (with Sydney Stevens)

Other Books by Dr. Barry Fox

Arthritis for Dummies (with Nadine Taylor)
The Arthritis Cure (with Dr. Jason Theodosakis and Brenda Adderly)
Maximizing the Arthritis Cure (with Dr. Jason Theodosakis and Brenda Adderly)
The Side Effects Bible (with Dr. Frederic Vagnini)
Syndrome X: The Silent Killer (with Dr. Gerald Reaven and Terry Kirsten Strom)
The 20/30 Fat and Fiber Diet Plan (with Dr. Gabe Mirkin)
What Your Doctor May Not Tell You about Hypertension (with Dr. Mark Houston and Nadine Taylor)
What Your Doctor May Not Tell You about Migraines (with Dr. Alexander Mauskop)

ALTERNATIVE CURES *THAT* REALLY WORK

ALTERNATIVE CURES *THAT* REALLY WORK

For the Savvy Health Consumer
A MUST-HAVE GUIDE
to More Than 100 Food Remedies, Herbs,
Supplements, and Healing Techniques

Ronald Hoffman, MD, and Barry Fox, PhD

RODALE

© 2006 by Barry Fox

All rights reserved. No part of this publication may be reproduced or transmitted in any form or by any means, electronic or mechanical, including photocopying, recording, or any other information storage and retrieval system, without the written permission of the publisher.

Rodale books may be purchased for business or promotional use or for special sales. For information, please write to:

Special Markets Department, Rodale Inc., 733 Third Avenue, New York, NY 10017

Printed in the United States of America

Rodale Inc. makes every effort to use acid-free ♾, recycled paper ♻.

Illustrations by Sandy Freeman

Book design by Tara Long

Library of Congress Cataloging-in-Publication Data
Hoffman, Ronald L.
   Alternative cures that really work : for the savvy health consumer—
a must-have guide to more than 100 food remedies, herbs, supplements, and
healing techniques / Ronald Hoffman and Barry Fox.
       p.   cm.
   Includes bibliographical references and index.
   ISBN-13 978–1–59486–452–0   hardcover
   ISBN-10 1–59486–452–7   hardcover
   ISBN-13 978–1–59486–453–7   paperback
   ISBN-10 1–59486–453–5   paperback
   1. Alternative medicine.   I. Fox, Barry.   II. Title.
R733.H615   2006
616—dc22   2006030524

Distributed to the book trade by Holtzbrinck Publishers

		8	10	9	7			hardcover
4	6	8	10	9	7	5	3	paperback

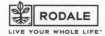

We inspire and enable people to improve their lives and the world around them

For more of our products visit **rodalestore.com** or call 800-848-4735

To all my courageous predecessors in the field of complementary medicine, whether now living or deceased, many of whom withstood scorn and derision for espousing "heretical" ideas. They would be gratified by the progress evinced in this book toward legitimizing the role played by diet, vitamins and minerals, herbs, and other natural therapies in preserving health and reversing disease.

–Dr. Ronald Hoffman

To my father, Arnold Fox, MD,
who always insisted that the patient comes first

–Dr. Barry Fox

CONTENTS

ACKNOWLEDGMENTS

From Dr. Ronald Hoffman: Thanks to my colleague and co-writer, Barry Fox, for his original contributions on how to analyze and rate scientific literature as it pertains to natural therapies. His clear vision inspired me to collaborate on this useful book, which will hopefully provide an authoritative guide to health practitioners and patients alike.

From Dr. Barry Fox: Thanks to my wife, Nadine Fox, who tirelessly read and reread the manuscript and made numerous excellent suggestions for improvement.

1

WHICH ALTERNATIVE CURES REALLY WORK?

Suppose you have osteoarthritis, with pain and stiffness that make it difficult for you to walk, or open a jar, or swing a tennis racquet.

The painkillers that your doctor gave you are tearing up your stomach, and you're worried about reports that they can increase the risk of heart disease. You'd like to find an effective alternative treatment, so you ask around. Your friends and coworkers offer numerous remedies, from copper bracelets to MSM to zinc. You're puzzled. Which of these approaches is backed by solid science? Not animal or laboratory studies, or a series of successful cases. Which is supported by clinical studies with human volunteers?

Or maybe you find yourself wrestling with a mild bout of depression. Your friends suggest homeopathy, mind-body therapies, reflexology, St. John's wort, and 5-HTP. Which of these therapies have proven their mettle in rigorous scientific studies? Which have been praised by the influential Cochrane reviews, or the Agency for Healthcare Research and Quality, or perhaps Germany's prestigious Commission E?

Unfortunately, that kind of information can be hard to find. It exists, but it's scattered about here and there, often buried under layers of myth and misinformation.

GROWING POPULARITY, GROWING CONFUSION

In the not-too-distant past, scientific Western medicine forged ahead of other healing systems, introducing antibiotics that could cure deadly infections, surgical procedures to set bones and remove cancers, pills to ease pain, and much more. In many ways, modern medicine is miraculous, helping to make our lives longer and healthier.

But as we've learned in the past several decades, standard Western medicine does not have all the answers. Physicians will admit they're not always successful in treating chronic pain and many other nagging, sometimes debilitating medical conditions. Some conditions remain incurable, despite all the modern medical advances at physicians' disposal. Even the powerful medicines they prescribe are two-edged swords that can trigger side effects ranging from annoying to deadly.

For these and other reasons, alternative medicine—sometimes called complementary medicine—is rapidly growing in popularity. Surveys show that over 40 million Americans use some form of alternative therapy, be it nutritional supplements, chiropractic, prayer, herbs, meditation, acupuncture, Ayurveda, or another approach. The field of alternative medicine continues to grow in numbers of adherents and practitioners as well as in prestige. Indeed, the National Institutes of Health responded to this burgeoning interest several years ago by opening a branch dedicated to alternatives called the National Center for Complementary and Alternative Medicine.

But not every alternative therapy is effective for every disease. Which raises the question: Which truly work? Not which might work, or which your mother's cousin's accountant once heard were good. Which alternatives have been proven by solid scientific evidence to be effective?

Test Your Knowledge

Unfortunately, there's a great deal of misinformation bandied about in magazine articles, flashed over the Internet, passed from person to person, and even promoted by some alternative healers. Despite the increasing popularity of alternative therapies, many laypeople and physicians simply don't know which therapies have scientific evidence to prove they are effective. Before reading on, take this quick true-false quiz.

T   F   Substances in green tea have been shown to reduce body fat.

T   F   Practicing yoga can help diabetics control their blood sugar.

T   F   Magnesium has been clinically proven to relieve migraines in certain people.

T   F   Dancing and playing board games reduce the risk of dementia.

T   F   X-ray evidence indicates that chondroitin can slow or stop the disease process that causes osteoarthritis.

T   F   Clinical evidence proves that chiropractic effectively relieves asthma.

T   F   Garlic destroys the *Helicobacter pylori* bacteria that can cause ulcers.

T   F   Acupuncture has been clinically proven to relieve tension headaches.

T   F   Glucosamine combats the symptoms of rheumatoid arthritis.

T   F   Studies show that naturopathy is as effective as standard medicine in treating back pain.

The first five statements are true, the next five are false. But surprisingly few people—including many physicians—know which therapies have scientific support and which do not.

RATING THE THERAPIES

To help you separate the wheat from the chaff, we've looked at the scientific evidence behind 110 different alternative therapies for 21 common ailments. Drawing on information from the National Library of Medicine, the World Health Organization, the Food and Drug Administration, the National Institutes of Health, numerous medical journals, and other sources, we've assessed the depth and breadth of scientific information in support of each

COCHRANE REVIEWS AND COMMISSION E

As you read through the discussions of studies in the chapters that follow, you'll notice that we sometimes refer to the Cochrane reviews and Germany's Commission E.

A Cochrane review is an extensive research paper published by the Cochrane Library, which examines the scientific evidence backing the use of specific treatments for various diseases. Cochrane reviews are believed to be very comprehensive and complete, making them authoritative sources of information.

Germany's Commission E is an official government body that could be described as the German FDA for herbs. Established some 30 years ago, it was charged with the task of investigating medicinal herbs. The commission has published a series of documents describing the use, safety, and effectiveness of several hundred herbs.

approach. To help summarize our analyses, we've rated each therapy on a scale ranging from one to five stars. Here's what the ratings mean. (We'll discuss the various types of trials in the next chapter.)

5 Stars = Convincing Evidence: Evidence of efficacy based on a significant body of good-quality clinical evidence (randomized, controlled clinical trials involving several hundred people with endpoints of clinical relevance), plus a positive review or recommendation from a major governmental or advocacy group such as the World Health Organization or the Food and Drug Administration (FDA).

4 Stars = Strong Evidence: Evidence of efficacy based on a significant body of good-quality clinical evidence (randomized, controlled clinical trials involving several hundred people with endpoints of clinical relevance), and/or a recommendation from Germany's Commission E.

3 Stars = Intriguing Evidence: Evidence of efficacy based on a modest body of good-quality clinical evidence (randomized, controlled clinical trials with endpoints of clinical relevance), plus supportive theoretical or population-based evidence.

2 Stars = Modest Evidence: Evidence of efficacy based on a small body of good-quality clinical evidence (randomized, controlled trials with endpoints of clinical relevance) or based primarily on uncontrolled clinical trials, cohort studies, and/or population studies.

1 Star = Preliminary Evidence: Evidence of efficacy based on nonrandomized, laboratory, animal, theoretical, and/or anecdotal evidence.

Five stars is the top rating, but the fact that a therapy earns five or even four stars does not necessarily mean that it will work for you. Just like the standard medicines physicians prescribe, individual alternative therapies work better for some people than for others.

On the other hand, a low rating does not necessarily mean that a therapy is not effective. It simply means that at the time this book was written, only a certain amount of scientific research conducted on humans was available, in English, for review. As new studies become available, a one-star therapy may move quickly up the rating scale.

Unfortunately, our rating system is not fair to certain alternative healing modalities such as homeopathy and Ayurveda. That's because homeopathic and Ayurvedic physicians carefully select individual remedies or regimens best suited to particular patients. It's difficult to evaluate the effectiveness of therapies that offer such an individualized approach with standard clinical trials, in which the goal is to give the same therapy to a large group of people. However, clinical trials are the backbone of our rating system. Thus, we've left Ayurveda out of this book entirely and discuss homeopathy only a few times.

WHICH BRAND IS BEST?

Purchasing an herbal or nutritional supplement can be a daunting task. Which of the two, five, perhaps a dozen brands sitting on the shelves is best?

Selecting a supplement can be difficult for at least three reasons. First, any herb or nutrient may take many forms. For example, we read about vitamin E in textbooks and hear that vitamin E did this or that in the latest study, but there is no single substance we can point to and say it's vitamin E. Instead, there are eight substances with vitamin E activity—that is, eight related compounds that do things vitamin E is credited with doing. Alpha-tocopherol is perhaps the best known of the eight. The others are beta-tocopherol, gamma-tocopherol, delta-tocopherol, alpha-tocotrienol, beta-tocotrienol, gamma-tocotrienol, and delta-tocotrienol. Most vitamin E supplements contain alpha-tocopherol—but an alpha-tocopherol-only supplement may not perform the same as a supplement containing some or all of the others.

Second, even where there is only one form of a supplement, there are often many "versions" of it. All St. John's wort, for example, is not the same. There is no standard "ingredient list" for this herb, and no agreement on how much of which of the many chemicals in St. John's wort should be included, so various manufacturers have produced differing extracts of St. John's wort. How can you tell which one really works?

Third, sad to say, some manufacturers use inferior materials and/or manufacturing procedures. The supplements they sell do not contain what the labels claim they do, or do not release their active ingredients well inside the digestive tract, or are contaminated with other substances that may interfere with the working of the active ingredient—or may be harmful in and of themselves.

How can you tell which brand to buy? Given all the confusion, it's often best to choose the brand used in the successful studies. That's why, in the discussion of studies in the coming chapters, we have indicated the name of the brand used, when that information is available. When it's not, we provide the name of the company supplying the materials for the study, if possible.

In studies where an herbal or nutritional supplement is compared to a standard medicine, we have included a brand name of the medicine in parentheses following the generic name. It's not necessarily the brand used in the study, for many drugs have more than one brand name. We simply chose one many people would be familiar with, so they could easily identify the medicine.

Despite its limitations, our rating system can help you sort through your options to find what might work best for you.

HOW TO USE THIS BOOK

In the chapters ahead, we'll be discussing alternative therapies for 21 separate ailments. It would be impossible to cover all the possible therapies for each ailment in a single book. Instead, we've selected the "hot" therapies, the ones we're asked about most. Some of them are backed by a substantial amount of scientific study, others by a moderate amount. Still others have relatively little backing, but they're the subject of great interest.

We suggest that you begin by reading Chapter 2 to learn a little about interpreting scientific studies. Next, turn to a chapter that addresses a condition you're interested in. There you'll find a brief explanation of the condition, plus an overview of the drugs and/or therapies usually recommended by conventionally trained medical doctors. Then comes the heart of the chapter: the list of common alternative therapies for the condition, followed by a brief discussion of the supporting scientific evidence and a rating for each.

When appropriate, we provide dosage instructions for an alternative therapy as well as information on possible side effects and interactions. The point is not to alarm you or suggest that alternative therapies are dangerous. Rather, it is to remind you that even the most seemingly innocuous therapies can have hidden and harmful consequences you should be aware of. In particular, interactions with standard medicines are unpredictable, not fully understood, and not yet fully catalogued. For this reason, you should speak with your doctor before embarking on an alternative therapy or changing your standard care in any way. The information in this book will be a good starting point for your conversation.

2

UNDERSTANDING MEDICAL STUDIES

Medical studies are filled with sometimes confusing terms such as epide-miological, randomized, double-blind, and placebo-controlled. They may seem confusing, but they're fairly easy to understand if you take them one by one.

THREE TYPES OF STUDIES INVOLVING HUMANS

Let's start with the types of studies. You can think of human health stud-ies as falling into three categories: counting, observing over time, and manipulating.

Counting studies do just that—they count the number of people who have a particular disease, who eat a certain amount of meat per year, who exercise regularly, who smoke, and so on. For a typical counting study, researchers might identify a certain group of people—such as men over the age of 50—and count various things about them. The data can be used to paint a picture of that group—telling us, for example, that the average male over 50 weighs 195 pounds, has mild pain in one knee, eats fish twice a week, was not exposed to asbestos at work, and has a total cholesterol of 237 mg/dL (milligrams per deciliter of blood). A counting study could go further, comparing one factor to another to find that men who eat fish three or more times a week have lower cholesterol than men who eat fish once a week or less.

Counting studies are known as population studies or epidemiological studies. They are statistical "snapshots" of a certain moment in time. They can link things to each other—like lower cholesterol and greater consump-tion of fish—but cannot prove that one causes the other.

For an observing-over-time study, researchers select a group of people—or maybe a couple of groups—and count many things about them. Then they watch to see what happens over the course of years, even decades. The most famous observing-over-time study is the Framingham Study, which began back in 1948. Researchers enlisted thousands of people living in Framingham, Massachusetts, then measured their weight and height, counted how much and what kinds of food they ate, kept records of their exercise habits and stress levels, and so on. As decades passed, the researchers recounted and recounted, developing thousands of "detail histories" that tracked the volunteers' lives and health.

An observing-over-time study can reveal information such as that people who began exercising in high school and continued to do so into middle age have less heart disease, or that those who eat diets rich in magnesium and riboflavin have fewer migraines. Observing-over-time studies are also known as cohort studies (in this context, a cohort is a group of people). If a counting study is like a snapshot, an observing-over-time study is like a movie showing events unfolding over a period of time. But like the counting studies, observing-over-time studies can only link things to each other; they cannot prove that one causes the other.

Manipulating studies are the only ones that can prove one thing causes another. For a manipulating study, researchers deliberately change something—what the people in the study eat, which medicines they take, how often they exercise, and so on. For example, researchers might give medicine X to people with elevated blood pressure and then watch to see whether their pressure drops over the course of a few days or weeks. Or a group of people with insomnia might take herb Y to see if it helps them sleep better. Manipulating studies are also called clinical trials, clinical studies, or experimental studies.

UNDERSTANDING CLINICAL TRIALS

In discussions of clinical trials, you may come across one or more of the following terms:

Placebo: A "fake treatment" designed to resemble the real thing. A typical placebo is a pill that's the same size, shape, and color as a real medicine but doesn't contain any active medicinal ingredients. Not all placebos are in pill form, however. In an acupuncture study, for example, the placebo may consist of deliberately inserting acupuncture needles in the wrong places. In a food study, some participants may be given muffins containing psyllium fiber, and others, muffins with wheat bran. In this case, the psyllium fiber is the "real thing" and the wheat bran muffin is the placebo.

Placebo effect: The phenomenon that often occurs when people are given any kind of treatment, even a worthless one. The body can translate the hope that things will be better into actual chemical/cellular/physiologic changes. These changes, in turn, can reduce the symptoms of a disease. It's common for 20 or 30 percent of the volunteers in a study to experience the placebo effect and feel better.

Placebo-controlled: Giving some study volunteers a real medicine and others a placebo. The placebo effect can skew study results and make even a worthless treatment seem effective, so researchers look to see if the real medicine can outperform a placebo. (Think of *controlled* as meaning "compared," so *placebo-controlled* means "compared to placebo.")

Controlled: Often times, a treatment being studied is compared not to a placebo but to another treatment. For example, a vitamin supplement may be pitted against a standard drug to see how well the supplement relieves migraines. In this case the study is "controlled" but it is not "placebo-controlled."

Blind: Not allowing someone to know who is getting a real medicine or a placebo until the end of a study. This is important, because if a participant knows she is getting a placebo she might stop taking it, or drop out of the study, or report that her sympt,oms are getting worse. Or, if a treating doctor knows which study volunteers are getting the real medicine and which the placebo, he might pay more attention to some patients than to others, give more credence to the symptoms of some patients than others, and so on.

Single-blind: When one group of people involved in a study does not know who is receiving the real medicine and who is getting the placebo. In a typical single-blind study, the physicians know which group is receiving the medicine and which the placebo, but the volunteers do not.

Double-blind: When two groups of people participating in a study do not know who is being treated with real medicine and who is getting a placebo. In a double-blind study, it's typically the participants and the treating doctors who are blinded.

Open-label: When nobody is blinded, so the volunteers, the treating doctors, and everyone else involved in the study knows that all the volunteers are taking the real medicine. Placebos are not used in open-label studies.

Randomized: If study volunteers are going to be divided into groups, it's vital that the groups be equal. That is, the people in the groups should be of approximately the same age, weight, cholesterol level, education level, and so on. They should also have the same "sickness" level. To make sure this happens, and to ensure that there is no deliberate or inadvertent prejudice in assigning people to the study groups, the volunteers are randomly assigned to the groups.

Crossover: When the volunteers in a study take both the real medicine and the placebo, one at a time and in different orders. For example, the participants may be divided into two groups. Group 1 takes the medicine for a month, then the placebo for a month, while Group 2 takes the placebo for a month followed by the medicine for a month. The volunteers would be blinded, so they wouldn't know when they were taking the real medicine or the placebo. Crossover studies are useful for eliminating confusion that might arise because of subtle differences between the two study groups. Since everyone has taken the real medicine and the placebo, although at different times, in a sense everyone belongs to both the "real medicine group" and the "placebo group."

Sample size: The number of people participating in a study. There is no set minimum or maximum number of people required for a study. Some studies involve only 10 or 20 volunteers, while others enroll thousands.

Study duration: How long a study lasts, which can vary greatly from one to the next. For example, a study examining how eating a certain food influences postprandial (after eating) blood sugar levels may run only a few hours, while one tracking the long-term effects of exercise may last for decades.

Long-term side effects: Side effects that can take months or even years to appear. They may be missed in studies lasting only a few weeks or months.

Endpoint: What the researchers are interested in seeing happen—that is, the objective of the study. For example, in a study of a treatment for elevated cholesterol, the endpoint might be a reduction in total cholesterol or in LDL cholesterol. There can be several endpoints. For a study of a treatment for prostate enlargement, the endpoints might be a reduction in the number of nighttime urinations, in the amount of time needed to begin urination, and in how much urine remains in the bladder upon completion of urination. A study also can have primary and secondary endpoints. For a study of an osteoarthritis treatment, the primary endpoint may be a halt to joint space narrowing as seen on x-rays, and the secondary endpoint could be improvement in the patients' subjective reports of pain.

A BRIEF WORD ON SIGNIFICANCE

When used in clinical trials, the word *significant* does not mean important, large, or noteworthy. Instead, it means statistically relevant. This, in turn, means that statistical methods have been used to demonstrate that the study results are not simply a matter of chance and that they almost certainly occurred for the reasons the researchers had hypothesized.

Results that are statistically significant are considered superior to nonsignificant results. But be wary when you read that something is significant, for results can be statistically significant yet not vital. For example, statistical analysis may demonstrate that treatment X significantly reduces cholesterol, but that reduction might be only 1 mg/dL. The drop in cholesterol level is statistically significant but not very large.

UNDERSTANDING REVIEW STUDIES AND META-ANALYSES

Medical evidence is like old *National Geographic* magazines: It keeps piling up, higher and higher and higher. As more and more studies—clinical trials, cohort studies, population studies, studies with animals, and studies conducted solely in test tubes—are performed, it becomes increasingly difficult to keep track of them all.

To complicate matters, it's quite common for studies of the same treatment to reach different conclusions. Sometimes the differences are small; perhaps one study indicates 10 milligrams is the optimal dose of supplement X while another suggests it's 11 milligrams. But oftentimes the differences are large, with some studies establishing that a therapy works and others demonstrating that it doesn't.

In an attempt to sort through such conflicting evidence, experts will write a review study. Typically, the review study describes the results of key studies, discusses why they may have arrived at different or conflicting results, and attempts to draw its own conclusion about the treatment in question. The review study is not based on new information; rather, it uses existing information.

A meta-analysis also tries to arrive at a new conclusion based on existing information. But instead of simply assembling and discussing individual clinical studies, it uses statistical methods to combine their results into one "giant" study.

IS THERE A "BEST" STUDY?

The various types of studies all provide valuable information. Sometimes only certain types of studies will work. A clinical trial won't tell you how many women age 60 and over have breast cancer, or how healthy the men who participated in collegiate athletics are once they reach their fifties. A population study is used to find the answer to the first question, while a cohort study is appropriate for the second.

When it comes to determining how effective a given treatment is, the clinical trial is considered best. It is the only type of study that can prove that a treatment does or does not work. There's even a hierarchy to clinical trials, with the open-label, nonrandomized, unblinded, noncontrolled study being the least persuasive, and the randomized, double-blind, placebo-controlled study being the most persuasive.

For even more definitive answers, researchers turn to the meta-analysis. This statistical blend of several clinical studies is believed to offer the definitive answer to the question: Is this treatment effective?

YOU'RE READY TO MOVE ON!

In the chapters that follow, the studies that serve as the basis for our one- to five-star remedy ratings were the most recently published in recognized medical and scientific journals or available in standard medical databases, in English, at the time this book was written. Other studies may have been conducted, but they were not available or did not meet our selection criteria.

That's all you need to know to understand the discussion of the studies in this book. You're ready to start reading about the scientific evidence supporting alternative therapies.

ALTERNATIVE APPROACHES TO

ALZHEIMER'S DISEASE

Ginkgo biloba ☆☆☆
Phosphatidylserine ☆☆☆
Vitamin E ☆☆☆
Idebenone ☆☆
Omega-3 fatty acids ☆☆

Alzheimer's disease (AD) is a form of dementia, a brain disorder that seriously interferes with a person's ability to carry out daily activities. It's the most common type of dementia found among older people, affecting the parts of the brain that control language, thought, and memory.

Identified in 1906 by a German doctor named Alois Alzheimer, AD has been called "the disease of plaques and tangles" as it involves a buildup of clumps of protein on the outside of brain cells (*amyloid plaques*) and twisted strands of another kind of protein inside the cells (*neurofibrillary tangles*). AD disrupts connections between brain cells and causes the death of the cells.

Currently affecting about 5 million Americans, AD usually begins after age 60, although it is not a normal part of aging. Symptoms last an average of 8 years from diagnosis to death, slowly worsening with time. AD eventually robs its victims of their personalities as well as their ability to walk, speak, eat, and even smile.

SYMPTOMS

The symptoms of AD appear gradually, beginning with brief memory lapses such as forgetting familiar words or names and losing or misplacing things. Symptoms can progress to trouble performing at work or in social situations, difficulty comprehending or remembering written material, and a decline in the ability to plan or organize. It may become difficult to perform such complex tasks as paying bills, driving, grocery shopping, doing arithmetic problems, or cooking a meal.

People in the middle stages of AD may find themselves unable to remember where they live or how to brush their teeth or dress themselves. They may fail to recognize familiar faces or places and forget the names of close relatives and friends.

In the later stages of AD, people may lose awareness of their surroundings, wander away from home, and become aggressive or anxious. Eventually, they may be unable to accomplish the most basic tasks, such as eating or going to the toilet. Toward the end of their lives they can require total care.

CAUSES

Scientists don't know exactly what causes AD. They do know that age and heredity can increase a person's risk of developing the disease.

STANDARD TREATMENTS

Although there is no cure for AD, there are certain medications that can improve cognitive function and slow mental decline. They include donepezil (Aricept), ENA-713 (Exelon), galantamine (Reminyl), memantine (Namenda), and tacrine (Cognex). With the exception of memantine, these drugs are effective only during the early to middle stages of the disease. The behavioral problems seen with AD may be treated with medications such as the antipsychotic risperidone (Risperidol), the selective serotonin reuptake inhibitors (SSRI) antidepressants (such as Prozac or Paxil), and anti-anxiety drugs from the benzodiazepine family (such as Valium).

RATING POPULAR ALTERNATIVE TREATMENTS FOR ALZHEIMER'S DISEASE

Ginkgo Biloba

Rating: ☆☆☆ = Intriguing Evidence

Ginkgo biloba comes from a tree native to Japan and China. Practitioners of traditional Chinese medicine have been using ginkgo for medicinal purposes for thousands of years.

Scientists do not fully understand ginkgo's mechanisms of action, but it may help reduce oxidative and free radical damage. Oxidants and free radicals occur in the body as a result of normal metabolism as well as exposure to smog and other toxins. Oxidants and free radicals can harm healthy tissues, which is why the body manufactures substances to "disarm" them. Oftentimes, however, oxidants and free radicals overwhelm the body's defense mechanisms, damaging cells and other tissues and possibly setting the stage for heart disease, cancer, and other ailments.

Ginkgo biloba also may help improve bloodflow to the heart, reduce the risk of dangerous blood clots, and boost the immune system. Extracts of ginkgo biloba are used to treat a variety of ailments, including headache, dizziness, PMS, and sexual problems, as well as Alzheimer's disease and other forms of dementia.

Ginkgo biloba is thought to help treat and possibly prevent Alzheimer's by guarding against oxidative damage to brain cells and helping to control the inflammation that may be linked to development of the disease. More than 50 studies and review articles have looked at ginkgo's effects on Alzheimer's. Here is a sampling:

♦ A 1997 study published in the *Journal of the American Medical Association* compared ginkgo biloba extract to a placebo in 202 people with mild to severe dementia associated with either Alzheimer's disease or multiple strokes.[1] For this randomized, double-blind study, the volunteers were assigned to receive either 120 milligrams of a European ginkgo biloba extract (EGb 761) or a placebo every day for 52 weeks. The patients' progress was tracked using the Alzheimer's Disease Assessment Scale–Cognitive subscale, the Geriatric Evaluation by Relative's Rating Instrument (GERRI), and other measurements. The results were positive, with the ginkgo biloba extract triggering "modest" improvements in the rating scales. The researchers concluded that this ginkgo biloba extract "appears capable of stabilizing and, in a substantial number of cases, improving the cognitive performance and the social functioning of demented patients for 6 months to 1 year."

♦ German researchers compared a ginkgo biloba extract to placebo in people with either dementia of the Alzheimer's type or dementia associated with multiple strokes.[2] One hundred fifty-six men and women, all age 55 or older, completed this randomized, double-blind study, which was published in *Pharmacopsychiatry* in 1996. The participants were assigned to receive either 240 milligrams of ginkgo biloba extract (EGb 761) or a placebo every day for 24 weeks. The researchers used the Clinical Global Impressions Scale, Syndrom-Kurztest, and other tools to track the participants' progress. By comparing beginning and ending scores on the scales as well as other data, the researchers concluded that the ginkgo biloba extract was clinically effective in treating both dementia of the Alzheimer's type and related to multiple strokes.

♦ Researchers from the Oregon Health Sciences University and the Portland Veterans Affairs Medical Center published a meta-analysis of ginkgo biloba/Alzheimer's disease studies in the *Archives of Neurology* in 1998.[3] They scoured the medical literature for randomized, double-blind, placebo-controlled studies that met their methodological criteria, using statistical methods to "marry" the four they found into a single, larger analysis. The researchers found that "there is a small but significant effect of 3- to 6-month treatment with 120 to 240 [milligrams] of G. biloba extract on objective measures of cognitive function" in Alzheimer's disease.

Summing Up the Evidence for Ginkgo Biloba

With a modest number of clinical studies supporting its use, it's fair to say that ginkgo biloba is a three-star treatment for Alzheimer's disease backed by intriguing evidence.

Other Names

Ginkgo biloba is known in various parts of the world by many names, including fossil tree, Japanese silver apricot, kew tree, and yinsing.

Available Forms

Ginkgo biloba is available in capsule, tablet, fluid extract, and tincture form.

How Much Ginkgo Biloba Is Typically Used

There is no standard dose of ginkgo biloba as a preventive or treatment for Alzheimer's disease. Supplemental doses in key studies ranged from 120 to 240 milligrams per day.

Possible Side Effects and Interactions

Supplementation with ginkgo biloba may cause headache, anxiety, loss of appetite, and rash. The herb also can interact with common pain relievers such as aspirin and ibuprofen and diabetes medications such as glipizide (Glucotrol), among other drugs. If you currently are taking any medication, be sure to consult your doctor before adding ginkgo biloba to your self-care regimen.

Phosphatidylserine

Rating: ☆☆☆ = Intriguing Evidence

A fatlike substance manufactured within the human body, phosphatidylserine has important duties in the brain. It helps brain cells maintain their proper internal environment, communicate with other cells, and store and retrieve information. Phosphatidylserine has been shown to increase levels of important brain chemicals (or neurotransmitters) such as serotonin and dopamine in people with Alzheimer's disease.

Some studies suggest that phosphatidylserine might help restore cognitive function in those with dementia of the Alzheimer's type or other forms. Among the studies are the following:

◆ German researchers enlisted 33 people with early dementia of the Alzheimer's type for their 1992 double-blind, crossover study comparing phosphatidylserine to placebo.[4] All of the volunteers took 300 milligrams of phosphatidylserine every day for 8 weeks followed by a placebo every day for 8 weeks, or the placebo followed by phosphatidylserine. The supplement was provided by Fidia Research Laboratories in Italy. While phosphatidylserine did not trigger improvement in all areas targeted by the researchers, it did produce "a small but significant improvement according to the clinicians' global judgment."

◆ Phosphatidylserine was compared to placebo in a randomized, double-blind study published in the *Psychopharmacology Bulletin* in 1988.[5] The 142 study participants, who ranged in age from 40 to 80, were assigned to take either 200 milligrams of phosphatidylserine (from Fidia Research Laboratories) or a placebo every day for 3 months. Their cognitive function was tested at the beginning and the end of the 3-month treatment period, and at several points during the 21 months following treatment. Cognitive progress or decline was tracked using the Randt

Memory Test, the Babcock Story Recall Test, and several other tools. The results were mixed, leading the researchers to conclude that oral supplemental doses of phosphatidylserine "may improve performance on selected cognitive variables." The researchers noted that severely impaired patients showed substantially greater improvement than those with lesser degrees of cognitive decline, suggesting that the supplement may help certain patients.

Summing Up the Evidence for Phosphatidylserine

It's difficult to make a definitive statement about the use of phosphatidylserine for Alzheimer's disease, since some of the studies that produced positive results were performed before clearly defined clinical diagnostic criteria were devised. This means, in effect, that only a modest number of newer studies are available for analysis. At this point, it is best to say that phosphatidylserine is a three-star treatment for Alzheimer's disease backed by intriguing evidence.

Available Forms

Phosphatidylserine is available in supplement form.

How Much Phosphatidylserine Is Typically Used

There is no standard dose of phosphatidylserine for Alzheimer's disease. Supplemental doses in studies have ranged from 200 to 300 milligrams per day.

Possible Side Effects and Interactions

Phosphatidylserine's side effects include insomnia and gastrointestinal upset. The supplement does not appear to interact in a significant way with standard medications. As with all supplements and drugs, be sure to read the label directions before using phosphatidylserine.

Vitamin E

Rating: ☆☆☆ = Intriguing Evidence

Vitamin E was discovered when scientists realized that a certain substance in food was necessary if laboratory animals were to bear young. This substance was given the scientific name *tocopherol*, which means "to bring forth children." Today we know that in addition to reproduction, vitamin E is necessary for the production of red blood cells and muscle tissue. It also functions as a powerful antioxidant.

What most people think of as a single vitamin is actually a "family" of eight substances that have vitamin E activity within the body. four of these substances are called tocopherols (alpha-, beta-, gamma-, and delta-tocopherol), and four are tocotrienols (alpha-, beta-, gamma-, and delta-tocotrienol). Vitamin E supplements typically are made from alpha-tocopherol.

The theory that certain vitamins—especially antioxidants such as vitamin E—can slow the progress of Alzheimer's disease has been tested over the course of many years, producing mixed results.

♦ A key study examining the efficacy of vitamin E supplements was performed by a team of American researchers and published in the *New England Journal of Medicine* in 1997.[6] Three hundred forty-one people with moderately severe Alzheimer's disease participated in this randomized, double-blind, placebo-controlled study comparing vitamin E to a drug called selegiline (Eldepryl). The volunteers were assigned to receive daily doses of 2,000 IU of vitamin E in the form of dl-alpha-tocopherol (manufactured by Hoffmann-LaRoche), 10 milligrams of selegiline, vitamin E plus selegiline, or a placebo. The treatment period lasted for 2 years, during which researchers kept track of the number of volunteers who were put in an institution, lost the ability to perform basic activities of daily life, developed severe dementia, or died. While both the vitamin and the drug slowed the rate of decline, an average of 670 days passed before one of the aforementioned events occurred in the vitamin E group, compared to 655 days in the selegiline group, 585 days in the vitamin E plus selegiline group, and only 440 days in the placebo group. The researchers concluded that "treatment with selegiline or alpha-tocopherol or both was beneficial in delaying the primary outcome of disease prevention."

♦ For a study published in the *American Journal of Clinical Nutrition* in 2005, researchers from Rush University Medical Center in Chicago looked at the kinds and amounts of vitamin E consumed by a group of 1,041 senior citizens.[7] Specifically, the researchers measured the amount of vitamin E, the alpha-tocopherol equivalents, and the individual tocopherols consumed from food, then used statistical methods to compare all three to the risk of developing Alzheimer's disease. The researchers found that larger intakes of vitamin E from food "were associated with a reduced incidence of Alzheimer disease." (Alpha-tocopherol equivalents measure the biological activity of the eight substances in the vitamin E family.)

Summing Up the Evidence for Vitamin E

Studies published in the *New England Journal of Medicine*, such as the one described on page 19, typically carry a lot of weight. However, since just a single study indicates that vitamin E may slow the progression of Alzheimer's disease, the evidence is intriguing but modest. And while this particular study found vitamin E to be effective for those with moderately severe Alzheimer's disease, other studies have suggested that vitamin E is not helpful for those with milder versions of Alzheimer's and that it does not lower the risk of developing the disease in the first place. To further complicate the issue, it's still unclear which form of the vitamin is effective or most effective and whether it is best consumed from food or taken in supplement form. At this point it is fair to say that vitamin E is a three-star treatment for Alzheimer's disease backed by intriguing evidence.

Available Forms

Among the food sources of vitamin E are wheat germ oil, almonds, corn oil, soybean oil, broccoli, pistachios, and kiwifruit. It is also available in supplement form.

How Much Vitamin E Is Typically Used

There is no standard dose of vitamin E for Alzheimer's disease. The dose used in the successful *New England Journal of Medicine* study was 2,000 IU per day, in the form of alpha-tocopherol.

Possible Side Effects and Interactions

The Food and Nutrition Board of the Institute of Medicine has set a tolerable upper limit of 1,000 milligrams of vitamin E per day for adults. Taking excessive amounts of supplemental vitamin E may interfere with the action of vitamin K and increase the risk of bleeding. In addition, vitamin E can interact with blood thinners such as warfarin (Coumadin, Jantoven), among other medications. Conversely, the body's ability to utilize vitamin E may be impaired by cholesterol- or blood-fat-lowering drugs such as colesevelam (WelChol). If you are taking any medication, be sure to consult your doctor before adding vitamin E to your self-care regimen.

Idebenone

Rating: ☆☆ = Modest Evidence

Idebenone is a synthetic "cousin" to coenzyme Q_{10}, a substance manufactured by the body that helps control blood pressure and prevent the conversion of "bad" LDL cholesterol into its more dangerous form. Believed to be an antioxidant and to play a role in cellular energy production, idebenone may guard against nerve damage while stimulating nerve growth. Idebenone is used as a treatment for a number of medical conditions, including liver disease, heart disease, and a neurological disorder called Friedreich's ataxia.

A modest body of evidence suggests that idebenone may be helpful in slowing the progression of Alzheimer's disease. For example:

♦ A 1997 study published in *Neuropsychobiology* compared two doses of idebenone to placebo in 247 people, ages 50 to 90, with probable Alzheimer's disease.[8] For this randomized, double-blind study, the volunteers were assigned to receive 90 milligrams of idebenone, 270 milligrams of idebenone, or a placebo every day for 6 months. The primary means of tracking the patients' progress was through changes in their scores on the Alzheimer's Disease Assessment Scale–Total. At the end of the 6-month treatment period, those who had been taking 270 milligrams of idebenone showed "statistically significant improvement" in their test scores. The researchers concluded that these results "demonstrate the efficacy of idebenone in improving signs of dementia."

♦ Researchers developed a complex design for a 1998 study conducted at 14 health centers in Germany.[9] The study compared two doses of idebenone to placebo for the first year, then different doses of idebenone to each other during the second year. Four hundred fifty people, ages 40 to 90, with probable Alzheimer's disease were randomly assigned to one of three groups:

◇ Group 1 received a placebo every day for 12 months, followed by 270 milligrams of idebenone every day for 12 months
◇ Group 2 received 270 milligrams of idebenone every day for 24 months
◇ Group 3 received 360 milligrams of idebenone every day for 24 months

The researchers used the Alzheimer's Disease Assessment Scale–Total, the Clinical Global Response scale, the Nurses' Observation Scale for Geriatric Patients, and other tools to assess the effectiveness of the various doses of idebenone. During the first year of treatment, when idebenone was compared to placebo, idebenone produced "statistically significant" improvement according to all scales. During the second year, when different doses of idebenone were compared to each other, there was continued improvement, with those on the larger dose of idebenone scoring higher on several scales than those on the lower dose. The researchers concluded that "idebenone exerts its beneficial therapeutic effects on the course of the disease by slowing down its progression."

♦ German researchers pitted idebenone head-to-head against tacrine (Cognex), a standard Alzheimer's drug, for a 2002 randomized, double-blind study.[10] Two hundred three people between the ages of 40 and 90, all with probable Alzheimer's disease, participated in the study. They were assigned to receive 360 milligrams of idebenone or up to 160 milligrams of tacrine every day for 60 weeks. At the end of the treatment period, "patients randomized to idebenone showed a higher benefit from treatment than patients randomized to tacrine." Table 3-1 on the next page compares how people responded to idebenone and tacrine on various scales.

Summing Up the Evidence for Idebenone

A relatively new supplement, idebenone is a two-star treatment for Alzheimer's disease backed by modest evidence.

Table 3-1: Both Idebenone and Standard Medication Trigger Improvement in Patients with Probable Alzheimer's Disease[11]

ASSESSMENT SCALES (LOWER SCORES ARE BETTER)	IDEBENONE GROUP		TACRINE GROUP	
	Beginning Score	Ending Score	Beginning Score	Ending Score
Alzheimer's Disease Assessment Scale– Total Score	41.55	34.51	41.52	30.44
Alzheimer's Disease Assessment Scale– Cognitive Subscore	30.23	26.4	30.93	24.81
Alzheimer's Disease Assessment Scale– Noncognitive Subscore	11.32	8.11	10.55	5.63
Clinical Global Impressions– Severity of Illness	5.22	4.43	5.19	4.53
Nurses Observation Scale for Geriatric Patients– Instrumental Activities of Daily Living Subscale	13.88	13.13	13.78	12.5

Available Forms

Idebenone is available in supplement form.

How Much Idebenone Is Typically Used

There is no standard dose of idebenone as a treatment for Alzheimer's. Supplemental doses in studies have ranged from 270 to 360 milligrams per day.

Possible Side Effects and Interactions

There have been no reports of significant side effects, or of interactions, with the dosages of idebenone used in studies. As with all supplements and drugs, be sure to read the label directions before using idebenone.

Omega-3 Fatty Acids

Rating: ☆☆ = Modest Evidence

Back in the 1970s, scientists wondered why Eskimos rarely developed heart disease despite the fact that their diets consisted almost entirely of very fatty fish. Research led the investigators to discover a group of heart-protective substances known as omega-3 fatty acids within the fat of the fish. The best known of the omega-3s are DHA (short for docosahexaenoic acid) and EPA (eicosapentaenoic acid).

Omega-3 fatty acids are found in the human brain, with high levels of DHA located in the mitochondria, cerebral cortex, and other areas that exhibit high levels of metabolic activity. This, plus interesting results of animal studies, led to the idea that omega-3 fatty acids may help slow the cognitive decline seen with Alzheimer's disease.

Only a few studies have tested this concept. They include the following:

♦ A study published in the *Archives of Neurology* in 2003 examined the effect of supplemental omega-3 fatty acids on the risk of developing Alzheimer's disease.[12] Researchers recruited 815 people ranging in age from 65 to 94, none with Alzheimer's disease, and tracked their mental health and lifestyle habits—including how much fish and omega-3 fatty acids they consumed—for an average of slightly more than 2 years. The study results showed that people who consumed at least one fish meal per week were 60 percent less likely to develop Alzheimer's disease than those who rarely or never ate fish. As for the specific omega-3 fatty acids, "only DHA . . . was protective against the development of Alzheimer's disease." The omega-3 known as alpha-linolenic acid also guarded against the onset of Alzheimer's disease, but only in those who had a certain genetic factor known as apolipoprotein E4 (apo ε4).

♦ For a 2002 cohort study published in the *British Medical Journal*, French researchers tracked the mental health and lifestyle habits of 1,674 senior citizens who did not have dementia.[13] Over a period of 2 to 7 years, the researchers monitored the volunteers' consumption of fish and seafood (to calculate the amount of omega-3 fatty acids consumed from food), and noted which volunteers developed Alzheimer's disease. The results indicated that "elderly people who eat fish or seafood at least once a week are at lower risk of developing dementia, including Alzheimer's disease."

◆ The Agency for Healthcare Research and Quality, part of the US Department of Health and Human Services, assessed the level of evidence supporting the use of omega-3 fatty acids for Alzheimer's disease in a 2005 report.[14] The authors of this report surveyed the scientific literature to find that "fish consumption was associated with a reduced risk of Alzheimer's dementia." However, only in one study did the link between fish consumption and a reduced risk of developing Alzheimer's disease reach statistical significance.

Summing Up the Evidence for Omega-3 Fatty Acids

Although omega-3 fatty acids have been the subject of investigation for many years, the existing evidence indicates that for Alzheimer's disease, they're a two-star treatment backed by modest evidence.

Available Forms

As Table 3-2 shows, the best sources of omega-3 fatty acids are cold-water fatty fish such as mackerel, salmon, herring, anchovies, tuna, and bluefish. As a general rule, the fattier the fish, the more omega-3s it contains. The human body can manufacture omega-3s from alpha-linolenic acid, which is found in walnuts and flaxseed. Omega-3 fatty acids are also available in supplement form, labeled fish oil, omega-3, EPA, DHA, or some combination of these.

Table 3-2: Fish Rich in Omega-3 Fatty Acids

Fish, Raw (3.5 oz)	EPA and DHA (grams)
Mackerel	2.30
Herring	1.55
Anchovy	1.45
Salmon, Chinook	1.35
Tuna	1.15
Bluefish	0.75
Swordfish	0.65

Amount of Omega-3 Fatty Acids Typically Used

There is no standard dose of omega-3 fatty acids to treat or prevent Alzheimer's disease. Some experts suggest eating 2 to 5 fatty fish meals per week—but the fish should not be fried because this preparation method destroys omega-3s.

Possible Side Effects and Interactions

The omega-3 fatty acids have been granted Generally Regarded as Safe (GRAS) status by the US government. They may prolong bleeding time, which could be a problem for those who have bleeding disorders, those who are taking medicines to thin the blood, or those who will be undergoing surgery soon. In addition, omega-3s may interact with aspirin, heparin, and other drugs that thin the blood. If you're taking any medication, be sure to consult your doctor before adding omega-3 fatty acids to your self-care regimen.

4

ALTERNATIVE APPROACHES TO

ANXIETY

Kava ☆☆☆☆
Valerian ☆☆☆☆
Tryptophan/5-HTP ☆☆☆

Anxiety is a feeling of fear, apprehension, unease, or agitation that occurs when you sense that some kind of danger or threat lies just around the corner. It may arise in response to something as specific as losing a job or a spouse or as general as life's daily uncertainties. Anxiety almost always influences the way you think, feel, and behave.

All of us experience anxiety from time to time. It is a normal and necessary reaction that increases alertness and gets the body ready for action. But when anxious feelings become overwhelming, occur frequently, last for an extended period, or interfere with the ability to function, they may be signs of an anxiety disorder.

SYMPTOMS

The anxiety disorders are a group of related illnesses that include generalized anxiety disorder, phobias, panic disorders, post-traumatic stress disorder, and obsessive-compulsive disorder. All of these illnesses involve unrealistic or excessive worry over a perceived threat. Whether this threat is real or imagined, large or small, the anxious feelings it causes can bring about a variety of physical, emotional, and behavioral symptoms, including:

- ◆ muscle tension
- ◆ rapid heartbeat
- ◆ shallow breathing

- difficulty concentrating
- dizziness, shakiness, or tremor
- eating more or less than usual
- upset stomach or "butterflies" in the stomach
- sleep disturbances
- excessive worrying
- tapping the feet or drumming the fingers
- nail biting
- "freezing" or feeling unable to act
- intense fear of failure or imperfection
- living in the future and predicting the worst outcome
- magnifying the significance of bad things that happen
- unrealistic fears of objects or situations
- avoidance of feared object or event
- a feeling of being out of control or unable to cope

Theories about the origins of anxiety abound, running the gamut from subconscious conflicts arising from childhood traumas to biochemical imbalances, to the idea that anxiety is a learned response to unpleasant situations. In most cases, anxiety is probably the result of some combination of all of these factors.

STANDARD TREATMENTS

The treatment of anxiety disorders typically involves psychotherapy, medication, or, more commonly both. The preferred form of psychotherapy is known as cognitive behavioral therapy (CBT), which has two components, as its name implies. The cognitive part of CBT aims to change the thinking patterns and eliminate the beliefs that keep unrealistic fears in place. The behavioral part seeks to change a person's reaction to anxiety-provoking situations, often by gradually exposing him or her to a feared object or situation under controlled circumstances until the fear eases or disappears altogether.

Medications can help keep the symptoms of anxiety under control, increasing a person's ability to concentrate more fully on the psychotherapy part of treatment. These medications can include antidepressants to regulate serotonin and other neurotransmitters; anticonvulsants and benzodiaze-pines to enhance the function of the important neurotransmitter GABA (gamma-aminobutyric acid), thereby inducing relaxation, pain relief, and sleep; and beta-blockers to reduce the body's ability to produce adrenaline.

Other standard treatments for anxiety include aerobic exercise to relieve muscle tension and burn stress hormones and to prompt the release of hor-mones called endorphins, which help lift mood; "hands-on" therapies such as massage, acupressure, and reflexology; and relaxation techniques such as deep breathing, yoga, meditation, tai chi, visualization, and prayer.

RATING POPULAR ALTERNATIVE TREATMENTS FOR ANXIETY

Kava

Rating: ☆☆☆☆ = Strong Evidence

Kava, an herb that comes from the South Pacific, has long been used as a tranquilizer and for ceremonial purposes by certain tribes. Kava contains substances called *kavalactones* that have sedative properties and, among other things, can relax skeletal muscles.

Several studies have investigated kava's ability to relieve anxiety, compar-ing it to some standard antianxiety medicines and to a placebo. In general, kava has proven to be superior to placebo for treating anxiety and compa-rable to tricyclic antidepressants (such as Asendin and Norpramin) and to low doses of benzodiazepines (such as Xanax).

♦ For a double-blind, randomized, placebo-controlled study, German researchers divided 40 patients suffering from nervous anxiety, tension, and restlessness into two groups.[1] One group was given 300 milligrams of a kava extract (Laitan 50), while the other was given a placebo, every day for 3 weeks. The researchers used the Hamilton Anxiety Scale and similar rating scales to monitor the patients' progress. The outcome was favorable, with the researchers reporting that the kava extract was "sig-nificantly more effective than placebo in the treatment of moderately severe anxiety disorders of nonpsychotic origin."

♦ In a 1997 double-blind, randomized, placebo-controlled study, 101 people suffering from anxiety of a nonpsychotic origin were divided into two groups and given either a kava extract containing 70 milligrams of kavalactones (Laitan 100) or a placebo.[2] Researchers used the Hamilton Anxiety Scale to track the patients' progress over the course of 25 weeks. The results were positive, with kava demonstrating "significant superiority" over the placebo, although kava's effects were not evident until the volunteers had been taking it for some 8 weeks. Side effects were rare and equally likely to occur in either group. According to the researchers, the study results suggested that kava should be considered as an alternative to tricyclic antidepressants or benzodiazepines for the treatment of anxiety disorders.

◆ For a study published in *Phytomedicine* in 2003, kava extract was compared to the standard antianxiety drugs buspirone (BuSpar) and opipramol (Insidon).[3] The 129 people who enrolled in the study—all suffering from generalized anxiety disorder—were given 400 milligrams of kava (identified as LI 150), 10 milligrams of buspirone, or 100 milligrams of opipramol every day for 8 weeks. The researchers used several scales measuring anxiety and quality of life to determine if the herbal extract and/or the medicines were working. They concluded that for this group of patients, the kava extract was "well tolerated and as effective as" the two drugs for the treatment of generalized anxiety disorder. Table 4-1 below shows how kava and the two drugs reduced the scores on four scales. Both the drugs and the herb produced substantial improvements in measures of anxiety.

Table 4-1: Kava as Effective as Two Standard Medicines for Anxiety[4]

SCALE	AT BEGINNING OF STUDY			AFTER 8 WEEKS		
	Kava	Buspirone	Opipramol	Kava	Buspirone	Opipramol
Hamilton Anxiety Scale	23.14	23.55	23.93	8.37	8.00	7.74
Boerner Anxiety Scale	13.00	13.10	12.33	5.79	5.62	5.12
Self-Rating Anxiety Scale	52.70	52.95	54.40	39.67	37.48	37.79
Self-Rating Scale for Well-Being	34.79	33.95	34.55	19.86	18.76	17.19

♦ A 2003 Cochrane review—published by the Cochrane Library, which explores existing scientific knowledge regarding a particular disease and its treatment(s)—looked at various studies to determine how kava extract compared to placebo in treating anxiety.[5] After examining 11 studies involving a total of 645 people, the authors concluded that "compared with placebo, kava extract appears to be an effective symptomatic treatment option for anxiety."

♦ A 2005 meta-analysis combined the results of 6 placebo-controlled, randomized studies to create a larger statistical look at the effects of a kava extract (Laitan 50) on anxiety.[6] The authors of the meta-analysis found that this particular kava extract is effective and should be considered an alternative to standard medicines such as benzodiazepines, selective serotonin reuptake inhibitors (SSRIs), and other antidepressants for treatment of nonpsychotic anxiety.

♦ Germany's Commission E, the government arm charged with evaluating medicinal herbs, has approved the use of kava to treat nervous anxiety, stress, restlessness, tension, and agitation.

Summing Up the Evidence for Kava

Given the positive Cochrane review and the approval from Germany's Commission E, it is fair to say that kava is a four-star treatment for anxiety backed by strong evidence.

Other Names

Kava's scientific name is *Piper methysticum.* It goes by several other common names, including kava-kava, kew, sakau, and yagona.

Available Forms

Kava is available in capsule, beverage, tablet, tincture, and extract form.

How Much Kava Is Typically Used

There is no standard dose of kava. Successful studies have used dosages of up to 400 milligrams per day.

Possible Side Effects and Interactions

Be aware that the FDA has issued a warning about the potential for severe liver injury related to the use of kava. It has asked physicians to review cases of liver toxicity to see if there was a history of kava intake.

Kava has a number of possible side effects, including blurred vision, nausea, loss of appetite, and shortness of breath. The herb can interact with blood thinners such as dalteparin (Fragmin) to increase the risk of bruising or bleeding. Taking kava with anticonvulsants such as diazepam (Valium) may increase the risk of mental impairment and depression. If you're on any medication, be sure to consult your doctor before adding kava to your self-care regimen.

Valerian

Rating: ☆☆☆☆ = Strong Evidence

Valerian, an herb with clusters of small white or pink flowers and a massive root system, is sometimes called "herbal Valium" because it relieves anxiety and insomnia, just like the drug. (It has also been called "stinky socks" because that's what it smells like!) The herb was used in ancient China, Greece, and other cultures. It also was listed in the US National Formulary (an agency providing standards for botanicals) until the 1940s, when it fell out of favor—possibly because of the development of new, powerful pharmaceutical sleeping aids.

Although valerian has long been recommended by herbalists to relieve anxiety, relatively few studies examining the herb's antistress properties have been published in English. Among the handful are the following:

♦ In a double-blind study, 48 young men and women ranging in age from 19 to 29 were randomly assigned to receive 100 milligrams of valerian extract; 20 milligrams of the antianxiety drug propranolol (Inderal); a combination of 100 milligrams of valerian extract and 20 milligrams of propranolol; or a placebo.[7] All of the volunteers were healthy—that is, none was suffering from anxiety before the study. They were put into stressful situations during the study, and their physiological and psychological responses were monitored. Valerian reduced the volunteers' subjective feelings of anxiety without causing them to feel sedated.

♦ For a 2002 study, 54 healthy volunteers were asked to complete a standardized mental stress test on two occasions.[8] After they took the test the first time, they were randomly assigned to receive 600 milligrams of valerian (identified as LI 156), 120 milligrams of kava (LI 150), or nothing every day for seven days. Then they repeated the test. Their blood pressure, heart rate, and subjective feelings of anxiety were measured while they were resting and while they were taking the test. Both valerian and kava caused the volunteers' heart rate reactions, blood pressure responsiveness, and self-reported stress levels to drop.

But would valerian help people who were already suffering from anxiety, not just healthy people in anxiety-producing situations?

♦ For a study presented in *Phytotherapy Research* in 2002, 36 people suffering from generalized anxiety disorder were randomly assigned to receive daily doses of valerian averaging 81.3 milligrams of valepotriates (the "active ingredient" in the herb); 6.5 milligrams of diazepam (Valium); or a placebo.[9] The volunteers in this preliminary study were treated for 4 weeks. When the researchers calculated the results, they found that both the herb and the medicine produced a significant drop in the severity of anxiety, as measured by the Hamilton Anxiety Scale.

Summing Up the Evidence for Valerian

Although there are not enough large-scale, double-blind studies to allow for a definitive conclusion, given the positive results of several smaller studies and a recommendation from Germany's Commission E for using valerian to treat restless states, it is fair to say that valerian is a four-star treatment for anxiety backed by strong evidence.

Available Forms

Valerian is available in capsule, tincture, liquid, extract, crude herb, and tea form.

How Much Valerian Is Typically Used

There is no standard dose of valerian. Supplemental doses may range from 400 to 900 milligrams per day.

Possible Side Effects and Interactions

When taken for long periods of time, valerian can cause side effects such as irregular heartbeat, headache, uneasiness, restlessness, and insomnia. Though rare, there have been reports of gastrointestinal problems and contact allergies.

Taking valerian with blood thinners such as fondaparinux (Arixtra) may increase the risk of bleeding, while mixing the herb with antidepressants such as bupropion (Wellbutrin) can trigger depression or mental impairment. If you're on any medication, be sure to consult your doctor before adding valerian to your self-care regimen.

Tryptophan/5-HTP

Rating: ☆☆☆ = Intriguing Evidence

Tryptophan is an essential amino acid that the body uses to increase serotonin levels and manufacture niacin. It was a popular treatment for insomnia and other ailments until the 1980s, when a contaminated batch from Japan caused many people to suffer from a serious pain syndrome. This episode prompted the Food and Drug Administration to ban supplements containing tryptophan.

5-HTP, otherwise known as 5-hydroxytryptophan, quickly took tryptophan's place in the supplement market. A close "cousin" to the amino acid, 5-HTP also increases the production of serotonin in the central nervous system. Serotonin, in turn, helps ease depression, anxiety, and the sensation of pain, among other things.

Several studies suggest that tryptophan/5-HTP may help reduce anxiety. Among them:

+ Thirty-nine people participated in a double-blind study that was published in the *British Journal of Psychiatry* in 2000.[10] Twenty suffered from panic disorder with at least weekly panic attacks, while the remaining 19 were healthy. All the volunteers followed a low-protein diet for 24 hours; then they were given either an amino acid drink containing 2.3 grams of tryptophan or an amino acid drink without tryptophan. (Consuming amino acids but not tryptophan causes blood levels of tryptophan to drop, thus triggering a tryptophan-deficient state.) Next, the volunteers were subjected to a "CO_2 challenge," a standard technique for inducing experimental panic. (In a CO_2 challenge, a person breathes regular air through a mask; at a preselected point in time, the regular air is replaced by 5 percent carbon dioxide.) Each volunteer went through the challenge twice—once after drinking the amino acid drink with tryptophan and once after consuming the drink without tryptophan. Afterward, they rated their psychological states using the Spielberger Trait Anxiety Inventory and similar rating scales. The results of the study indicated that "acute tryptophan depletion increased anxiety responses" in people with panic disorder, but not in the healthy volunteers.

◆ A similar study looked at the effects of the CO_2 challenge in 24 people with panic disorder and 24 without after they had been given either 200 milligrams of 5-HTP or a placebo.[11] The data indicate that compared to placebo, 5-HTP "significantly reduced the reaction to the panic challenge in panic disorder patients, regarding subjective anxiety, panic symptom score, and number of panic attacks."

◆ British researchers tested the effects of tryptophan depletion for a 2004 study published in *Biological Psychiatry*.[12] All 14 volunteers in this double-blind, placebo-controlled, crossover study suffered from social anxiety disorder, and all were being treated with SSRIs (such as Prozac). The volunteers were instructed to perform anxiety-raising tasks twice—once after the use of dietary means to trigger tryptophan depletion and once after a placebo procedure that mimicked the tryptophan depletion but did not alter blood levels of the amino acid. The results indicated that "anxiety was significantly increased on the depletion day compared with the control day," suggesting that lack of tryptophan is linked to increased anxiety.

Summing Up the Evidence for Tryptophan/5-HTP

Given the fair amount of research on the effects of both tryptophan and 5-HTP, it seems reasonable to say that tryptophan/5-HTP is a three-star treatment for anxiety backed by intriguing evidence.

Available Forms

5-HTP is available in supplement form.

How Much 5-HTP Is Typically Used

There is no standard dose of 5-HTP as a treatment for anxiety. Supplemental doses may range from 150 to 300 milligrams per day.

Possible Side Effects and Interactions

Among 5-HTP's possible side effects are nausea, diarrhea, and breathing difficulties. Taken in large doses, it may trigger serotonin syndrome, characterized by confusion, agitation, rapid heart rate, changes in blood pressure and mental status, and even coma—all caused by elevated levels of serotonin in the brain. Similarly, 5-HTP may interact with antidepressants such as sertraline (Zoloft) to trigger serotonin syndrome. If you're taking any medication, be sure to consult your doctor before adding 5-HTP to your self-care regimen.

5

ALTERNATIVE APPROACHES TO

ASTHMA

Antioxidants ★★★☆
Caffeine ★★★☆
Omega-3 fatty acids ★★★☆
Homeopathy ★★☆
Pycnogenol ★★☆

Asthma is the narrowing of the airways in the lungs (the bronchi) in response to certain triggers, to the point where getting a decent breath becomes difficult if not impossible. During an asthma attack, the muscular walls of the bronchi go into spasm, and their linings swell and become inflamed, significantly narrowing the airways. The swelling causes the bronchi linings to produce extra mucus, which narrows the airways even further. Sometimes the mucus clumps together, forming a plug that partially or completely blocks an airway.

You can get a better idea about what goes on during an asthma attack if you think of your airways as a garden hose turned on full blast. Now imagine what would happen if you were to step on that hose. Suddenly, less water can flow through. And while you're stepping on the hose, its inner lining begins to swell, allowing even less water to flow through. Then suppose you were to pour a bottle of rubber cement into the blocked hose with the swollen lining. If anything can still flow through this constricted, gloppy mess, it's miracle. That's asthma.

Asthma affects up to 300 million people worldwide and kills over 180,000 per year.[1] Unfortunately, it's becoming even more common. Between 1980 and 1996, the number of Americans suffering from asthma more than doubled to almost 15 million; in 2002, that figure increased to 20 million. It's projected that there will be 28 million asthma cases in the United States by 2020. One-third of those who suffer from asthma are children.[2]

Even more frightening is the fact that fatalities associated with asthma are on the rise. While approximately 4,000 Americans died from asthma in 2002, experts predict twice that number by the year 2020.[3]

SYMPTOMS

The symptoms of asthma are shortness of breath (especially when exhaling), feeling the need to take another breath before completing the current one, coughing (often the first indication of an impending asthma attack), wheezing (a whistling sound in the airways caused by the accumulation of mucus), and tightness in the chest. In more severe cases, the person will instinctively sit up and lean forward in order to use his or her neck and chest muscles to assist with breathing.

CAUSES

Researchers believe that the airway spasms seen in asthma are often the result of an allergic reaction to an inhaled substance, such as dust, animal dander, cigarette smoke, pollen, mold, smog, or some other environmental pollutant. Allergies are common among those with asthma; at least 70 percent of asthma sufferers also have at least occasional bouts of allergic rhinitis—that is, hay fever.[4] When asthma is caused by allergens, it's called *allergic asthma*, a condition that affects approximately 60 percent of US asthma sufferers.

The irritation of the airways that triggers bronchial spasms also can be brought on by nonallergens—the most common being exercise, emotional stress, cold air, viral infections, and medications. The odds of developing asthma are higher for those who have a parent with allergies or asthma; whose diets are high in food additives, preservatives, or other chemicals that sensitize the body; who are undernourished; or who have been exposed to large amounts of environmental pollutants.

STANDARD TREATMENTS

The standard treatments for asthma include antihistamines to calm the inflammation response; decongestants and antiallergy sprays to shrink swollen nasal passages; synthetic steroid sprays to fight inflammation and calm the allergic response; bronchodilators to relax bronchial tube spasms; and inhaled anti-inflammatory drugs to soothe inflamed membranes.

RATING POPULAR ALTERNATIVE TREATMENTS FOR ASTHMA

Antioxidants

Rating: ☆☆☆ = Intriguing Evidence

Antioxidants—including vitamin C, vitamin E, alpha-lipoic acid, and lycopene—help correct and combat the damage caused by oxidation. To chemists, oxidation means the loss of an electron. To the rest of us, it means electron-hungry substances running rampant through the body's tissues, desperately snatching electrons from other substances to satisfy themselves. Unfortunately, this electron-stealing behavior can damage molecules, cells, and tissues, increasing the risk of developing a number of diseases. Antioxidants help prevent this by keeping oxidation under control. The body manufactures some antioxidants; we get others from foods.

It is believed that antioxidants may help manage and prevent oxidation-induced inflammation and thus reduce symptoms of asthma. Some studies seem to corroborate this theory.

♦ For a 2000 study published in *Thorax*, Italian researchers analyzed data collected from several thousand children who had been participating in the "Italian Studies on Respiratory Disorders in Children and the Environment."[5] Parents of more than 4,000 children were asked to indicate how often their children consumed citrus fruit or kiwi or drank freshly squeezed citrus juice. (Citrus fruit and kiwi were singled out because citrus fruit, eaten mostly in the winter, is "the most important source of vitamin C" in the Italian diet, and kiwi contains a large amount of vitamin C.) A year after supplying the dietary information, the parents were asked to indicate how often their children suffered from wheezing or shortness of breath during the previous 12 months. After analyzing the data, the researchers concluded that there was "a clear association between a low intake of oranges and other vitamin C–containing fruits during winter and an increased risk of wheezing symptoms in children."

Table 5-1 below shows how symptoms of asthma fall as the consumption of citrus fruit and kiwi rises.

Table 5-1: Intake of Vitamin C–Rich Fruit Linked to a Lessening of Asthma Symptoms[6]

SYMPTOMS	PERTENTAGE RISK OF DEVELOPING SYMPTOMS			
	Less Than 1 Vitamin C–Rich Fruit a Week	1-2 Vitamin C–Rich Fruits per Week	3-4 Vitamin C–Rich Fruits per Week	5-7 Vitamin C–Rich Fruits per Week
Wheezing	9.9%	7.4%	7.5%	6.6%
Wheezing and shortness of breath	6.8%	4.8%	5.1%	4.6%
Wheezing due to exercising	2.3%	1.5%	1.5%	1.7%
Severe wheezing	2.2%	1.6%	1.3%	1.2%
Nighttime cough	21.3%	18.4%	17.9%	16.1%
Chronic cough	12.1%	10.0%	11.4%	9.3%
Rhinitis	16.3%	14.0%	13.2%	12.3%

♦ Israeli researchers tested the effects of the antioxidant lycopene in 20 people with exercise-induced asthma for a 2000 study published in *Allergy.*[7] For this double-blind, placebo-controlled, crossover study, the volunteers' lung function was measured before and after they had exercised for 7 minutes on a treadmill. They were randomly assigned to receive 1 week's treatment with daily doses of either 30 mg of lycopene (Lyc-O-Mato) or a placebo. At the end of the treatment period, the exercise sessions and lung function tests were repeated. Then the volunteers were "crossed over" to the other treatment for a week and tested again. The researchers reported that while the placebo had no beneficial effect, lycopene treatment "significantly protected" 55 percent of the volunteers from exercise-induced asthma. The researchers concluded that their findings "clearly support the assumption that in most patients, dietary supplementation with lycopene protects against" exercise-induced asthma.

Summing Up the Evidence for Antioxidants

A fair number of population and clinical studies have linked increased consumption of antioxidants with a reduction in the risk of suffering from asthma attacks. Although there are conflicting reports, and questions concerning exactly which antioxidants—and in which dosages—are best suited to which groups of people, there is enough research to conclude that antioxidants are a three-star treatment for asthma backed by intriguing evidence.

Available Forms

Antioxidants such as vitamin C and lycopene are found in various foods. They're also available in supplement form.

Amount of Antioxidants Typically Used

There is no standard dose of antioxidants for asthma. Typical therapeutic dosages of vitamin C for other ailments range up to 1,000 milligrams per day. The dose of lycopene in the aforementioned study was 30 milligrams per day.

Possible Side Effects and Interactions

The Food and Nutrition Board of the Institute of Medicine has set a tolerable upper limit of 2,000 milligrams of vitamin C per day for adults. Among vitamin C's possible side effects are diarrhea, nausea, and heartburn. As for other antioxidants, possible side effects can vary from one to the next.

Antioxidants also may interact with a number of medicines. For example, taking vitamin C with pain pills or estrogen preparations such as estradiol (Climara) may raise blood levels of these drugs, along with the risk of side effects, while combining C with HIV medications such as saquinavir (Fortovase) may lower blood levels of the drug. As with all supplements and drugs, you should take antioxidants only according to directions and under a physician's supervision.

Caffeine

Rating: ☆☆☆ = Intriguing Evidence

Found in coffee, tea, and certain other popular beverages, caffeine has been both praised and reviled. It is a popular remedy for headaches, low blood pressure, and other ailments and is used by many people to enhance mental alertness and athletic performance. But it also can contribute to irregular heartbeat, anxiety, and insomnia, and it may interfere with blood sugar control in people with diabetes.

The pros and cons of caffeine have been debated for many years, and the arguments most likely will continue for years to come. However, several small studies have indicated that caffeine can provide modest, temporary relief of asthma symptoms. Of note are these:

♦ For a double-blind study published in the *New England Journal of Medicine* in 1984, 23 people ages 8 to 18—all with asthma—were given either caffeine or the asthma drug theophylline in amounts calculated according to body weight.[8] Both caffeine and the drug significantly improved several markers of respiratory health, with the researchers noting that caffeine's ability to widen the breathing tubes "did not differ significantly" from that of the drug. The researchers concluded that caffeine is an effective means of widening the breathing tubes in young people.

♦ The Cochrane Database of Systematic Reviews issued a review of the effects of caffeine on asthma in 2001.[9] Six separate randomized, crossover studies involving 55 people were included in the review. Noting that all six studies were "of high quality," the authors concluded that "caffeine appears to improve airway function modestly in people with asthma for up to four hours."

Summing Up the Evidence for Caffeine

There seems to be general agreement that caffeine can provide a modest amount of temporary relief from certain symptoms of asthma in some people. This makes caffeine a three-star treatment for asthma backed by intriguing evidence.

Available Forms

Caffeine is found in coffee, tea, caffeinated sodas, and other beverages, as well as in chocolate and in tablet and powder form.

How Much Caffeine Is Typically Used

There is no standard dose of caffeine. Supplemental doses used in the studies are in the neighborhood of 5 milligrams of caffeine per kilogram of body weight, or about 264 milligrams of caffeine for a 120-pound person. (A kilogram equals 2.2 pounds, so simply divide your weight by 2.2, then multiply by 5 to figure out how many milligrams of caffeine would be considered a standard dose for you.)

Possible Side Effects and Interactions

Caffeine can cause rapid heartbeat, stomach irritation, insomnia, nervousness, anxiety, and tremors. In addition, it may interact with diabetes medicines such as glipizide (Glucotrol), causing blood sugar to either rise or fall, and with antibiotics such as ciprofloxacin (Cipro), causing blood levels of the drug to rise and thus raising the risk of side effects. If you're taking any medication, be sure to consult your doctor before adding therapeutic amounts of caffeine to your self-care regimen.

Omega-3 Fatty Acids

Rating: ☆☆☆ = Intriguing Evidence

The omega-3 fatty acids—the best-known of which are EPA (eicosapentaenoic acid) and DHA (docosahexaenoic acid)—have anti-inflammatory properties. For this reason, they're helpful as treatments for conditions in which inflammation plays a role, such as heart disease, rheumatoid arthritis, and chronic pain.

In recent years, medical scientists have learned that inflammation is a factor in the development of asthma, raising the possibility that omega-3s could help prevent and/or treat this condition. Some studies suggest that this is indeed the case:

♦ Japanese researchers tested the effects of omega-3 fatty acids in 29 children with asthma for a double-blind study presented in the *European Respiratory Journal* in 2000.[10] The children in the study were randomly assigned to receive 10 months of treatment with daily doses of either fish oil capsules containing EPA and DHA (manufactured by Nippon Suisan Kaisha Ltd.) or a placebo containing olive oil. The dosage of EPA and

DHA varied with the children's body weight. The children were in a long-term treatment hospital, so the researchers could observe them and the severity of their symptoms several times a day. The results were positive, with consumption of omega-3 fatty acids lowering asthma scores (which reflect the severity of asthma symptoms). Figure 5-1 below shows the asthma scores for the omega-3 fatty acid and placebo groups from the beginning of the study—the zero point—through month 10. The placebo group begins with a much lower score, but the line representing the omega-3 fatty acid group moves under the placebo line by month 4 and tends to remain there. While the placebo line moves up and down quite a bit, the general trend for the omega-3 fatty acid line is down, suggesting that consumption of omega-3s helps reduce the severity of asthma attacks.

Figure 5-1: Omega-3 Fatty Acids Lower Asthma Scores Better Than Placebo[11]

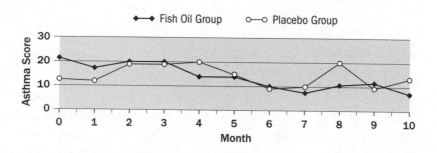

♦ A paper published in the journal *Nutrition* in 2005 described the results of a case-control study investigating whether diet had an impact on asthma.[12] Fifty-four people with asthma, average age 23, and 54 without asthma, average age 27, enrolled in the study. All of the volunteers recorded what they ate for 3 days. Then the researchers looked for correlations between diet and disease. They found "a positive association between omega-3 fatty acids . . . and FEV1"—which stands for forced expiratory volume in 1 second, a measure of how much air a person can expel from the lungs in 1 second. FEV1 is a standard test to measure lung function.

♦ Fourteen people participated in a 2000 study comparing the effects of perilla seed oil, which contains omega-3 fatty acids, to placebo.[13]

(Perilla is an herb that has traditionally been used to treat asthma, nausea, and other ailments.) The volunteers—who ranged in age from 22 to 84 and had moderately severe asthma—were randomly assigned to receive 4 weeks of treatment with either 10 to 20 grams of perilla seed oil per day or a corn oil placebo. The results were positive, with the perilla oil producing significant improvements in forced expiratory volume and other measures of respiratory health. The researchers concluded that "perilla seed oil-rich supplementation is useful for the treatment of asthma."

♦ A 2004 review published in the *Journal of Alternative and Complementary Medicine* surveyed the scientific literature and concluded that supplementing the diet with omega-3 fatty acids "may be a viable treatment modality and/or adjunct therapy" for asthma.[14]

Summing Up the Evidence for Omega-3 Fatty Acids

Although there are conflicting reports, the results of a fair number of clinical and population studies indicate that consumption of omega-3 fatty acids from foods and/or supplements has a protective effect against symptoms of asthma. Thus, it is fair to say that omega-3 fatty acids are a three-star treatment for asthma backed by intriguing evidence.

Available Forms

The best sources of omega-3 fatty acids are cold-water fatty fish such as mackerel, salmon, herring, anchovies, tuna, and bluefish. As a general rule, the fattier the fish is, the more omega-3s it contains. The human body can manufacture omega-3s from alpha-linolenic acid, which is found in walnuts and flaxseed. Omega-3 fatty acids are also available in supplement form, labeled as fish oil, omega-3, EPA, DHA, or some combination of these.

Amount of Omega-3 Fatty Acids Typically Used

There is no standard dosage of omega-3 fatty acids for asthma. The therapeutic dosages for a variety of ailments range up to 500 milligrams of EPA and 480 milligrams of DHA per day.

Possible Side Effects and Interactions

The omega-3 fatty acids are found in common foods and have been granted Generally Regarded as Safe (GRAS) status by the US government. Among their possible side effects are belching, heartburn, and nausea. Omega-3s also may prolong bleeding time, which may be a problem for those who have bleeding disorders, those who are taking medicines to thin the blood, or those who will be undergoing surgery soon.

Along the same line, omega-3 fatty acids may interact with aspirin, heparin, and other drugs that thin the blood, increasing the risk of bleeding. If you're taking any medication, be sure to consult your doctor before adding omega-3 supplements to your self-care regimen.

Homeopathy

Rating: ☆☆ = Modest Evidence

Developed by a German physician in the 18th century, homeopathy is based on the idea that "like cures like." Therefore, instead of using drugs to suppress symptoms of a disease, homeopathy seeks to strengthen a patient's natural defenses by introducing a tiny amount of a substance that, in larger doses, would cause symptoms of a certain disease in a healthy person. For example, a homeopathic physician might treat asthma by giving a patient a minuscule dose of a substance that causes breathing difficulties, in an attempt to strengthen the body's respiratory mechanism. The closest analogy to the homeopathic approach in standard Western medicine is the vaccine, which "teaches" the body how to fight off a particular germ by giving it a weakened or dead version of the germ.

Whereas in standard Western medicine the same drug may be prescribed for many patients with similar symptoms or diseases, in homeopathic medicine the physician tailors a patient's treatment to his or her individual characteristics and symptoms.

A small number of studies have shown that homeopathy can be helpful in treating asthma. For example:

♦ Cuban researchers performed a randomized, double-blind study on 28 adults and 34 children with asthma.[15] The participants were assigned to receive either individualized homeopathic treatment or a placebo. The results were positive, with 97.4 percent of the homeopathy group improving, and 87.2 percent able to reduce their dosages of standard medicine. In the placebo group, only 12.5 percent showed improvement, and none reduced their dosage of standard medicine.

♦ A 1994 study published in *Lancet* described the effects of homeopathy on 28 people with allergic asthma.[16] The volunteers were randomly assigned to receive either homeopathic immunity treatment or a placebo. (For homeopathic immunity treatment, patients are given a tiny homeopathic dose of the substance to which they are allergic. In this study, most of the volunteers were allergic to dust mites.) Everyone also continued with their standard medical care. The results were positive, with 9 of the 11 receiving homeopathy improving, compared to only 5 of the 13 receiving the placebo.

♦ The same *Lancet* article also reported on the results of an extensive meta-analysis of three homeopathy/asthma studies, involving a total of 202 patients. Data produced by the statistical merging of these studies found "a clear indication of a mean [average] advantage of homeopathy over placebo."

Summing Up the Evidence for Homeopathy

Rating the effectiveness of homeopathic treatment is difficult because the treatment is, by design, very individualized. It's virtually impossible to say that a particular homeopathic medicine either works or doesn't work, or that one homeopathic medicine is superior to another. With respect to asthma, there is a paucity of well-designed studies analyzing the effect of homeopathy on asthma. With all this in mind, it's fair to say that homeopathy is a two-star treatment for asthma backed by modest evidence.

Finding a Homeopathic Physician

For more information about homeopathy, or to find a qualified practitioner, contact the National Center for Homeopathy at www.homeopathic.org.

Pycnogenol

Rating: ☆☆ = Modest Evidence

Pycnogenol is the registered trademark for a proprietary extract taken from the bark of the French Maritime pine tree. Containing catechins, flavonoids, and other nutraceuticals, Pycnogenol is believed to have anti-inflammatory and immune-stimulating properties. It has been used to treat allergies, diabetes, pain, and a number of other conditions.

A small number of studies suggest that Pycnogenol might be helpful in treating asthma. For example:

+ A 2001 study conducted at the Mashhad University of Medical Sciences in Iran, in conjunction with the College of Public Health and School of Medicine at the University of Arizona, looked at the effects of Pycnogenol on 26 people suffering from asthma.[17] For this randomized, double-blind crossover study, the volunteers were assigned to receive up to 200 milligrams of Pycnogenol (1 milligram per pound of body weight) or a placebo every day for 4 weeks. Then the groups switched treatments and took the other substance for another 4-week period. The results were intriguing, with asthma symptom scores significantly improving when the volunteers took Pycnogenol. FEV1 scores also improved significantly after Pycnogenol was taken but not after the placebo was administered. The study's authors reported that the volunteers typically responded "favorably to Pycnogenol when compared to the placebo, most saying they noted improvement in their breathing ability."[18]

+ A double-blind study published in the *Journal of Asthma* in 2004 involved 60 boys and girls, average age 14, with mild to moderate asthma.[19] The volunteers were randomly assigned to receive either Pycnogenol (1 milligram per pound of body weight) or a placebo every day for 3 months. Those taking Pycnogenol showed a greater reduction in their asthma symptoms and a greater improvement in their lung function tests than those taking the placebo.

Summing Up the Evidence for Pycnogenol

These studies, combined with laboratory research into Pycnogenol's possible mechanisms of action against asthma, are intriguing. Still, it's too early to make a definitive statement about Pycnogenol's merits as a treatment for asthma. Suffice it to say that Pycnogenol is a two-star treatment backed by modest evidence.

Available Forms

Pycnogenol is available as an oral supplement.

How Much Pycnogenol Is Typically Used

There is no standard dose of Pycnogenol. Studies have used supplemental doses of up to 200 milligrams per day.

Possible Side Effects and Interactions

Pycnogenol may aggravate the symptoms of multiple sclerosis, rheumatoid arthritis, and other autoimmune ailments because of its immune-stimulating properties. In addition, Pycnogenol may interact with immunosuppressant drugs such as cyclosporine (Sandimmune), which are vital to preventing rejection of transplanted organs. If you're taking any medication, be sure to consult your doctor before adding Pycnogenol to your self-care regimen.

6

ALTERNATIVE APPROACHES TO

COLDS

Androgarphis	☆☆☆
Echinacea	☆☆☆
Zinc	☆☆

The common cold is a viral infection of the nose and throat that may also involve the sinuses and the bronchial tubes. It can be a mild annoyance that lasts for a few days, or it can drag on for as long as a few weeks. The infection can also trigger a more serious, longer-lasting problem such as a sinus infection, a middle ear infection, asthma, bronchitis, or pneumonia.

SYMPTOMS

The first symptom of a cold is often a sore throat, followed by sneezing, a runny nose, fatigue, and in some cases, fever. Nasal secretions typically begin as clear, watery, and abundant; within a few days, they start to thicken, become opaque, and may turn yellow to yellow-green. The secretions plug up the nose, making breathing difficult, and can irritate the throat, causing a cough.

The symptoms of a cold usually last from 4 to 10 days, though postnasal drip and coughing can continue for up to 3 weeks.

CAUSES

The common cold begins with infection by a virus. The most likely culprit is the rhinovirus, of which there are more than 100 types. No matter what the type, the virus is typically spread by the hands of someone who has come into contact with the nasal secretions of a person who's infected, since the virus is contained in these secretions. Another (less likely) way of spreading the virus is by inhaling droplets that have been propelled into the air by the coughing or sneezing of a person who's infected. When the virus comes into contact with an opening in the body such as the eyes, nose, or mouth, it can invade and cause a cold.

STANDARD TREATMENTS

The standard treatment for a cold includes rest, drinking plenty of fluids, inhaling steam from a vaporizer to loosen secretions, and staying warm and comfortable. Over-the-counter cold remedies may help ease the symptoms of a cold but will not cure it. These remedies include analgesics for pain; antihistamines to clear blocked nasal passages and reduce sneezing; decongestants to lessen congestion; cough suppressants to reduce coughing; throat lozenges to ease sore throat pain; and expectorants to break up mucus so that it's easier to expel. An infected person can reduce the chance of spreading a cold by washing his or her hands frequently, coughing or sneezing into tissues, staying home from work or school to avoid infecting others, and using disinfectants to clean objects shared with others.

RATING POPULAR ALTERNATIVE TREATMENTS FOR THE COMMON COLD

Andrographis

Rating: ☆☆☆ = Intriguing Evidence

The leaves, flowers, and juice of the andrographis plant (*Andrographis paniculata*)—an herb native to India, Sri Lanka, and adjacent areas—have a long history of use for medicinal purposes. In Traditional Chinese Medicine, andrographis is recommended to improve cardiovascular, urinary, and digestive health. During the great flu epidemic of 1919 to 1920, countless sufferers in India were treated with this herb, which has also been used as a remedy for common allergies, anorexia, snakebite, colic, diabetes, and numerous other ailments. Some scientific evidence suggests that andrographis may be able to stimulate the immune system, relieve the symptoms of upper respiratory infections, and reduce fever and pain.

Several studies have indicated that andrographis may be helpful for easing the symptoms of the common cold. These include the following:

♦ For a 2004 study, Russian and Swedish scientists enlisted 130 children ranging in age from 4 to 11 and suffering from the common cold.[1] The children were divided into three groups and given one of these treatments for 10 days: an andrographis preparation (brand name Kan Jang) plus standard therapy; an echinacea preparation (Immunal) plus standard therapy; or standard therapy. The results were positive, with the effects of andrographis being "particularly pronounced" in reducing the amount of nasal congestion and nasal secretion. In addition, "the use of standard medication was significantly less" among those taking andrographis compared to those taking the echinacea or receiving only standard treatment. Table 6-1 below shows how the amount of nasal secretions dropped in the andrographis, echinacea, and control groups.

Table 6-1: Andrographis Reduces Nasal Secretions Better Than Echinacea or Placebo[2]

SYMPTOMS	NASAL SECRETIONS (GRAMS PER DAY)			
	Day 1	Day 3	Day 5	Day 8
Andrographis group	3.23	2.51	1.26	0.30
Echinacea group	2.51	2.41	1.91	1.23
Control group	3.11	2.60	2.70	1.47

♦ A study involving 158 Chilean adults suffering from the common cold was published in *Phytomedicine* in 1999.[3] The men and women in this double-blind, placebo-controlled study were randomly assigned to receive 1,200 milligrams of an andrographis preparation (Kan Jang) or a placebo every day for 5 days. All of the volunteers evaluated their symptoms on days 0, 2, and 4 of the study. At the end of day 2, those taking the andrographis reported a significant decline in tiredness, sleeplessness, sore throat, and nasal secretions. By day 4, the intensity of all symptoms had improved significantly in the andrographis group. The researchers noted that there were no adverse effects, and concluded that andrographis "had a high degree of effectiveness in reducing the prevalence and intensity of the symptoms in uncomplicated common cold beginning at day two of treatment." Table 6-2 below shows how this andrographis preparation compared to placebo in reducing cold symptoms.

Table 6-2: Andrographis Superior to Placebo in Reducing Cold Symptoms[4]

SYMPTOMS	ANDROGRAPHIS GROUP		PLACEBO GROUP	
	Day 0	Day 3	Day 0	Day 3
Cough intensity	3.87	1.67	3.22	2.48
Cough frequency	3.25	1.35	2.95	2.37
Expectoration	2.17	1.28	2.12	2.18
Nasal secretion	8.10	1.53	8.22	4.40
Headache	3.11	1.19	3.06	2.72
Fatigue	7.06	2.60	7.14	4.07
Earache	1.62	0.76	1.62	2.00
Sleep disturbance	6.81	2.22	6.92	5.28

♦ A double-blind, placebo-controlled study, published in *Phytotherapy Research* in 1995, involved 59 men and women ranging in age from 18 to 60.[5] Those who took 1,200 milligrams of an andrographis preparation (Kan Jang) saw their cold symptoms subside or resolve faster than those taking the placebo. Table 6-3 on the next page shows the differences in the symptoms between the andrographis group and the placebo group at the beginning of the study and on day 4. The symptoms were measured on a scale of 0 to 3, with 0 being no symptoms and 3 being severe symptoms. Note that on day 0 the symptom scores were roughly equal in both the andrographis and placebo groups, but by day 4 the andrographis group had lower scores in every symptom category.

Table 6-3: Improvement in Cold Symptoms Triggered by Andrographis Compared to Placebo[6]

SYMPTOMS	ANDROGRAPHIS GROUP		PLACEBO GROUP	
	Day 0	Day 4	Day 0	Day 4
Strength of disease	1.91	0.94	1.96	1.71
Tiredness	2.15	1.15	2.17	1.67
Shivering	2.06	0.73	2.14	1.46
Sore throat	1.72	0.76	1.70	1.25
Muscular aches	2.06	0.82	2.04	1.60
Rhinitis	1.78	1.32	1.76	1.60
Sinus pain and headaches	1.78	1.33	1.86	1.57
Lymphatic swellings	1.09	0.88	1.03	1.21

◆ In 2004, Thai researchers published a systematic review and meta-analysis of the effect of andrographis on upper respiratory tract infections in the *Journal of Clinical Pharmacy and Therapeutics*.[7] This statistical merging encompassed three studies involving a total of 433 patients with upper respiratory tract infections. Some of these people had colds, while others had other kinds of respiratory infections. After analyzing the results, the researchers concluded that andrographis extract, either alone or in combination with Siberian ginseng (*Acanthopanax senticosus*) extract, "may be more effective than placebo and may be an appropriate alternative treatment of uncomplicated acute upper respiratory tract infection."

Summing Up the Evidence for Andrographis

Andrographis has been subjected to a fair amount of study, both in the laboratory and in people. Much of this research has utilized an herbal preparation known as Kan Jang, a standardized fixed combination of andrographis extract and Siberian ginseng extract. The weight of evidence suggests that andrographis can partially relieve cold symptoms in many people, leading to the conclusion that andrographis is a three-star treatment for the common cold backed by intriguing evidence.

Other Names

Andrographis is known to scientists as *Andrographis paniculata* and in various parts of the world as bhunimba, chuan xin lian, creat, Indian echinacea, kirta, sambilata, and takila.

Available Forms

Andrographis is available in tablet, capsule, and extract form.

How Much Andrographis Is Typically Used

There is no standard dose of andrographis. A typical supplemental dose for preventing the common cold is 200 milligrams of standardized andrographis extract (containing 4 to 5.6 milligrams of andrographolide) for 5 days a week. For treating cold symptoms, a typical dosage is 400 milligrams of andrographis, three times a day.

Side Effects and Interactions

Andrographis can cause vomiting, loss of appetite, headache, and rash. It may increase the risk of bruising or bleeding if taken with heparin (Hepalean) or other drugs that thin the blood. It also may interact with benazepril (Lotensin) and other medicines for elevated blood pressure, causing blood pressure to drop too much. If you're taking any medication, be sure to consult your doctor before adding andrographis to your self-care regimen.

Echinacea

Rating: ☆☆☆ = Intriguing Evidence

The word *echinacea* actually refers to three species of the same plant, all native to Missouri, Nebraska, and Kansas. American Indians used echinacea to treat cough, sore gums, snakebite, and a number of other ailments. It became a popular cold remedy in the late 1800s and was listed on the US National Formulary of Medicines from 1916 to 1950.

Beginning in the 1930s, as one new antibiotic after another emerged from research laboratories, echinacea gradually faded from public awareness. That has changed as natural remedies have come back into vogue over the last couple of decades. Echinacea has been studied as an adjunct treatment for colds and other upper respiratory tract infections as well as for urinary tract infections. It also has been used as an immune system stimulant in people with HIV/AIDS.

Several modern studies have indicated that echinacea can help reduce the severity and/or duration of cold symptoms. For example:

♦ Researchers from Canada and Austria investigated the efficacy of Echinilin, a brand-name formulation taken from freshly harvested *Echinacea purpurea* plants, as a treatment for the common cold.[8] For this double-blind trial, 282 adults in good health were randomly given either the echinacea preparation or a placebo and instructed to begin taking their pills as soon as cold symptoms appeared. One hundred twenty-eight of the volunteers caught a cold and took their pills for 7 days, while using a 10-point scale to record the severity of their symptoms. The results were positive, with the daily symptom score tallying 23.1 percent lower in those taking echinacea compared to those taking the placebo. The researchers concluded that use of this particular standardized echinacea extract "resulted in reduced symptom severity in subjects with naturally acquired upper respiratory tract infection."

♦ German researchers published the results of a similar study involving 80 men and women in 2001.[9] The volunteers for this double-blind, placebo-controlled trial were recruited when they showed the first signs of a cold, then randomly assigned to take either *E. purpurea herba* (brand name Echinilin) or a placebo. The researchers were primarily interested in seeing how many days the cold would last. The results were positive, with the colds in the echinacea group averaging 6.0 days, compared to 9.0 days in the placebo group. Table 6-4 on the next page shows how long individual symptoms lasted in both groups.

Table 6-4: Echinacea Shortens the Duration of Cold Symptoms[10]

SYMPTOMS	NUMBER OF DAYS SYMPTOMS LASTED	
	Echinacea Group	Placebo Group
Sneezing	4.70	6.13
Runny nose (rhinorrhea)	6.24	8.95
Nasal congestion	6.99	9.94
Sore throat	3.05	5.37
Cough	4.11	6.03
Headache	3.74	5.53
Malaise	5.76	8.24
Chills	1.60	1.45

♦ Ninety-five people who had runny noses, scratchy throats, or other early symptoms of a cold or the flu participated in a randomized, double-blind study published in the *Journal of Alternative and Complementary Medicine* in 2000.[11] The volunteers were assigned to drink either 5 to 6 cups of echinacea tea (Echinacea Plus) or a placebo tea every day. Researchers used a questionnaire to determine the extent and duration of the participants' symptoms. They concluded that treating with echinacea "at early onset of cold or flu symptoms was effective for relieving these symptoms in a shorter period of time than a placebo."

Several researchers have reviewed the scientific literature in an attempt to make a definitive statement on the use of echinacea for the common cold.

♦ For a 1999 review published in the *Journal of Family Practice*, the authors had searched for all randomized, blinded, placebo-controlled studies involving echinacea, whether published or not.[12] They found nine studies on echinacea and four on the prevention of upper respiratory tract infections (including colds). After noting that the methodological quality of most of the studies was modest, the researchers concluded, "Evidence from published trials suggests that echinacea may be beneficial for the early treatment of acute URIs" (upper respiratory infections, including colds).

♦ The authors of a 2000 review study, published in *Biochemical Pharmacology*, drew this conclusion after examining the literature: "The consensus of the studies . . . is that echinacea is indeed effective in reducing the duration and severity of symptoms, but that this effect is noted only with certain preparations of echinacea."[13]

♦ The prestigious Cochrane Library issued a review of the use of echinacea for the common cold, concluding that "the majority of the available studies report positive results. However, there is not enough evidence to recommend a specific echinacea product or echinacea preparations for the treatment or prevention of common colds."[14]

Summing Up the Evidence for Echinacea

These last two review studies point out some of the problems with the use of echinacea as a treatment for the common cold. First, while many studies show that echinacea effectively reduces the severity and/or length of cold symptoms, others do not. Second, with three varieties of echinacea and multiple preparations of each, it's difficult to say which are effective and which one—if any—is superior. To complicate matters, the active ingredients in echinacea and their mechanisms of action have yet to be pinpointed and scientifically defined. So it's not surprising that the relationship between echinacea and colds is confusing and that recent studies published in prestigious journals such as the *New England Journal of Medicine*[15] and the *Annals of Internal Medicine*[16] have concluded that the herb is not effective against cold symptoms.

Germany's Commission E has approved the use of *E. purpurea* for the common cold, while the World Health Organization has endorsed *E. augustifolia* as a treatment.[17] Normally, these two recommendations would entitle echinacea to a high rating. But given the dueling studies, it is best to be conservative and limit the herb to three-star status.

Other Names

The scientific names of the three species of echinacea are *E. augustifolia*, *E. pallida*, and *E. purpurea*. The herb is known by other names in various parts of the world, including American cone flower, black Susan, black Sampson, Indian head, Missouri snakeroot, red sunflower, and scurvy root.

Available Forms

Echinacea is available as a dried root, fluid extract, juice, tea, and tincture.

How Much Echinacea Is Typically Used

There is no standard dose of echinacea. To treat the common cold, supplemental daily doses for adults may range from 1 to 3 grams of dried root or 400 to 900 milligrams of dry powder extract.

Possible Side Effects and Interactions

Echinacea's side effects include fever, nausea, and constipation. In some people, it may trigger an allergic reaction.

Taking echinacea with cholesterol-lowering drugs such as atorvastatin (Lipitor) may increase the risk of liver damage. The herb also may interfere with the actions of drugs such as daclizumab (Zenapax), which help prevent organ rejection in those who've received organ transplants. If you're taking any medication, be sure to consult your doctor before adding echinacea to your self-care regimen.

Zinc

Rating: ☆☆☆ = Intriguing Evidence

Although the human body contains just a few grams of the mineral zinc, the mineral is absolutely essential to health since it participates in more than 100 enzyme reactions. Zinc helps synthesize proteins, metabolize carbohydrates, utilize vitamin A, heal wounds, and strengthen bones. A zinc deficiency can cause delayed sexual maturity, impotence, lack of appetite, loss of hair, diarrhea, and other problems.

Zinc has been used to treat acne, poor fertility, and impaired immune function, as well as to improve athletic performance. Back in 1974, scientists noted that zinc could inhibit the replication of the rhinovirus implicated as the cause of the common cold.[18] Since then, numerous studies have tested zinc's effects on cold symptoms. For example:

♦ For a 1996 randomized, double-blind study presented in the *Annals of Internal Medicine,* researchers recruited 100 adults who had experienced cold symptoms for 24 hours or less.[19] The volunteers were assigned to take either zinc lozenges containing 13.3 milligrams of zinc gluconate (supplied by the Quigley Corporation) or a placebo every 2 hours while awake for as long as they had symptoms. They also rated their symptoms—such as headache, nasal congestion, and nasal drainage—on a scale of 0 (no symptoms) to 3 (severe symptoms). The results were positive, with symptoms in the zinc group resolving in an average of 4.4 days, compared to 7.6 days in the placebo group.

♦ One hundred two student volunteers recruited at the University of Texas participated in a randomized, double-blind study published in *Current Therapeutic Research* in 1998.[20] All of the volunteers, who ranged in age from 18 to 54, had cold symptoms. Those in one group were given lozenges containing 9 milligrams of zinc, while the rest were given a placebo. Both groups were instructed to take one lozenge every 1.5 hours while awake during the first day, then every 2 hours while awake after that until their symptoms had disappeared. They also were asked to rate their symptoms on a scale of 0 (no symptoms) to 3 (severe symptoms) every day. The results were positive and statistically significant, with symptoms lasting an average of 3.8 days in the zinc group compared to 5.1 days in the placebo group. Table 6-5 below summarizes the differences between the zinc and placebo groups.

Table 6-5: Zinc Outperforms Placebo in Reducing Cold Symptoms[21]

	Zinc Group (Average)	Placebo Group (Average)
Number of days all cold symptoms lasted	3.8	5.1
Number of days longest-lasting cold symptom lasted	5.3	7.1
Average severity rating	1.41	1.50

♦ A randomized, double-blind study published in the *Annals of Internal Medicine* in 2000 compared zinc to placebo for treating the symptoms of the common cold.[22] Fifty volunteers from the Detroit Medical Center, who had experienced cold symptoms for 1 day or less, were assigned to take either lozenges containing 12.8 milligrams of zinc acetate or a placebo every 2 to 3 waking hours until their symptoms resolved. The volunteers rated the severity of their symptoms daily on a scale of 0 to 3. The results were positive, with the researchers noting that "administration of zinc lozenges was associated with reduced duration and severity of cold symptoms, especially cough." Table 6-6 below compares the average length of the overall and individual symptoms in the zinc and placebo groups.

Table 6-6: Improvement in Cold Symptoms Triggered by Zinc Compared to Placebo[23]

SYMPTOMS	AVERAGE NUMBER OF DAYS SYMPTOMS LASTED	
	Zinc Group	Placebo Group
Overall symptoms	4.5	8.1
Sore throat	2.0	3.0
Nasal discharge	4.1	5.8
Nasal congestion	3.3	4.7
Sneezing	2.7	4.4
Cough	3.1	6.3
Scratchy throat	2.8	2.8
Hoarseness	2.0	1.2
Muscle ache	1.4	1.5
Fever	0.4	0.2
Headache	2.0	2.4

Summing Up the Evidence for Zinc

The "zinc wars" have raged through the medical literature, with several studies in prestigious mainstream medical journals showing that the mineral helps reduce the average duration and severity of cold symptoms—and several other studies in equally important journals arguing the opposite. Some have criticized the negative research, saying that the studies involved zinc lozenges that did not dissolve properly to release the mineral or that they used the wrong form of zinc. Others have said that the methodology of the positive studies was flawed and allowed for bias, skewing the results.

While zinc appears to be able to reduce the duration and severity of cold symptoms, the most effective form of zinc, the best delivery vehicle (type of lozenge), and the optimal dosage have yet to be determined. Thus, it is fair to conclude that zinc is a three-star treatment for the common cold backed by intriguing evidence.

Available Forms

Among the food sources of zinc are oysters, chicken leg, pork tenderloin, plain yogurt, pecans, and cashews. The mineral also is available in supplement form.

How Much Zinc Is Typically Used

The Recommended Dietary Allowances of zinc are 11 milligrams for men ages 19 and older and 8 milligrams for women ages 19 and older. The studies involving zinc as a treatment for cold symptoms have used dosages of up to 13.3 milligrams every 2 hours while awake.

Possible Side Effects and Interactions

The Food and Nutrition Board of the Institute of Medicine has set a tolerable upper intake for zinc of 40 milligrams per day for adults. Taking excessive amounts of zinc can lower levels of "good" HDL cholesterol and weaken the immune system. In addition, zinc may hamper the absorption of antibiotics such as ciprofloxacin (Cipro), reducing blood levels of the drug. If you're taking any medication, be sure to consult your doctor before adding therapeutic doses of zinc to your self-care regimen.

7

ALTERNATIVE APPROACHES TO

CONSTIPATION

Biofeedback ☆☆☆
Prebiotics/probiotics ☆☆

Constipation is defined as infrequent or uncomfortable bowel movements, a not-too-serious problem that strikes everyone from time to time. But it can become serious if it develops into a chronic condition that persists for months or even years.

Constipation occurs when the transit time of stool slows as it moves through the large intestine. This allows greater than usual amounts of water to be reclaimed from it and sent back into circulation. As a result, the stool becomes hard and dry, so it's difficult and uncomfortable to pass.

While constipation is defined, in part, as "infrequent bowel movements," there is no set number of bowel movements that is considered "normal" or "abnormal." Some perfectly healthy people have as many as two or three bowel movements a day, while others have as few as two or three a week. The onset of constipation is most likely indicated by a sudden decline in the frequency of bowel movements, coupled with drier, harder stool.

SYMPTOMS

The most common symptoms of constipation are less frequent bowel movements; harder, drier stools that are difficult to pass; a feeling that the rectum has not been thoroughly emptied after a bowel movement; abdominal and rectal pain; nausea; lack of appetite; and straining during a bowel movement—which, in turn, can cause hemorrhoids and a temporary rise in blood pressure.

CAUSES

One fairly common cause of constipation is pelvic floor dyssynergia (also known as functional constipation), in which the muscles in the rectum and anus contract rather than relax while straining during defecation. Other conditions that can contribute to constipation include an underactive thyroid gland, Parkinson's disease, high blood levels of calcium, an inactive colon, nerve or spinal cord injuries, and changes in the levels of neurotransmitters (brain chemicals) such as serotonin.

Various lifestyle factors—such as dehydration, lack of dietary fiber, aging, and lack of exercise—can slow the transit time of stool. So can certain drugs, among them aluminum hydroxide (Alu-Cap), certain antihypertensives (Zebeta), anticholinergic drugs (Atropine), bismuth subsalicylate (Pepto-Bismol), iron salts (eFeratab), and most sedatives (Valium).

STANDARD TREATMENTS

The best way to treat constipation is to prevent it from occurring in the first place by eating a high-fiber diet, drinking plenty of fluids, and getting an adequate amount of exercise. Doing so is especially important when taking medications that can cause constipation, which, in some cases, might require taking a gentle laxative. Laxatives containing bulking agents such as psyllium and bran produce softer stool and promote natural intestinal contractions.

If constipation has already settled in, the usual recommendation is to combine the lifestyle changes above with a stool softener or a stimulant laxative. Stool softeners help increase the amount of water in the stool so that it's easier to pass, while stimulant laxatives irritate the intestinal walls, promoting intestinal contractions that push the stool along.

Another treatment option is an osmotic agent, which is typically used to clear the intestines before administering colonoscopies or bowel x-rays. The osmotic agents work by drawing large amounts of water into the stool while distending the intestinal walls, which stimulates contractions.

Enemas are a mechanical way of clearing the rectum and lower part of the intestine by introducing a small amount of fluid into the rectum to lubricate and flush out the stool.

RATING POPULAR ALTERNATIVE TREATMENTS FOR CONSTIPATION

Biofeedback

Rating: ☆☆☆ = Intriguing Evidence

Biofeedback allows patients to "see" what's happening in a certain part of the body and to gain some measure of control over it. This therapy is often recommended to people suffering from stress, insomnia, headaches, and muscle injuries to help them learn to relax certain muscles, slow their breathing, or otherwise adjust a body function.

During a biofeedback session, electrodes coming from a machine may be attached to the skin over certain muscles. As the patient contracts and relaxes those muscles, he or she receives audio and/or visual feedback from the machine. This feedback tells the patient whether he or she is effectively slowing her breathing or relaxing a particular muscle, or otherwise achieving the desired result.

Biofeedback has been used for quite some time to treat fecal incontinence (uncontrolled passing of stool) by strengthening muscles in the pelvic area. Noting its success in stopping unwanted bowel movements, researchers decided to find out if biofeedback would help relieve constipation.

There are several techniques for applying the principles of biofeedback to the problem of constipation. One is sensory training, in which a water-filled balloon is inserted into the rectum and then withdrawn slowly. Patients are instructed to ease the passage of the balloon by focusing on the sensations it triggers as it moves. They may also be asked to expel the balloon as if it were feces, to improve bowel function.

Another technique, called electromyography, uses probes or electrodes to register activity as the patient practices relaxing certain pelvic muscles while pushing, and watches the results of his or her efforts on a monitor. And in manometry, balloons or probes are used to measure pressure in the anal canal as the patient relaxes and contracts certain pelvic muscles.

All of these techniques are designed to eliminate any "wayward" muscle contractions that may be interfering with bowel evacuation.

♦ In 1997 researchers from the University of Iowa published the results of their study involving 25 patients suffering from obstructive defecation (significant difficulty in expelling stool or an inability to do so).[1] Over the course of six sessions, manometry was used to guide patients through pelvic muscle relaxation training and simulated defecation maneuvers. The results were positive, with straining effort and laxative consumption decreasing. Sixty percent of the volunteers reported a 75 percent or greater increase in satisfaction with bowel habits after training, while 32 percent reported a 50 percent or greater increase.

◆ In 1998 researchers from St. Mark's Hospital in London presented the results of their study involving 100 people who had been suffering from idiopathic constipation, or constipation for which there is no known cause.[2] Their average age was 40, and a third of them had been living with constipation since childhood. This was a retrospective study, meaning that it was done by gathering the records of patients who had already undergone biofeedback training, then conducting follow-up interviews an average of 23 months after they'd completed their treatment. Over half of the patients reported that they had been helped by biofeedback. Their subjective judgments were supported by these facts: The use of oral laxatives fell from 66 percent of participants before treatment to 38 percent afterward; the use of enemas fell from 24 percent to 13 percent; and the use of suppositories fell from 28 percent to 16 percent. According to the researchers, their study "has shown that biofeedback is a successful treatment for constipation [that] patients and their doctors judge to have been unresponsive to other treatments." Table 7-1 below shows some of the results of biofeedback training.

Table 7-1: Percentage of Patients with Symptoms of Constipation Before and After Biofeedback[3]

Symptoms	Prior to Biofeedback Training Course	After Biofeedback Training Course	Upon Questioning an Average of 23 Months Later
Straining	86%	61%	56%
Rectal or vaginal digitation	48%	28%	31%
Feeling of incomplete evacuation	85%	63%	64%
Pain (mild to severe)	84%	68%	64%
Bloating (mild to severe)	86%	76%	72%

+ Forty-nine patients, average age 39, with idiopathic constipation were given an average of five biofeedback sessions.[4] After completing treatments, the number who had stools that were either hard or pelletlike fell from 30 to 7; who needed to strain at stool, from 26 to 9; who needed to digitate (that is, press their fingers against the perineum or adjacent areas to stimulate bowel movement or to remove feces), from 19 to 9; who had abdominal bloating, from 39 to 11; and who used laxatives, from 34 to 9. The number who had fewer than 3 bowel movements per week—a sign of constipation for many people—dropped from 27 to 9.

+ For a review study published in *Applied Psychophysiology and Biofeedback* in 2004, researchers from the Department of Medicine at the University of North Carolina at Chapel Hill searched the scientific literature to find all of the published papers on biofeedback and constipation.[5] They identified 38 different studies—a mix of randomized and nonrandomized, controlled and uncontrolled—and analyzed the findings to see if they could make a definitive recommendation for biofeedback as a treatment for constipation. They concluded that for pelvic floor dyssynergia/functional constipation, the "success rate per subject is significantly higher for biofeedback treatment than for standard medical care," and that biofeedback is a "valuable adjunct to medical management."

+ Another review of the literature, published in the *British Medical Journal* in 2004,[6] criticized the quality of the research but concluded that "biofeedback training seems to be a good treatment for lower gastrointestinal disturbances, especially for pelvic floor dyssynergia" and accompanying constipation.

Summing Up the Evidence for Biofeedback

There are a fair number of studies pointing to the usefulness of biofeedback for constipation, but they are open-label trials. That is, the researchers and participants knew participants were receiving biofeedback, so the placebo effect may have come into play. This limits the usefulness of the studies, leading to the conclusion that biofeedback is a three-star treatment for constipation backed by intriguing evidence. (Note, however, that it seems to be more helpful for idiopathic constipation and dyssynergia than for constipation related to slow transit time.)

Where to Get Biofeedback Training

Biofeedback training should be performed by a medical doctor or a trained biofeedback technician working under a physician's supervision. Upon the successful completion of training, you should be able to relax or contract the appropriate muscles, or otherwise achieve the desired result on your own, without the use of biofeedback devices. The Biofeedback Certification Institute of America posts a list of certified biofeedback technicians on its Web site (www.bcia.org).

Prebiotics and Probiotics

Rating: ☆☆ = Modest Evidence

Prebiotics are substances that encourage the growth of probiotics like *Lactobacillus acidophilus* inside the body. In a sense, prebiotics serve as raw materials for the manufacture of probiotics. They include inulin, FOS (fructo-oligosaccharides), and GOS (galacto-oligosaccharides), among others.

Probiotics are living microorganisms that, when consumed in sufficient amounts, produce health benefits beyond simple nutritional assistance. The probiotics found in cultured dairy products (such as the *Lactobacillus acidophilus* found in yogurt) have long been used for nutrition and health; indeed, they are even mentioned in the Bible and ancient Hindu texts. The basic idea behind probiotic therapy is to "seed" the intestines with the kind of helpful microorganisms that naturally populate a healthy gut.

Both prebiotics and probiotics can help lower cholesterol and blood fats, ease lactose intolerance, strengthen the immune system, and otherwise improve health. Some studies have found that prebiotics and probiotics can alleviate the symptoms of constipation. Among them:

♦ *Prebiotics*: A study reported in the *American Journal of Clinical Nutrition* in 1997 compared the effects of the prebiotic inulin to lactose, a sugar used as a treatment for constipation.[9] Twenty-five elderly women with constipation were enrolled in the study. Ten were given inulin (brand name Raftiline) and 15 were given lactose. Both groups received dosages that began at 20 grams per day and increased to 40 grams per day during the 19-day study period. The results were positive, with inulin significantly increasing the amount of the prebiotic bifidobacteria found in the feces and producing a better laxative effect than lactose. The researchers noted that inulin "improved constipation in 9 of 10 subjects" and "reduced functional constipation with only mild discomfort."

♦ *Prebiotics*: Finnish researchers looked at the effects of the prebiotics known as *GOS (galacto-oligosaccharides)* in 14 women, average age 79, who had constipation.[10] For 2 weeks of this double-blind, crossover study, the volunteers were given either yogurt containing 9 grams of GOS (brand name Elix'or) or regular yogurt without GOS. During an additional 2 weeks, the groups switched treatments, with the GOS group receiving "regular" yogurt and the "regular" yogurt group receiving the GOS yogurt. While the study participants were consuming the GOS yogurt, the frequency of bowel movements increased from an average of 5.9 per week to an average of 7.1 per week. The researchers concluded that "9 [grams] of GOS daily seemed to relieve constipation in most of the elderly subjects, mainly by making defecation easier."

♦ *Probiotics*: Researchers from the German Institute of Human Nutrition investigated the effects of a beverage containing probiotics on 70 men and women suffering from chronic constipation.[11] For this randomized, double-blind study, the volunteers were assigned to receive either 65 milliliters of a beverage containing the probiotic *Lactobacillus casei* Shirota or a placebo drink every day for 4 weeks. Those who drank the probiotic beverage reported a "significant improvement" in the severity of their constipation, beginning with the second week of treatment. The researchers concluded that "probiotic foodstuffs may be recommended as an adjunctive therapy for chronic constipation."

♦ *Probiotics*: In 2004 Finnish researchers reported the results of their study involving a mix of probiotics.[12] Twenty-eight elderly people suffering from constipation were recruited to help test the effects of three different drinks. For the first 3 weeks all 28 volunteers drank the plain orange juice. For the next 4 weeks they were divided into three groups, with one group receiving the plain juice, another group, the juice plus *Lactobacillus reuteri*, and the third group, the juice plus *Lactobacillus rhamnosus* and *Propionibacterium freudenreichii* every day. For the final 3 weeks, everyone drank the plain juice once again. The researchers noted the frequency of defecation, the use of laxatives, the pH of the feces, and other indicators of bowel status. Among the volunteers who drank the juice plus *Lactobacillus rhamnosus* and *Propionibacterium freudenreichii*, the frequency of bowel movements increased by 25 percent. While this is a positive sign, it was not accompanied by a decrease in laxative use, leading the researchers to conclude that the combination of probiotics produced "some relief" from constipation. (Similar results were not seen in those who drank the juice plus *Lactobacillus reuteri*.)

Summing Up the Evidence for Prebiotics and Probiotics

Although there are several studies looking at the effects of prebiotics on constipation, several of them are open-label studies subject to influence by the placebo effect. As for probiotics for the treatment of constipation, there are not enough studies, and the few that exist used different types and amounts of probiotics. Thus, given the evidence available at this point, it's fair to say that prebiotics and probiotics are a two-star treatment for constipation backed by modest evidence.

Available Forms

Among the food sources of prebiotics are onions, Jerusalem artichokes, garlic, and chicory root. They're also available in supplement form. Probiotics may be found in certain brands of yogurt and other foods. They're also available in capsule, tablet, and powder form.

How Much Is Typically Used

There is no standard dose of prebiotics or probiotics. For probiotics, doses of up to 10 billion colony-forming units may be taken two or three times a week.[13]

Possible Side Effects and Interactions

Taking prebiotics or probiotics can cause gastrointestinal discomfort and flatulence. As with all supplements and drugs, be sure to read the product labels carefully before adding prebiotics and/or probiotics to your self-care regimen.

8

ALTERNATIVE APPROACHES TO
CORONARY HEART DISEASE

Omega-3 fatty acids	☆☆☆☆☆
B vitamins	☆☆☆☆
Garlic	☆☆☆☆
Magnesium	☆☆☆
Alcoholic beverages	☆☆
Olive oil	☆☆
Nuts	☆☆

Heart disease—a major killer of Americans and one of the leading causes of disability—is also known as coronary heart disease (CHD) because it involves the narrowing of the *coronary arteries*, which feed fresh blood to the heart muscle. When these blood vessels become narrow, brittle, or clogged, they can't supply enough blood for the heart to work properly.

The narrowing, stiffening, and clogging of the coronary arteries (called *atherosclerosis*) is due to the build-up of *plaque* on their inner walls. Plaque is a thick, waxy substance made up of cholesterol, fat, smooth muscle cells, and cellular debris that makes artery walls rigid and unable to expand when necessary. The build-up of plaque can narrow a coronary artery to the point where it's completely clogged, or a piece of plaque may break off and float "downstream" until it gets caught in a smaller blood vessel, causing a blockage. Thick, sticky blood that's full of clotting substances can also contribute to blockages.

When a coronary artery becomes blocked, the area of the heart muscle that it serves is starved of oxygen and nutrients. The heart muscle becomes damaged or even dies, an event we refer to as a heart attack. Almost all heart attacks result from atherosclerosis in the coronary arteries combined with the formation of one or more clots.

SYMPTOMS

Heart disease can progress undetected for many years before it produces any obvious symptoms. When the disease is well-advanced, however, it can cause *angina*—pain that originates in the chest and radiates to the neck and jaw, shoulders and arms, back, or upper abdomen. There may also be shortness of breath, a squeezing or crushing sensation in the chest, heart palpitations or irregular heartbeat, fatigue, light-headedness, fainting, nausea, and sweating.

CAUSES

Many factors contribute to heart disease. Among them are high blood levels of total cholesterol, oxidized LDL cholesterol, C-reactive protein, or homocysteine; low blood levels of HDL cholesterol; high blood pressure; diabetes; obesity; smoking; stress; and lack of physical activity—all of which, fortunately, can be controlled. Factors that can't be controlled include having a family history of heart disease or stroke; being African-American, Mexican-American, or Native American; being male; being postmenopausal; and aging.

STANDARD TREATMENTS

Standard medical treatment for heart disease begins with a low-fat, low-cholesterol diet, regular exercise, and weight loss when necessary. If these measures don't work, drugs that lower cholesterol and/or blood fats—such as the popular statin drugs (Lipitor or Zocor)—may be prescribed.

In more severe cases of heart disease, surgery may be recommended. Angioplasty is a surgical procedure in which a thin tube is threaded through the blood vessels until it reaches the clogged artery in the heart. There a balloon on the tip of the tube is inflated, which presses the plaque against the inner walls of the artery and physically widens them, allowing more blood to flow through. In some cases, a coiled piece of metal (a *stent*) is left inside the artery to help keep it open.

Perhaps the best known of the surgical procedures for heart disease is the coronary bypass. In a bypass, a blood vessel is taken from another part of the body and attached to a coronary artery, rerouting the blood flow through that artery and bypassing the blocked or severely narrowed section.

RATING POPULAR ALTERNATIVE TREATMENTS FOR HEART DISEASE

Omega-3 Fatty Acids

Rating: ☆☆☆☆☆ = Convincing Evidence

Back in the 1970s, scientists wondered why Eskimos rarely had heart disease despite the fact that their diets—which consisted almost entirely of very fatty fish—were very high in fat. Research led the investigators to discover a group of heart-protective substances within the fat of the fish called omega-3 fatty acids. The best known of the omega-3s are DHA (docosahexaenoic acid) and EPA (eicosapentaenoic acid).

Scientists have found that in humans, the higher the level of omega-3s in body tissues and the blood, the lower the risk of developing heart disease. That's because the omega-3s reduce total cholesterol and triglyceride levels, increase "good" HDL cholesterol, decrease atherosclerosis, and inhibit the formation of blood clots that can trigger a heart attack.

Numerous population studies have linked a diet rich in fish (and the omega-3 fatty acids they contain) to better heart health. For example:

♦ A 2002 study published in the *Journal of the American Medical Association* followed nearly 85,000 women participating in the Nurses' Health Study for 16 years. Those who ate two to four servings of fish a week cut their risk of developing heart disease by 30 percent.[1]

♦ A team of American researchers examined data from a 30-year study tracking the health and habits of 1,822 men, ranging in age from 40 to 55.[2] They found "an inverse association between fish consumption and death from coronary heart disease," meaning that the more fish the men ate, the less likely they were to die from heart disease. Specifically, eating at least 35 grams of fish (a little more than 1 ounce) per day reduced the relative risk of death from coronary heart disease and heart attack by more than 35 percent, as compared to eating no fish.

Other studies have linked omega-3 fatty acids from *any* source to better heart health, including this one:

♦ Researchers from Brigham and Women's Hospital, Harvard Medical School, and the University of Washington presented the results of their study in the journal *Circulation* in 2005.[3] They examined data that had been collected over the course of 14 years from more than 45,000 men, none of whom had heart disease when the study began. The researchers found that omega-3 fatty acids, whether from seafood or plant sources, could reduce the risk of coronary heart disease.

While population studies have linked increased consumption of omega-3 fatty acids to a lower risk of heart disease, they don't prove that the former causes the latter. Only experimental studies can do that, and several have put omega-3 fatty acids to the test:

♦ In 1989 researchers presented results from DART (the Diet and Rein-farction Trial) in the journal *Lancet*.[4] More than 2,000 men who had recovered from a heart attack were randomly assigned to receive dietary advice based on one of three different strategies:

◊ Fat advice—reduce overall fat intake, increase polyunsaturated fat intake
◊ Fish advice—eat at least two portions of fatty fish, such as salmon or trout, per week
◊ Fiber advice—eat 18 grams of cereal fiber per day

The "winning advice" turned out to be the instructions to eat fish. During the 2-year period after the men had been advised to increase their intake of fatty fish to between 200 and 400 grams per week, their risk of dying from any cause decreased. The greatest drop was in the risk of suffering a fatal heart attack. The researchers noted, "The results suggest that fatty fish (and fish oil) reduces mortality in men after [heart attack], by about 29 [percent] during the first 2 years."

♦ Indian researchers tested the effects of omega-3 fatty acids in a randomized, double-blind study with people who had suffered heart attacks.[5] An average of 18 hours following symptoms of a heart attack, the 360 participants were randomly assigned to receive daily doses of fish oil containing 1.08 grams of EPA; mustard oil containing 2.9 grams of alpha-linolenic acid, which converts to an omega-3 fatty acid in the body; or a placebo. A year later, those who had been taking the fish oil or the mustard oil had significantly fewer heart problems than those in the placebo group. And the fish oil group had significantly fewer deaths due to heart disease compared to the placebo group, a result not seen with the mustard oil. The researchers concluded, "The findings of this study suggest that fish oil and mustard oil, possibly due to the presence of [omega-3 fatty acids], may provide rapid protective effects" in those who have suffered a heart attack.

♦ A large open-label, controlled trial testing the effects of omega-3 fatty acids on heart disease enlisted 11,324 people who had recently survived a heart attack.[6] The volunteers were randomly assigned to receive 1 gram of omega-3 fatty acids (EPA and DHA) per day, 300 milligrams of vitamin E per day, both, or neither. After following the participants for 3½ years, the researchers concluded that treatment with omega-3 fatty acids significantly lowered the rate of death as well as of nonfatal heart attacks and strokes, while vitamin E did not have similar effects.

♦ For a 2002 meta-analysis appearing in the *American Journal of Medicine*, Swiss researchers combed the scientific literature to identify 11 randomized, controlled trials testing the effects of omega-3 fatty acids in people with coronary artery disease.[7] These studies involved a total of 7,951 patients receiving omega-3 fatty acids, plus 7,855 patients in control groups. After statistically merging the information from the various studies, the researchers concluded that omega-3 fatty acids from food or supplements reduce the risk of death due to heart attacks as well as deaths due to all causes in people with coronary heart disease.

♦ An American Heart Association Scientific Statement appearing in the journal *Circulation* in 2002 noted, "Omega-3 fatty acids have been shown in epidemiological and clinical trials to reduce the incidence of [cardiovascular disease]. Large-scale epidemiological studies suggest that individuals at risk for [coronary heart disease] benefit from the consumption of plant- and marine-derived omega-3 fatty acids."[8]

♦ In 2004 the Agency for Healthcare Research and Quality, part of the US Department of Health and Human Services, issued a report stating that "a number of studies offer evidence" supporting the hypothesis that consuming fish or fish oil reduces the risk of heart attack, stroke, or other negative outcomes associated with cardiovascular disease.[9]

Summing Up the Evidence for Omega-3 Fatty Acids

Given this wealth of information from population and experimental studies, it is safe to conclude that omega-3 fatty acids are a five-star treatment for coronary heart disease backed by convincing evidence.

Available Forms

The best sources of omega-3 fatty acids are cold-water fatty fish such as mackerel, salmon, herring, anchovies, and tuna. As a general rule, the fattier a fish is, the more omega-3s it contains. The human body can manufacture omega-3s from alpha-linolenic acid, which is found in walnuts and flaxseed. Omega-3 fatty acids are also available in supplement form, labeled as fish oil, omega-3, EPA, DHA, or some combination of these.

Amount of Omega-3 Fatty Acids Typically Used

There is no standard dosage of omega-3 fatty acids. The American Heart Association offers these suggestions:

♦ If you don't have heart disease, eat at least two servings per week of a variety of fish—preferably the fatty kind like salmon, which contains omega-3 fatty acids.

♦ If you have heart disease, get at least 1 gram of DHA or EPA per day, from foods or supplements.

♦ If you need to lower your blood fats, take 2 to 4 grams of EPA and DHA per day, under your physician's care.

Possible Side Effects and Interactions

The omega-3 fatty acids are found in common foods and have been granted Generally Regarded as Safe (GRAS) status by the US government. Possible side effects include prolonged bleeding time, which may be a problem for those who have bleeding disorders, those who are taking medicines to thin the blood, or those who will be undergoing surgery soon. Along the same line, omega-3s may interact with aspirin, heparin, and other drugs that thin the blood, increasing the risk of bleeding. If you're taking any medication, be sure to consult your doctor before adding omega-3 supplements to your self-care regimen.

B Vitamins

Rating: ☆☆☆☆ = Strong Evidence

The B vitamins are a group of related substances—including thiamin, riboflavin, niacin, vitamins B_6 and B_{12}, pantothenic acid, biotin, and folic acid—with numerous functions in the body. The argument for the use of folic acid and vitamins B_6 and B_{12} for heart health is based on the fact that a lack of these three specific nutrients is associated with a rise in blood levels of an amino acid called homocysteine. Too much homocysteine, in turn, is associated with an increased risk of coronary artery damage, heart attack, and stroke.

Several studies have found that these three B vitamins do indeed protect against heart disease:

◆ Pakistani researchers looked for a link between B vitamins and homocysteine in 224 people who'd had heart attacks and 126 others who hadn't.[10] Blood samples were drawn from the volunteers, and the amounts of folic acid, vitamin B_6, vitamin B_{12}, and homocysteine in each sample were determined. As shown in Figure 8-1 on the next page, the average levels of folic acid and B_6 were lower in the blood of the heart attack patients than in the healthy volunteers, while the average level of B_{12} was significantly lower. In addition, those who'd suffered heart attacks were significantly more likely to have actual deficiencies in folic acid, B_6, and B_{12}. Homocysteine levels were higher among those who had suffered heart attacks, but the difference was not statistically significant. The researchers concluded that major deficiencies of folic acid, vitamin B_6, and vitamin B_{12}, combined with mildly elevated homocysteine, may increase the risk of coronary heart disease.

Figure 8-1: Heart Attack Patients More Likely to Be Deficient in B Vitamins

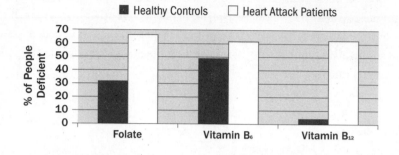

◆ A 2004 study published in *Pharmacological Research* tested the effects of folic acid supplementation in 30 people who had recently suffered heart attacks and had elevated levels of homocysteine.[11] The volunteers were randomly assigned to receive 3 months of treatment with daily doses of 15 to 30 milligrams of folic acid, or 15 to 30 milligrams of folic acid plus 900 milligrams of vitamin E. The results were positive, with folic acid reducing homocysteine levels by 41 percent and producing significant improvement in the function of the arterial linings. (Vitamin E did not improve either the homocysteine level or arterial function.)

◆ Canadian researchers tested the effects of folic acid alone and combined with antioxidants for a randomized, double-blind study published in the *Journal of the American College of Cardiology* in 2000.[12] The 75 participants in this study, all of whom had coronary artery disease, were assigned to receive one of three treatments: folic acid only (5 milligrams of folic acid per day); folic acid plus antioxidants (5 milligrams of folic acid, 2,000 milligrams of vitamin C, and 800 IU of vitamin E per day); or placebo. One of the hallmarks of coronary artery disease is endothelial dysfunction, caused by damage to the interior arterial linings. As a result, the arteries may not be able to expand and contract as necessary to accommodate bloodflow. Ultrasound was used to assess the study participants' endothelial function. The results were positive; compared to placebo, folic acid treatment reduced homocysteine levels and significantly improved endothelial functioning in key arteries.

Summing Up the Evidence for B Vitamins

A large number of population studies have linked B vitamin deficiencies to heart disease, and a fair amount of experimental evidence indicates that B vitamin supplements can lower homocysteine levels and improve the functioning of coronary arteries. It is safe to say that B vitamins are a four-star treatment for coronary heart disease backed by strong evidence.

Available Forms

Food sources of folic acid include leafy green vegetables and dried peas and beans; of vitamin B_6, bananas, oatmeal, and garbanzo beans; and of vitamin B_{12}, beef liver, rainbow trout, and sockeye salmon. The B vitamins are available in supplement form.

Amount of B Vitamins Typically Used

There is no standard dose of B vitamins for heart disease. Supplemental doses for lowering elevated homocysteine may range up to 30 milligrams of folic acid per day, 200 milligrams of vitamin B_6 per day, and 500 micrograms of vitamin B_{12} per day.

Possible Side Effects and Interactions

The Food and Nutrition Board of the Institute of Medicine has set tolerable upper intakes of 100 milligrams for vitamin B_6 and 1,000 micrograms of folic acid, per day, for adults. There is no tolerable upper intake for vitamin B_{12}.

Among folic acid's side effects are rash and abdominal cramps. In addition, it may inhibit the effectiveness of drugs for cancer, such as methotrexate (Trexall), and drugs for seizures, such as primidone (Mysoline).

Vitamin B_6 can cause nausea and headache. It also may lower blood levels of seizure medicines, such as phenobarbital, and may reduce the effectiveness of Parkinson's medications, such as levodopa (Dopar).

Vitamin B_{12}'s side effects include diarrhea and itching. It is not known to interfere with the actions of medications when taken in therapeutic amounts.

As with all supplements and drugs, be sure to read the label directions carefully before taking B vitamin supplements. And if you're taking any medication, consult your doctor before adding B vitamins to your self-care regimen.

Garlic

Rating: ☆☆☆☆☆ = Strong Evidence

Garlic has a long history as a healing herb in cultures throughout the world. It was used by Egyptian healers to keep their slaves healthy; by Dr. Albert Schweitzer in Africa to treat cholera, typhus, and other ailments; and by Russian physicians during World War II to disinfect battlefield wounds. Today, the herb is a popular treatment for colds, allergies, diarrhea, arthritis, and a number of other ailments. Garlic appears to fight bacteria and viruses, stimulate the immune system, and support general good health.

Numerous studies over the past several decades have investigated garlic's protective effects against coronary heart disease. The herb has several helpful actions, including lowering elevated blood pressure and blood fats, guarding against age-related damage to the arteries and veins, and reducing the risk of dangerous blood clots.

Garlic's ability to lower blood pressure is explored in detail in Chapter 13. This discussion will focus on reducing cholesterol and other risks.

Garlic and Cholesterol

Several studies have focused on garlic's cholesterol-lowering ability, including the following:

♦ A team of researchers from Loma Linda University School of Medicine presented the results of their garlic/cholesterol study in *Nutrition Research* in 1987.[13] Thirty-two men and women, ages 45 to 68 and with total cholesterol levels ranging from 220 to 440 mg/dL (milligrams per deciliter of blood), participated in this randomized study. The volunteers were given either 4 milliliters of liquid garlic extract (brand name Kyolic AGE) or placebo every day for 6 months. The results were positive, with total cholesterol falling by an average of 44 points in the garlic group, compared to 10 points in the placebo group. The researchers also monitored blood fats (triglycerides), looking to see whose would drop by 10 percent or more. This happened in 10 of the 15 taking garlic, compared to only 3 of the 12 taking the placebo. Table 8-1 on the next page shows the beginning and ending cholesterol levels for the volunteers taking garlic.

Table 8-1: Aged Garlic Extract Reduces Total Cholesterol[14]

VOLUNTEER NUMBER	TOTAL CHOLESTEROL LEVEL		
	Beginning of Study (mg/dL)	6 Months Later (mg/dL)	Increase/Decrease (mg/dL)
1	226	188	-38
2	240	182	-58
3	236	202	-34
4	280	232	-48
5	267	184	-83
6	286	224	-62
7	340	352	+12
8	410	414	+4
9	440	320	-120
10	288	210	-78
11	270	216	-54
12	368	374	+6
13	388	342	-46
14	254	262	+8
15	296	234	-62
Average for the entire group	306	262	-44

♦ As reported in the *American Journal of Clinical Nutrition* in 1996, 56 men with elevated cholesterol levels were enlisted for a double-blind, crossover study comparing aged garlic extract to placebo.[15] The volunteers ranged in age from 32 to 68 and had total cholesterol levels ranging from 220 to 290 mg/dL (milligrams per deciliter of blood). After being advised to follow a standard cholesterol-lowering diet, the volunteers were randomly assigned to receive either 7.2 grams of aged garlic extract or a placebo every day. After 6 months, they switched to the other treatment for an additional 4 months. Analysis of the study data showed that total cholesterol levels were 6.1 percent lower and LDL cholesterol levels were 4.0 percent lower during administration of the aged garlic than during administration of the placebo. The researchers concluded that "dietary supplementation with aged garlic extract has beneficial effects on the lipid profiles" of men with moderately elevated cholesterol levels.

♦ Forty-three people with elevated cholesterol participated in a double-blind Australian study published in the *Journal of the American College of Nutrition* in 2001.[15] For 12 weeks the volunteers were randomly assigned to receive daily doses of either 880 milligrams of garlic powder, equivalent to 10.4 grams of fresh garlic, or a placebo. (The garlic was manufactured by Pharmaction Pty Ltd.) The results were positive, with the garlic group showing statistically significant reductions of 4.2 percent in total cholesterol and 6.6 percent in LDL cholesterol. These decreases were small, but they compared well to the placebo group, which had small increases in total cholesterol and LDL.

Garlic and Other Heart Disease Risks

A number of studies have examined the effects of garlic on the likelihood of developing other risk factors for heart disease. For example:

♦ *Garlic and plaque growth*: Researchers from the Harbor–UCLA Medical Center tested the effects of garlic on plaque accumulation in coronary arteries.[17] The presence of too much plaque in an artery can increase the risk of arterial blockage and heart attack; conversely, slowing or stopping the rate of plaque accumulation can help reduce the risk of heart attack. All 19 volunteers in this double-blind, randomized study had, or were at high risk for developing, coronary artery disease. They were assigned to receive 1 year of treatment with either 4 milliliters of garlic extract (Kyolic AGE) or placebo. Electron-beam tomography was used to calculate the calcium score, a measure of plaque growth. The average calcium score rose by 22 percent in the placebo group, compared to only 7.4 percent in the garlic group. According to the researchers, these results demonstrate the potential of this aged garlic extract "to inhibit the rate of progression of coronary calcification, as compared to placebo over one year."

♦ *Garlic and endothelial dysfunction*: German researchers tested the effect of garlic on endothelial function in a blinded crossover study.[18] The endothelium is the lining of an artery; healthy endothelial function is important, for poor function is associated with coronary artery disease and elevated blood pressure. The volunteers in this study were pretreated with either garlic or placebo for 6 weeks. Then the researchers gave the participants the amino acid methionine to deliberately increase their homocysteine levels, and monitored the effects on the linings of the arteries. In round two of the study, the volunteers switched treatments and again received methionine to raise their homocysteine levels. The results were positive, indicating that 6 weeks of pretreatment with aged garlic extract "significantly diminished the adverse effects" of elevated homocysteine on the endothelium.

♦ *Garlic and platelet "stickiness"*: Platelets—tiny disc-shaped objects in the blood—are designed to stick to each other and to other substances in the bloodstream when a blood vessel is ruptured. Unfortunately, platelets can aggregate—that is, stick together—at the wrong time, forming clots that can clog coronary arteries and trigger a heart attack. The ability of garlic to help prevent unwanted platelet aggregation was tested in a 2000 study published in the *Journal of Nutrition*.[19] Twenty-three healthy men and women, ranging in age from 22 to 45, participated in this open study. After having their blood drawn, they were treated with 5 milliliters of aged garlic extract (Kyolic AGE) every day for 13 weeks. The garlic extract supplementation "significantly inhibited both the total percentage and initial rate of platelet aggregation."

Review Study of Garlic

♦ A 2004 review published in the *FASEB Journal* reviewed a number of studies of garlic's effects on the cardiovascular system.[20] All of the studies were randomized, double-blind, and placebo-controlled; lasted between 1 month and 1 year; and had between 19 and 80 subjects. Dosages of garlic (Kyolic AGE) equivalent to 4 milliliters ranged from 1.2 to 3.6 grams per day. This review found that aged garlic extract triggered reductions of 65 percent in plaque formation, 10 to 25 percent in platelet aggregation, and 38 percent in the oxidation of LDL to its more dangerous form. The authors concluded that aged garlic extract "may be useful and beneficial for the treatment and prevention of cardiac atherosclerosis."

Summing Up the Evidence for Garlic

Many studies indicate that garlic can lower cholesterol, reduce blood pressure, lessen the tendency of the blood to clot at the wrong time, and otherwise reduce the risk of coronary artery disease. In all fairness, some studies have come to the opposite conclusion. This confusion may be due to differences in garlic preparations (dried, powdered, time-release, aged or not aged, and so on); amounts of allicin or other substances in the various extracts studied; dosages; study lengths; and other variables. Even after taking all of this into consideration, it is fair to say that garlic is a four-star treatment for coronary heart disease backed by strong evidence.

Available Forms

Garlic is available at the grocery store in the form of raw cloves (a single raw clove contains about 3 grams of garlic), chopped bottled garlic, or garlic powder. It is also found in supplement form at health food and vitamin stores, either by itself or in combination with other ingredients.

How Much Garlic Is Typically Used

There is no standard dose for garlic. Several successful studies used dosages between 4 and 5 milliliters of aged garlic extract per day.

Possible Side Effects and Interactions

Garlic's side effects include dizziness, headache, irritation of the gastrointestinal tract, thinning of the blood, prolongation of bleeding time—and, of course, "garlic breath." (Some garlic supplements are specially formulated to eliminate garlic breath.) In addition, garlic may interact with antidiabetes drugs such as glipizide (Glucotrol), increasing the risk of low blood sugar as well as with drugs for elevated blood pressure such as amlodipine (Norvasc), causing blood pressure to fall too low. If you're taking any medication, be sure to consult your doctor before adding therapeutic amounts of garlic to your self-care regimen.

Magnesium

Rating: ☆☆☆ = Intriguing Evidence

The mineral magnesium is used by every cell in the body, participating in more than 300 biochemical reactions to help produce energy, manufacture fats and proteins, bind calcium to tooth enamel, and flush excess ammonia from the body, among other things. Only a small amount of the mineral is found in the bloodstream. But should you run short of magnesium, you may develop muscle tremors, gastrointestinal problems, generalized weakness, personality and mood changes, and other symptoms.

It's long been known that magnesium plays a vital role in the health of the cardiovascular system. An outright deficiency of magnesium has been shown to damage the arteries in the heart, which encourages the build-up of plaque.[21] Population studies have shown that people consuming low amounts of magnesium have a greater risk of developing elevated blood pressure. Magnesium deficiency has also been linked to a greater incidence of cardiovascular disease in people with diabetes.[22]

Several studies indicate that supplemental magnesium may help in controlling some of the effects of coronary artery disease. Among them:

♦ A 2003 study published in the *American Journal of Cardiology* examined the effects of magnesium on 187 men and women, average age 63, who were suffering from coronary artery disease.[23] The volunteers in this randomized, double-blind study were assigned to take either 730 milligrams of magnesium (brand name Magnosolv-Granulat) or a placebo every day for 6 months. Various tests, including treadmill and bicycle exercise tolerance tests, were performed at the beginning of the study and again at the end of the 6-month study period. The researchers reported that the magnesium treatment resulted "in a significant improvement in exercise tolerance, exercise-induced chest pain, and quality of life."

♦ Fifty men and women with coronary artery disease participated in a randomized, double-blind study published in the journal *Circulation* in 2000.[24] The volunteers, average age 67, were assigned to receive either 730 milligrams of magnesium (Magnosolv-Granulat) or a placebo every day for 6 months. At the beginning and end of the study, the 50 men and women underwent treadmill and other tests to measure the health of their cardiovascular systems. The results were positive, with the magnesium treatment triggering a significant improvement in the function of the lining of an important artery (the brachial artery) and in the ability of the volunteers to tolerate exercise.

♦ A 1999 study presented in the *American Journal of Cardiology* looked at the effects of magnesium on blood clots (platelet-dependent thrombosis).[25] Forty-two people with coronary artery disease—average age 68 and on standard medical therapy—participated in this randomized, double-blind crossover study. They were assigned to receive either 800 to 1,200 milligrams of magnesium oxide or a placebo every day for 3 months, then switched to the other treatment for another 3 months. The results were positive, with the average incidence of clotting (specifically, platelet-dependent thrombosis) dropping by 35 percent when the volunteers were taking magnesium.

Summing Up the Evidence for Magnesium

With a fair amount of evidence suggesting that magnesium helps combat coronary artery disease in more than one way, it is fair to say that the mineral is a three-star treatment for coronary heart disease backed by intriguing evidence.

Available Forms

Among the food sources of magnesium are Florida avocados, toasted wheat germ, pumpkin seeds, cooked soybeans, spinach, dry-roasted almonds, peanuts, and cashews. The mineral also is available in supplement form.

How Much Magnesium Is Typically Used

There is no set dose of magnesium for heart disease. Dosages used in the studies ranged from roughly 730 to 1,200 milligrams per day.

Possible Side Effects and Interactions

The Food and Nutrition Board of the Institute of Medicine has set a tolerable upper intake for magnesium of 350 milligrams per day for adults. Taking too much can cause diarrhea, lethargy, and weakness. In addition, magnesium may interact with aminoglycoside antibiotics such as streptomycin to trigger neuromuscular weakness, and may reduce the absorption of quinolone antibiotics such as ciprofloxacin (Cipro). If you are taking any medication, be sure to consult your doctor before adding supplemental magnesium to your self-care regimen.

Alcoholic Beverages

Rating: ☆☆ = Modest Evidence

Various forms of alcohol have been with us since prehistoric people first drank fermented fruit juice. And while its negative effects have long been known, 20th-century researchers began to wonder if the French habit of consuming large amounts of wine could be a factor in their low rates of cardiovascular disease. Numerous studies performed over the past three or four decades have indeed shown that drinking moderate amounts of wine can guard against heart disease and certain kinds of stroke, make the blood less likely to clot, and raise "good" HDL cholesterol.

Here's a brief overview of some of the many population studies linking moderate consumption of alcohol to a reduced risk of coronary heart disease:

♦ Researchers examined data collected from 38,077 male health professionals whose health and habits had been traced for a dozen years and reported their findings in the *New England Journal of Medicine* in 2003.[26] They concluded that "among men, consumption of alcohol at least three to four days per week was inversely associated with the risk of myocardial infarction." In other words, moderate alcohol consumption was approved to protect the men against heart attacks.

♦ A 2001 study published in the *Journal of the American Medical Association* tracked for an average of 3.8 years more than 1,900 men and women who had been hospitalized after suffering a first heart attack.[27] The data indicated that "moderate alcohol consumption" in the year before the heart attack was linked to a better chance of survival in the years immediately after it. The researchers concluded that moderate alcohol consumption is associated with a lower risk of suffering a heart attack and a lower long-term risk of death following a heart attack.

♦ Researchers from the American Cancer Society, University of Oxford, and World Health Organization examined data that had been collected from 490,000 men and women and published their findings in the *New England Journal of Medicine* in 1997.[28] The men and women ranged in age from 30 to 104, and their health and habits were followed for 9 years. The researchers concluded that "the rates of death from all cardiovascular disease were 30 to 40 percent lower among men . . . and women . . . reporting at least one drink daily than among nondrinkers."

♦ In a study reported in the *American Journal of Cardiology* in 1997, researchers from the Kaiser Permanente Medical Center in Oakland, California, tracked the health and habits of 128,934 adults living in

Oakland and San Francisco.[29] Analysis of the data led the researchers to conclude that "drinking ethyl alcohol apparently protects against coronary disease."

♦ Researchers from Harvard Medical School and Brigham and Women's Hospital used data on the health and habits of more than 87,000 female nurses who had been tracked from 1976 to 1984 for their study, which was published in the *New England Journal of Medicine* in 1988.[30] They found that "among middle-aged women, moderate alcohol consumption decreases the risk of coronary heart disease." (They added, however, that it may raise the risk of brain hemorrhage.)

♦ In 2001 the American Heart Association published a Science Advisory in the journal *Circulation*.[31] The organization noted, "There are more than 60 prospective studies that suggest an inverse relation between moderate alcohol beverage consumption and [coronary heart disease]. A consistent coronary protective effect has been observed for consumption of 1 to 2 drinks per day of an alcohol-containing beverage." Of course, the American Heart Association does not recommend drinking alcohol as a means of protecting the heart; it simply notes that if you already drink in moderation, you may be enjoying some benefits. The advisory goes on to note that drinking more than one to two alcoholic beverages per day is associated with an overall increased risk of death.

Summing Up the Evidence for Alcoholic Beverages

Although several large-scale observational studies have linked moderate alcohol consumption to a decreased risk of coronary heart disease, we do not have the "gold standard" evidence that can be derived only from clinical trials. And we likely never will, given the ethical problems that arise when people are asked to consume alcohol for a study. With this in mind, it is safe to say that there is modest evidence to support the protective effects of alcoholic beverages against coronary heart disease, making alcohol a two-star treatment.

Important Points to Consider

Of course, the previous studies should *not* be interpreted as a license to consume alcohol. First of all, they are observational studies, not clinical trials.

While the researchers tracked the behaviors of a group of people and linked this information to health status, they did not prove that moderate alcohol consumption has any effect on the development of heart disease. This can be done only with an experimental study in which one group is given a moderate amount of alcohol, another is not, and both are followed for some time to see which group (if either) develops the disease.

Second, all such studies have emphasized that only *moderate* amounts of alcohol consumption may be helpful. An alcohol intake of more than two drinks per day for a man or one drink per day for a woman no longer falls into the "moderate" category.

Third, a "drink" or a "serving" of alcohol is not a six-pack or a pitcher. A serving of alcohol is defined as 12 ounces of regular beer *or* 5 ounces of wine *or* 1.5 ounces of 80-proof distilled spirits.

Finally, health experts agree that there's no need to start drinking or to increase the amount you already drink in order to obtain these "heart-healthy" benefits. You can do the same thing with careful diet, weight loss, exercise, and other lifestyle measures.

Possible Side Effects and Interactions

Excessive alcohol consumption can lead to a variety of health and social problems. If you don't already drink, don't start. If you do already drink, don't increase your consumption in the hope of reducing your risk of developing heart disease.

Olive Oil

Rating: ☆☆ = Modest Evidence

Pressed from the fruit of the olive tree (*Olea europaea*), olive oil has been used to treat elevated blood pressure and cholesterol, heart disease, diabetes, migraines, constipation, and numerous other ailments. It is also used as a cooking and salad oil, and to make soap and other commercial products.

A high intake of olive oil has been suggested as an explanation for the low rate of coronary heart disease seen in Mediterranean countries. But it is less clear whether the credit belongs to the olive oil or to the diet. In an attempt to answer this question, some studies have focused specifically on olive oil and its effects on coronary heart disease:

◆ Spanish researchers performed a study of olive oil and coronary disease, which appeared in the *International Journal of Epidemiology* in 2002.[32] One hundred seventy-one people admitted to the hospital after suffering their first heart attacks were matched with 171 people of similar age and gender who were in the hospital for other reasons. The researchers interviewed all 342 participants, inquiring as to their diets, exercise habits, and other heart disease risk factors. Statistical analysis of the results revealed that those who consumed the most olive oil (an average of 54 grams or about 4½ tablespoons per day) were 82 percent less likely to suffer a first heart attack, compared to those who consumed the least olive oil (an average of 7 grams or about 2 teaspoons per day). The researchers concluded that "olive oil may reduce the risk of coronary disease."

◆ Another Spanish study—this time a randomized, crossover, controlled clinical trial reported in *Atherosclerosis* in 2005—was performed on 40 males, average age 67, with stable coronary heart disease.[33] The researchers found that consuming 50 milliliters (slightly more than 3 tablespoons) of virgin olive oil every day for 3 weeks resulted in lower levels of oxidized LDL (the more dangerous form of LDL) and greater activity of one of the body's major antioxidants (glutathione peroxidase)—plus lower systolic blood pressure. In other words, virgin olive oil helped control free radicals, improve antioxidant activity within the body, and lower blood pressure—all of which help ward off coronary heart disease.

Summing Up the Evidence for Olive Oil

These studies are intriguing, and consistent with the known fact that the olive oil–based Mediterranean diet is heart-healthy. At this point, however, the science behind olive oil as a means of heart protection is limited by the lack of large-scale clinical trials. Thus, it is fair to say that olive oil is a two-star treatment for coronary heart disease backed by modest evidence.

How Much Olive Oil Is Typically Used

There is no standard dose of olive oil. In certain studies, amounts as high as 54 grams (about 4½ tablespoons) per day were found to be helpful.

Possible Side Effects and Interactions

Olive oil can trigger biliary colic in those with gallstones or gallbladder disease. In addition, olive oil may interact with medicines for diabetes, such as glimepiride (Amaryl), causing blood sugar to fall too low. If you're taking any medication, be sure to consult your doctor before adding therapeutic doses of olive oil to your self-care regimen.

Nuts

Rating: ☆☆ = Modest Evidence

Some people shy away from nuts because they tend to be high in fat. However, much of the fat is monounsaturated or polyunsaturated, the types that can help rein in cholesterol levels. Nuts also contain fiber, magnesium, and B vitamins.

Numerous studies have demonstrated that eating nuts can help reduce cholesterol levels. For our purposes here, we're interested in only those studies that show nuts can reduce the risk of developing or dying from heart disease. Several large-scale observational studies have done just that, including the following:

- Researchers involved in the Adventist Health Study observed more than 30,000 Seventh-day Adventists—all residents of California—from 1977 to 1982, monitoring their health and dietary and lifestyle habits. To check the effects of nuts on heart health, the researchers excluded people who already had heart disease or diabetes, and focused on the 26,000-plus who did not.[34] They found that people who consumed nuts more than 1 to 4 times per week had substantially fewer fatal heart attacks, compared to those who ate nuts less than once a week.
- The Iowa Women's Health Study collected data from 34,000-plus postmenopausal women who did not have coronary heart disease (CHD) at the beginning of the study.[35] Analysis of the data revealed that "frequently consumption may offer postmenopausal women modest protection against the risk of death from all causes and from CHD."
- The Nurses' Health Study followed some 86,000 registered nurses for several years.[36] Those who ate at least 5 ounces of nuts per week showed a 35 percent drop in the risk of a nonfatal heart attack, compared to those who ate 1 ounce of nuts per month or less.

◆ The Physicians' Health Study tracked 21,000 male doctors for many years, finding that as the consumption of nuts increased, the risk of dying from heart disease decreased significantly.[37]

Summing Up the Evidence for Nuts

The results of these and other observational studies were positive. Remember, however, that while observational studies link habits to health and give us a good idea of what is helpful, they do not prove anything. Only experimental studies can do that, and so far, most of the experimental studies have looked at the effects of nuts on cholesterol, not on the risk of death due to heart disease. Still, these large-scale studies are impressive enough to give a strong indication that nuts are a two-star treatment for coronary heart disease backed by modest evidence.

Amount of Nuts Typically Used

There is no standard dose of nuts. One study found good results when participants ate 5 ounces (about 1¼ cups) of nuts per week.

Possible Side Effects

Some people can experience a life-threatening allergic reaction when exposed to certain kinds of nuts. If this should happen to you, be sure to seek emergency medical care without delay.

ALTERNATIVE APPROACHES TO

DEPRESSION

SAMe	☆☆☆☆
St. John's wort	☆☆☆☆
Omega-3 fatty acids	☆☆☆
5-HTP	☆☆
Chromium	☆☆
Saffron	☆☆

Feeling sad, hopeless, or "down in the dumps" from time to time is normal, especially when life becomes difficult. But when the "down" feelings strike for no apparent reason or linger longer than 2 weeks; when your energy level and motivation go down the tubes; when you can't sleep or you sleep too much; when life seems to lose its luster, you may be suffering from a major depressive episode.

Surprisingly common, depression severe enough to warrant medical attention affects about 10 percent of the US population, one-third of whom have long-lasting (chronic) depression.[1] Untreated, a typical episode of depression lasts about 6 months but may go on for 2 years or longer.[2] Depression seems to have a particular affinity for women, affecting more than 12 million adult females in the United States.[3] That's almost twice as many women as men.

SYMPTOMS

Derived from the Latin word *deprimere*, which means "pressing down," depression can seem like a heavy weight sitting on your head, although symptoms may vary greatly from one person to the next. While some people experience overwhelming feelings of sadness, grief, worthlessness, or hopelessness, others may simply feel agitated and "antsy." Then there are those who feel nothing at all—no pleasure, no sadness, just a sense of being absolutely flat and lethargic.

Some people with depression experience no dramatic emotional changes, just physical ones like fatigue, chronic headache, decreased libido, weight loss or gain, and vague physical discomforts. Appetite changes at either end of the spectrum are common; while some people don't feel hungry at all, others find they can't stop eating. Other common symptoms of depression include isolation, sleep problems, a loss of libido, and feelings of anxiety, low self-esteem, and loneliness.

CAUSES

Many physical conditions can bring about depression, including anemia, cancer, diabetes, childbirth, hormonal imbalances, nutritional deficiencies, and chronic infections. So can certain medications. But the most common cause of major depressive disorder is believed to be changes in the amounts and functions of neurotransmitters (brain chemicals), which then destabilize the brain circuitry.

The brain consists of trillions of nerve cells, and electrical messages constantly rocket through these cells at lightning speed. Because most of the nerve cells don't actually touch each other, an electrical message must be "ferried" across a gap between two nerve endings—a job that is accomplished by neurotransmitters. Those that have the greatest effect on mood and emotions are dopamine, norepinephrine, and, perhaps most importantly, serotonin. Low levels of serotonin have been linked to a laundry list of conditions, including depression, anxiety, obsessive-compulsive disorder, sleep disorders, seasonal affective disorder (SAD), bulimia, alcohol abuse, drug abuse, mania, and mood swings.

STANDARD TREATMENTS

The cornerstone of treatment for depression is medication, and several kinds of drugs may be prescribed. The current favorites are the selective serotonin reuptake inhibitors (SSRIs) such as fluoxetine (Prozac), sertraline (Zoloft), and paroxetine (Paxil). The SSRIs are designed to normalize serotonin function and increase the availability of this important neurotransmitter. Other classes of antidepressant drugs include the monoamine oxidase inhibitors (phenelzine), the psychostimulants (dextroamphetamine), and the tricyclics (nortriptyline), as well as newer drugs such as bupropion, nefazodone, and venlafaxine.

RATING POPULAR ALTERNATIVE TREATMENTS FOR DEPRESSION

SAMe

Rating: ☆☆☆☆ = Strong Evidence

SAMe (short for S-adenosyl-L-methionine) is a natural substance manufactured in the body from the amino acid methionine. Among other things, SAMe helps the body produce neurotransmitters, hormones, and proteins. When given in large doses of up to 1 gram per day, SAMe can help combat depression. It does this in part by increasing the production of serotonin, which helps regulate mood. Studies involving SAMe include the following:

♦ In 1988 researchers from the University of California, Irvine, published the results of their small, brief, double-blind study in the *American Journal of Psychiatry*.[4] This study examined the effects of SAMe on 18 adults suffering from major depression. The volunteers were randomly assigned to two groups. The first group received an intravenous infusion of up to 400 milligrams of SAMe per day, plus a placebo capsule. (The SAMe preparation was provided by BioResearch S.p.A.) The second group received a placebo infusion plus up to 150 milligrams of the standard antidepressant imipramine (Tofanil), in capsule form, per day. After 14 days of treatment, 66 percent of those taking SAMe showed "clinically significant improvement in depressive symptoms," compared to only 22 percent of those taking the drug.

♦ A 2002 paper published in the *American Journal of Clinical Nutrition* reported the results of two separate double-blind studies that looked at the effects of SAMe on depression.[5] Both studies were randomized and double-blind, and both compared SAMe to the standard antidepressant imipramine in people who had been diagnosed with major depression. For the first study, 281 volunteers were randomly assigned to receive oral doses of up to 1,600 milligrams of SAMe or up to 150 milligrams of imipramine per day. For the second study, 295 participants were randomly assigned to receive daily injections of 400 milligrams of SAMe plus a placebo capsule, or daily oral doses of up to 150 milligrams of imipramine plus a placebo injection.

The researchers used the Hamilton Rating Scale for Depression and similar rating tools to measure the effects of treatment. In both studies, both treatments reduced symptoms of depression significantly and roughly equally. The researchers concluded, "The antidepressive efficacy of 1,600 milligrams of SAMe [per day] orally and 400 milligrams of SAMe [per day] intramuscularly is comparable with that of 150 milligrams of imipramine [per day] orally, but SAMe is significantly better tolerated." As Table 9-1 below shows, SAMe was as effective as the drug in reducing the symptoms of depression, as measured by two different rating scales.

Table 9-1: Oral and Injectable SAMe Comparable to Standard Drug for Reducing Depression[6]

	SAMe	Imipramine
Study 1 with Oral SAMe		
Reduction in Hamilton Rating Scale for Depression Score	-12.6	-13.1
Reduction in Montgomery-Asberg Depression Rating Score	-14.9	-15.0
Study 2 with Injected SAMe		
Reduction in Hamilton Rating Scale for Depression Score	-12.6	-13.1
Reduction in Montgomery-Asberg Depression Rating Score	-14.5	-14.3

♦ For a 2004 study published in the *Journal of Clinical Pharmacology*, researchers from Harvard Medical School and the Baylor Institute of Metabolic Disease in Dallas tested the effects of SAMe in combination with standard antidepressants on people whose symptoms had not been resolved by these medications.[7] The participants in this open trial were

30 adults who had major depressive disorders despite treatment with fluoxetine (Prozac), paroxetine (Paxil), citalopram (Celexa), or venlafaxine (Effexor). The volunteers were given daily doses of 800 to 1,600 milligrams of SAMe (brand name Nature Made), and continued taking their medications. The results of this study were positive, with scores on the Hamilton Depression-17 scale falling from an average of 17.7 to 10.0, and scores on the Montgomery-Asberg Depression Rating scale dropping from an average of 23.2 to 13.9. Other indicators of depression improved as well. The researchers concluded, "The combination of SAMe with antidepressants deserves further scrutiny as a potentially safe and effective addition to the growing armamentarium of treatment approaches to resistant depression."

♦ A 1994 meta-analysis of 13 clinical trials comparing SAMe to placebo or standard antidepressants concluded, "The efficacy of SAMe in treating depressive syndromes and disorders is superior to that of placebo and comparable to that of standard tricyclic antidepressants."[8]

♦ These findings were confirmed and expanded in a 2002 report presented by the Agency for Healthcare Research and Quality.[9] This report, which used 28 studies to develop a meta-analysis, found that SAMe was superior to placebo. And when SAMe was compared to standard antidepressants, there was no statistically significant difference. In other words, SAMe produced about the same effect as standard antidepressant medications.

Summing Up the Evidence for SAMe

The use of SAMe as a treatment for mild to moderate depression is supported by numerous studies—although many of these looked at small number of patients—and a positive finding from the Agency for Healthcare Research and Quality. Thus, it's fair to say that SAMe is a four-star treatment for depression backed by strong evidence.

Available Forms

SAMe is available in capsule or tablet form.

How Much SAMe Is Typically Used

There is no standard dose of SAMe. Supplemental doses may range from 400 to 1,600 milligrams per day.

Possible Side Effects and Interactions

SAMe can cause anxiety, insomnia, and gastrointestinal upset. In addition, it may interact with antidepressants such as clomipramine (Anafranil) to trigger agitation, tremors, rapid heartbeat, and other symptoms of serotonin syndrome (the result of elevated levels of serotonin in the brain).

SAMe should not be taken by those suffering from bipolar disorder and should be used by those with depression only under a physician's supervision.

St. John's Wort

Rating: ☆☆☆☆ = Strong Evidence

St. John's wort is a small yellow wildflower found in Europe, where it is widely prescribed for depression and anxiety, as well as for irregular heartbeat, exhaustion, headache, and a number of other ailments. We don't know exactly how it works, but we do know that St. John's wort contains two chemicals—hypericin and hyperforin—that may alter levels of serotonin and other neurotransmitters in the brain.

The effect of St. John's wort on depression has been the subject of numerous studies. Here's an overview of several key trials, including a few that compared St. John's wort to Prozac and Zoloft, two widely prescribed antidepressants:

♦ *St. John's wort vs. placebo:* German researchers enrolled 39 men and women suffering from mild depression in a 4-week randomized, double-blind study.[10] The participants were divided into two groups and given daily doses of either 900 milligrams of a St. John's wort extract (brand name Jarsin 300) or a placebo. At the beginning of the study, halfway through, and at the end, the patients' depth of depression was assessed using the Hamilton Rating Scale for Depression and other rating tools. By the end of the 4-week study, there was "significant improvement" in the St. John's wort group as compared to the placebo group. Specifically, 70 percent of those taking St. John's wort were free of depression symptoms after 4 weeks, compared to 47 percent of those taking the placebo.

♦ *St. John's wort vs. imipramine:* A report published in the *British Medical Journal* in 1999 presented the results of a randomized, double-blind study comparing St. John's wort extract to placebo and to the antidepressant imipramine.[11] Two hundred sixty-three men and women suffering from moderate depression were divided into three groups and given daily doses of 1,050 milligrams of St. John's wort extract (brand name STEI 300), 100 milligrams of imipramine, or placebo. The researchers measured the participants' progress using the Hamilton Rating Scale for Depression, the Hamilton Anxiety Scale, the Clinical Global Impressions Scale, and other rating tools. The results were positive, with the researchers reporting that St. John's wort extract "was more effective than placebo and at least as effective as 100 [milligrams of] imipramine daily in the treatment of moderate depression." They concluded that St. John's wort extract "is safe and improves quality of life."

♦ *St. John's wort vs. Zoloft:* In 2000 a team of researchers reported the results of their study comparing St. John's wort extract to the antidepressant sertraline (Zoloft).[12] For this randomized, double-blind study, 30 men and women suffering from mild to moderate depression were given daily doses of either St. John's wort extract (LI 160, provided by Lichtwer Pharma US) or sertraline. For the first week of the study, they received either 600 milligrams of the herb or 50 milligrams of the drug; then for the next 6 weeks, the dosages increased to 900 milligrams of the herb or 75 milligrams of the drug. Both treatments eased the patients' depression, with scores on the Hamilton Rating Scale for Depression and the Clinical Global Impression Score falling in both groups. The researchers concluded that in this small study, St. John's wort extract "was at least as effective as sertraline in the treatment of mild to moderate depression."

♦ *St. John's wort vs. Prozac:* In 1999 German researchers published the results of a study pitting St. John's wort extract head-to-head against the very popular antidepressant fluoxetine (Prozac).[13] One hundred forty-nine elderly men and women suffering from mild to moderate depressive episodes participated in this randomized, double-blind study. They were divided into two groups, with one group taking 800 milligrams of St. John's wort extract per day and the other taking 20 milligrams of fluoxetine per day. (The herb was given the laboratory designation LoHyp-57.) Over the course of the 6-week study, the researchers tracked the patients' progress on the Hamilton Rating Scale for Depression. They found the St. John's wort extract to be "both statistically and clinically equivalent to fluoxetine" in treating mild to moderate depressive episodes in this group of patients.

♦ *St. John's wort vs. Prozac*: St. John's wort extract also was compared to fluoxetine in a larger randomized, double-blind study involving 240 people with mild to moderate depression.[14] The participants were divided into two groups. For 6 weeks, one group took St. John's wort extract, the other fluoxetine. (The herb was given the laboratory designation ZE 117 and was provided by Zeller AG.) By the end of the study, scores on the Hamilton Rating Scale for Depression were slightly lower in those taking St. John's wort compared to those taking fluoxetine. The researchers concluded that the herb and the drug "are equipotent with respect to all main parameters used to investigate antidepressants in this population." In other words, St. John's wort extract was as effective as fluoxetine in this group of volunteers.

♦ An article published in the journal *Phytomedicine* in 2005[15] reviewed the results of 16 nonrandomized, observational studies involving 34,804 people taking St. John's wort. Most of these studies lasted 4 to 6 weeks and focused on people suffering from mild to moderate depression. Between 65 and 100 percent of these patients responded to treatment with St. John's wort; in the two studies that lasted nearly a year apiece, the response rate ranged from 60 to 69 percent. The authors of this review concluded that St. John's wort extract is "well tolerated and . . . effective in the routine treatment of mild to moderate depressive disorders."

Several meta-analyses have examined the efficacy of St. John's wort in relieving symptoms of depression. Among them:

♦ A team of German and American researchers published the results of their meta-analysis in the *British Medical Journal* in 1996.[16] This meta-analysis combined the results of 23 randomized clinical studies involving more than 1,700 patients suffering primarily from mild to moderately severe depressive disorders. As the researchers concluded, there is evidence that extracts of St. John's wort "are more effective than placebo for the treatment of mild to moderately severe depressive disorders."

♦ A 2002 meta-analysis published in *Psychopharmacology* was based on three randomized, double-blind, placebo-controlled studies involving 544 people suffering from mild to moderate depression.[17] In all three studies the volunteers received either 900 milligrams of a

St. John's wort extract (WS 5570 or WS 5572, supplied by Dr. Willmar Schwabe Pharmaceuticals) or a placebo every day for 6 weeks. After combining and analyzing the data, the researchers concluded that the St. John's wort extract's "therapeutic profile was . . . found to be similar to the profile of selective serotonin reuptake inhibitors." In other words, the herbal extract was as effective at treating mild to moderate depression as the class of drugs that includes fluoxetine (Prozac) and sertraline (Zoloft).

St. John's wort has proven to be a successful treatment for mild to moderate depression in enough clinical trials to earn approval from Germany's Commission E for use in treating depressive moods. Of course, not all of the studies of St. John's wort have gleaned positive results. In fact, two studies published in the *Journal of the American Medical Association* in 2001[18] and 2002[19] found that St. John's wort was not effective in treating major depression. However, alternative health experts quickly pointed out that the patients in both of these studies were suffering from major depression, while St. John's wort is generally recommended for mild to moderate depression. Thus it was argued that the studies were unfair because they were testing the herb as a treatment for something it was not expected to cure.

♦ The question of whether St. John's wort is an effective treatment for people suffering from major depression was revisited by German researchers in a paper published in the *British Medical Journal* in 2005.[20] For this study, which compared the effectiveness of St. John's wort extract to the drug paroxetine (Paxil), 251 adults suffering from moderate to severe major depression were randomly assigned to receive either St. John's wort or paroxetine, which belongs to the same class of drugs (the SSRIs) as fluoxetine (Prozac). Each person took either 900 milligrams of St. John's wort extract (WS 5570, supplied by Dr. Willmar Schwabe Pharmaceuticals) or 20 milligrams of paroxetine every day for 6 weeks—unless there was no improvement after 2 weeks, in which case the dose of either treatment was doubled. The researchers used the Hamilton Total Depression Scores, the Beck Depression Inventory, and similar tools to measure the patients' progress. The results were positive, with the Hamilton scores falling by 56 percent in the St. John's wort group, compared to 45 percent in the paroxetine group. The researchers concluded that for treating moderate to severe major depression, St. John's wort extract is "at least as effective as paroxetine and is better tolerated."

Summing Up the Evidence for St. John's Wort

Using St. John's wort for mild to moderate depression is supported by more than 20 randomized, double-blind, placebo-controlled studies. The herb also garnered a positive recommendation from Germany's Commission E. Thus, despite the inevitable studies producing negative outcomes, it's fair to say that St. John's wort is a four-star treatment for depression backed by strong evidence.

Other Names

St. John's wort's scientific name is *Hypericum perforatum L.* It goes by several other common names, including amber, goatweed, John's wort, Klamath weed, rosin rose, and witches herb.

Available Forms

St. John's wort is available in capsule, tincture, and cream form.

How Much St. John's Wort Is Typically Used

There is no standard dose of St. John's wort. Supplemental doses may be as high as 900 milligrams of St. John's wort extract, preferably taken as 300-milligram doses three times a day.

Possible Side Effects and Interactions

St. John's wort has been used extensively in Germany to treat depression, and there have been no reports of serious toxicity problems. Among the herb's possible side effects are constipation, restlessness, fatigue, dizziness, rash, and increased sun sensitivity. St. John's wort may reduce the effectiveness of estrogen or estradiol-based medicines used to prevent pregnancy or to relieve menopausal symptoms. When taken in combination with antidepressants such as fluoxetine (Prozac), the herb may trigger rapid heartbeat, flushing, agitation, and other symptoms of serotonin syndrome. If you're on any medication, be sure to consult your doctor before adding St. John's wort to your self-care regimen.

Omega-3 Fatty Acids

Rating: ☆☆☆ = Intriguing Evidence

The omega-3 fatty acids—found in cold-water fatty fish and other foods—were originally noted for their ability to protect against coronary heart disease. As research into these "good fats" continued, scientists noted that the omega-3s are concentrated in the brain, and that depressive orders are less common in areas where large amounts of fish oil are consumed.[21] This prompted them to investigate a possible link between omega-3 fatty acids and depression.

The studies below suggest that omega-3 fatty acids—specifically eicosapentaenoic acid (EPA) and docosahexaenoic acid (DHA)—may be helpful in treating some forms of depression:

♦ A randomized, double-blind study led by a Harvard Medical School researcher compared omega-3 fatty acids to placebo in 30 people with bipolar disorder.[22] The men and women volunteering for the study ranged in age from 18 to 65. One group took 9.6 grams of omega-3 acids (EPA and DHA) a day during the course of the 4-month study period, while the other group took olive oil, which served as the placebo. The study participants also continued with their standard treatment. The results were positive, with the omega-3 fatty acids leading to "significant symptom reduction and a better outcome when compared to placebo." The researchers concluded that "omega-3 fatty acids were well tolerated and improved the short-term course of illness in this preliminary study."

♦ An Israeli study published in the *American Journal of Psychiatry* in 2002 examined the effects of one particular omega-3 fatty acid, EPA, on 17 women and three men suffering from recurrent major depressive disorder.[23] For this 4-week, double-blind study, the volunteers were randomly assigned to receive either 2 grams of EPA (brand name E-EPA) or a placebo every day. The researchers tracked the patients' scores on the Hamilton Rating Scale for Depression to see if EPA would lift their depression. The results were positive, with the average Hamilton score falling by 12.4 points in the EPA group, compared to only 1.6 points in the placebo group. The Hamilton score dropped by 50 percent for 6 of 10 in the EPA group, compared to 1 of 10 in the placebo group. Table 9-2 on the next page shows the scores for the individual patients. The 10 patients who took EPA are listed first, followed by those who took the placebo.

Although individual results varied considerably, those in the EPA group tended to see larger drops in their scores than those in the placebo group.

Table 9-2: Effects of EPA and Placebo on Hamilton Rating Scale for Depression Score[24]

PATIENT	TREATMENT	HAMILTON RATING SCALE FOR DEPRESSION SCORE				
		Beginning of Study	Week 1	Week 2	Week 3	Week 4
1	EPA	25	24	18	11	7
2	EPA	21	21	12	10	9
3	EPA	24	24	17	17	17
4	EPA	18	18	18	13	13
5	EPA	26	26	18	18	20
6	EPA	24	24	24	21	21
7	EPA	26	26	18	15	12
8	EPA	26	26	14	9	6
9	EPA	22	21	8	8	2
10	EPA	28	28	19	15	9
11	Placebo	20	20	18	18	18
12	Placebo	23	23	21	21	23
13	Placebo	19	22	22	22	20
14	Placebo	27	27	23	23	25
15	Placebo	21	21	21	14	14
16	Placebo*	29	29	34	–	–
17	Placebo	26	26	29	29	29
18	Placebo	20	11	1	0	0
19	Placebo	21	21	21	25	25
20	Placebo	24	24	25	25	26

*This patient dropped out of study.

♦ Researchers from Swallownest Court Hospital in England tested the effects of different doses of the omega-3 fatty acid EPA in their 2002 study, which appeared in the *Archives of General Psychiatry*.[25] This randomized, double-blind study involved 60 men and women suffering from persistent depression—that is, depression that lingered despite treatment with standard medications. The patients were assigned to receive 12 weeks of treatment with 1, 2, or 4 grams of EPA per day, or a placebo. The researchers tracked the patients' depth of depression by using the Hamilton Rating Scale for Depression, the Montgomery-Asberg Depression Rating Scale, and the Beck Depression Inventory. Those taking 1 gram of EPA per day fared the best, showing significantly greater improvement on all three rating scales than those taking the placebo. Taking 2 grams of EPA per day seemed to trigger no improvement, and 4 grams per day only slight improvement. The researchers concluded that 1 gram of EPA per day "was effective in treating depression in patients who remained depressed despite adequate standard therapy."

Summing Up the Evidence for Omega-3 Fatty Acids

Although there are a large number of studies investigating the effects of the omega-3 fatty acids—especially EPA—on depression, there are not enough large-scale, scientifically sound trials to produce a definitive answer. Thus, given the information available at this time, it is fair to say that omega-3 fatty acids are a three-star treatment for depression backed by intriguing evidence.

Available Forms

The best food sources of omega-3 fatty acids are cold-water fatty fish such as mackerel, salmon, herring, anchovies, and tuna. As a general rule, the fattier a fish is, the more omega-3s it contains. The human body can manufacture omega-3s from alpha-linolenic acid, which is found in walnuts and flaxseed. Omega-3 fatty acids are also available in supplement form, labeled as fish oil, omega-3, EPA, DHA, or some combination of these.

Amount of Omega-3 Fatty Acids Typically Used

There is no standard dose of omega-3 fatty acids. Some studies have shown that taking 1 gram of EPA per day can ease symptoms of depression.

Possible Side Effects and Interactions

The omega-3 fatty acids are found in common foods and have been granted Generally Regarded as Safe (GRAS) status by the US government. They can prolong bleeding time, which may be a problem for those who have bleeding disorders, those who are taking medicines to thin the blood, or those who will be undergoing surgery soon.

Along the same line, the omega-3 fatty acids may increase the risk of bruising and bleeding when taken with drugs that thin the blood, such as aspirin and heparin (Hep-Lock). They also may interact with medicines for elevated blood pressure, such as atenolol (Tenormin), causing the blood pressure to drop too low. If you're taking any medication, be sure to consult your doctor before adding therapeutic amounts of omega-3s to your self-care regimen.

5-HTP

Rating: ☆☆ = Modest Evidence

5-HTP, otherwise known as 5-hydroxytryptophan, increases the production of serotonin in the central nervous system. Serotonin, in turn, helps ease depression, anxiety, and the sensation of pain, among other things.

A relatively large number of studies have examined whether 5-HTP relieves the symptoms of depression. Many of these were conducted before the release of Prozac and other SSRIs, which relieve depression by increasing the available amount of serotonin in the brain. For example, one double-blind study involving 40 people found that 200 milligrams of 5-HTP per day was better than a placebo, and almost as effective as the antidepressant clomipramine (Anafranil), at relieving depression.[26]

Japanese researchers conducted several studies on 5-HTP and depression in the 1970s, which produced findings such as these:

- In an open-label study, 24 people hospitalized for moderate to severe depression were taken off all antidepressant medication for at least 7 days, then given 300 milligrams of 5-HTP per day for 2 weeks.[27] Seven of the 24 responded with "clear-cut improvement in their depression," while another two showed mild improvement.
- Fifty-nine people suffering from bipolar and other types of depression were given 150 to 300 milligrams of 5-HTP daily.[28] Forty patients

showed "favorable responses" to treatment, and 13 of those were "markedly improved."

♦ According to a 2002 review study by the Cochrane Library, the available evidence suggests that 5-HTP is "better than placebo at alleviating depression," although the authors criticized the overall quality of the existing studies.[29]

Summing Up the Evidence for 5-HTP

Given what we know to date, it's fair to say that 5-HTP is a two-star treatment for depression backed by modest evidence.

Available Forms

5-HTP is available in supplement form.

How Much 5-HTP Is Typically Used

There is no standard dose of 5-HTP. Supplemental doses may range from 150 to 300 milligrams per day.

Possible Side Effects and Interactions

5-HTP's side effects include nausea, diarrhea, and breathing difficulties. Large doses may trigger serotonin syndrome, as could interaction with antidepressants such as sertraline (Zoloft). If you're taking any medication, be sure to consult your doctor before adding 5-HTP to your self-care regimen.

Chromium

Rating: ☆☆ = Modest Evidence

Chromium is a trace mineral, which means that only a small amount of it (about 6 milligrams) is found in the body. We don't yet fully understand what chromium does or how it works, but we do know that it plays an important role in the body's handling of insulin, the metabolism of carbohydrates and fat, and the action of several enzymes. A shortfall of chromium can interfere with the body's ability to utilize blood sugar and can be the cause of unexplained weight loss. Chromium has been used to treat diabetes and elevated cholesterol, to bulk up muscle mass, and to increase athletic performance.

A small amount of research has suggested that chromium may influence the body's response to serotonin. This led to the suggestion that the mineral may be helpful for those with depression, particularly the type known as atypical depression. Atypical depression has five key characteristics: mood reactivity, hypersomnia (excessive sleeping), hyperphagia (increased appetite or weight gain), leaden paralysis, and rejection sensitivity. Among the studies that examined chromium's effect on certain symptoms of atypical depression are the following:

♦ A 2005 study published in the *Journal of Psychiatric Practice* looked at the effects of chromium in 110 people, ages 18 to 65, with atypical depression.[30] The volunteers in this double-blind study were randomly assigned to receive 400 to 600 micrograms of elemental chromium in the form of chromium picolinate (brand name Chromax) or a placebo every day for 8 weeks. The researchers measured the depth of the volunteers' depression by using the Hamilton Rating Scale for Depression and the Clinical Global Impressions Improvement Scale. Although the depression scores improved in both groups, those who had been taking chromium showed fewer symptoms of atypical depression, such as increased appetite and carbohydrate cravings. The authors concluded that chromium picolinate may be "beneficial for patients with atypical depression who also have severe carbohydrate craving[s]."

♦ Fifteen people with major depressive disorder of the atypical type participated in a 2003 study published in *Biological Psychiatry*.[31] For this randomized, double-blind study, the volunteers were given 400 to 600 micrograms of chromium picolinate or a placebo every day for 8 weeks. Seventy percent of those taking the chromium responded to treatment, compared to 0 percent of those taking the placebo. A response was defined as at least a 66 percent drop in the Hamilton Rating Scale for Depression score. The researchers concluded, "The results of this pilot study suggest benefit, along with relative freedom from side effects, for chromium picolinate in atypical depression; its effect, moreover, was often rapid."

Figure 9-1 below shows the drop—which signifies improvement—in the depression scores for the 10 people taking chromium. Though not everyone showed improvement, for 7 of the 10 people the second bar (representing their score after taking chromium) was lower than the first bar (representing their score before taking the mineral).

Figure 9-1: Chromium Produces Drop (Improvement) in Hamilton Rating Scale for Depression Score[32]

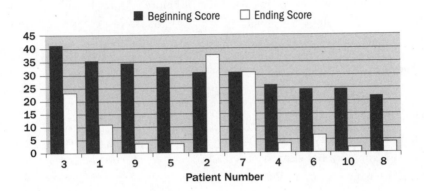

Summing Up the Evidence for Chromium

Based on the body of research available for analysis, it is reasonable to say that chromium is a two-star treatment for atypical depression backed by modest evidence.

Available Forms

Chromium is found in foods such as broccoli, grape juice, English muffins, mashed potatoes, orange juice, bananas, and green beans. It is also available in supplement form.

How Much Chromium Is Typically Used

Chromium supplements come in several forms, including chromium picolinate and chromium chloride. The most important factor is how much elemental chromium the supplements contain. (Check the label.) A typical daily dose for depression may range from 600 to 1,000 micrograms of elemental chromium.

Possible Side Effects and Interactions

Taking chromium in supplement form can cause headaches, mood swings, and sleep disturbances. Some experts believe that taking more than 300 micrograms of elemental chromium every day for several months may be toxic to the liver, while others have suggested that long-term use may damage cellular DNA.

Chromium supplements may interact with diabetes medicines such as glyburide (DiaBeta), causing blood sugar to fall too low. If you're taking any medication, be sure to consult your doctor before adding chromium supplements to your self-care regimen.

Saffron

Rating: ☆☆ = Modest Evidence

The flowers, seeds, and oil taken from this native plant of Iran and India have a long history as a treatment for diarrhea, stomach problems, appetite loss, insomnia, and skin disorders. Saffron has many other uses as well, including as a spice, a food colorant, a dye, and a fragrance for cosmetics and soaps.

The idea of saffron as a treatment for depression is relatively new. All three studies of interest were performed by researchers at the Tehran University of Medical Sciences in Iran.

♦ *Saffron vs. placebo*: This randomized, double-blind study involved 35 adults with mild to moderate depression.[33] They were assigned to receive either 30 milligrams of saffron (supplied by Novin Zaferan Company) or a placebo every day for 6 weeks. The depth of their depression was tracked using the Hamilton Rating Scale for Depression. According to the researchers, those taking saffron "experienced statistically significant benefits [to] their mood after 6 weeks [of] treatment."

♦ *Saffron vs. imipramine:* Thirty adults were enlisted for this randomized, double-blind study comparing the effects of saffron to the standard antidepressant imipramine (Tofranil).[34] The volunteers ranged in age from 18 to 55, and all had been diagnosed with depression. They were assigned to receive either 30 milligrams of saffron (Novin Zaferan Company) or 100 milligrams of imipramine every day for 6 weeks. The patients' emotional status was checked at the beginning of the study, and again at weeks 1, 2, 3, 4, and 6. Both groups of patients showed significant improvement, with saffron proving to be as effective at relieving depression as imipramine. This led the researchers to conclude that "saffron may be of therapeutic benefit in the treatment of mild to moderate depression."

♦ *Saffron vs. fluoxetine:* This study upped the ante by comparing saffron to fluoxetine (Prozac), which is considered to be one of the most successful antidepressant medications.[35] For this 2005 double-blind trial, 40 adults suffering from mild to moderate depression were randomly assigned to receive either 30 milligrams of saffron (Novin Zaferan Company) or 20 milligrams of fluoxetine every day for 6 weeks. The herb proved to be just as effective as the drug in reducing depression, with the researchers concluding that this dose of saffron was "similar to fluoxetine in the treatment of mild to moderate depression."

Summing Up the Evidence for Saffron

Currently there are only three studies of note examining saffron's effect on mild to moderate depression, leading to the conclusion that saffron is a two-star treatment for depression backed by modest evidence.

Other Names

Saffron is known to scientists as *Crocus sativus*, and in various parts of the world by different names, including autumn crocus, croci stigma, Indian saffron, kum kuma, true saffron, and Spanish saffron.

Available Forms

Saffron is available in powdered form in health food stores and some grocery stores.

How Much Saffron Is Typically Used

There is no standard dose of saffron. The aforementioned studies discussed used dosages of 30 milligrams of saffron per day.

Possible Side Effects and Interactions

Saffron's side effects include dizziness, nausea, facial flushing, and slow heart rate. It may be lethal in extremely large doses of 20 grams or more. As with all supplements and drugs, be sure to follow directions carefully when adding therapeutic amounts of saffron to your self-care regimen.

10

ALTERNATIVE APPROACHES TO

DIABETES

Pycnogenol	☆☆☆☆
Alpha-lipoic acid	☆☆☆
Blond psyllium	☆☆☆
Chromium	☆☆☆
Cinnamon	☆☆
Fenugreek	☆☆
Glucomannan	☆☆
Guar gum	☆☆
Vanadium	☆☆
Bitter melon	☆
Gymnema sylvestre	☆

Diabetes is a chronic condition in which the body is unable either to produce or to utilize insulin, the hormone that ferries glucose from the bloodstream into the cells of bodily tissues. Cells burn glucose for energy, or store it as glycogen or fat for later use. But when insulin is in short supply, or it isn't working as it should, glucose can't enter cells and instead builds up in the bloodstream.

When blood glucose rises above 180 mg/dL (milligrams per deciliter), it begins to spill into the urine and make it sweet—a phenomenon observed by the ancient Romans, who noted that ants seemed to be attracted to the urine of certain people. The Greeks observed that those with sweet urine seemed to produce liquid almost as fast as they consumed it; whatever they drank just ran right through them, as if through a siphon. Thus, the condition earned its name *diabetes mellitus—diabetes* being the Greek word for siphon, and *mellitus* (MEL-lih-tuhs), the Latin word for sweet.

There are several types of diabetes, the most common being type 1 and type 2. In type 1, a faulty or damaged pancreas manufactures little or no insulin, so blood glucose has no way to enter most of the body's hungry cells. In type 2, the pancreas manufactures normal amounts of insulin, but the body's cells become resistant to its effects, so insulin can't do its job properly (a condition known as *decreased insulin sensitivity*). The outcome of both types of diabetes is basically the same: The cells don't get enough fuel, while glucose in the bloodstream rises to unhealthy levels. The lack of cellular fuel leads to symptoms such as weakness, fatigue, intense hunger, and unexplained weight loss. The excessive blood glucose can cause serious body-wide complications, including damage to the kidneys, eyes, nerves, heart, skin, and blood vessels.

CAUSES

Type 1 diabetes—which often begins in childhood and affects about 10 percent of those with diabetes—is the result of an autoimmune disorder in which the body attacks itself and destroys the beta cells of the pancreas, where insulin is formed. The destruction of the beta cells most likely results from an inherited tendency coupled with exposure to a virus or some other environmental trigger.

Type 2 diabetes is much more common than type 1, affecting about 75 percent of diabetics, or approximately 8 to 10 million people. It typically begins at about age 40 and usually is due to an inherited tendency combined with obesity and/or lack of exercise.

SYMPTOMS

Symptoms of both types of diabetes include frequent hunger, excessive thirst, frequent urination, dehydration, fatigue, weakness, weight loss, and—in women—persistent vaginal infections. According to the American Diabetes Association, the diagnosis of diabetes can be made if:

- blood glucose is greater than or equal to 200 mg/dL 2 hours after ingesting 75 grams of glucose by mouth
- fasting blood glucose is greater than or equal to 126 mg/dL
- blood glucose is 200 mg/dl and the symptoms of diabetes are present

STANDARD TREATMENTS

The standard treatment for diabetes, whether type 1 or type 2, begins with proper diet and regular exercise. With type 1, daily injections of insulin are also necessary. With type 2, the most important treatment is usually weight loss, coupled with an increase in physical activity. Then if high blood glucose levels persist, a medication such as metformin (Glucophage) or glipizide (Glucotrol) is prescribed. In some cases, insulin injections may be necessary.

RATING POPULAR ALTERNATIVE TREATMENTS FOR DIABETES

Pycnogenol

Rating: ☆☆☆☆ = Strong Evidence

Pycnogenol is the registered trademark for a proprietary extract of the bark of the French Maritime pine tree. Pycnogenol contains catechins, flavonoids, and other nutraceuticals that are believed to give it anti-inflammatory, antioxidant, and immune-stimulating properties. It has served as a treatment for a number of conditions, including allergies, pain, and diabetes.

In addition to lowering blood sugar, Pycnogenol appears to attack several of the problems associated with diabetes, including leaking blood vessels in the eyes that can cause vision loss (diabetic retinopathy); elevated blood pressure; and poor performance of the inner linings of the blood vessels throughout the body (endothelial dysfunction). Several studies have looked at Pycnogenol's effects on some of these diabetes-related problems:

♦ *Controlling blood sugar*: A study conducted in China looked at the effects of Pycnogenol on blood sugar. Thirty men and women between ages 28 and 64, all with mild type 2 diabetes, participated.[1] They were given 50 milligrams of Pycnogenol daily for 3 weeks; then 100 milligrams for 3 weeks; then 200 milligrams for 3 weeks; and finally 300 milligrams for 3 weeks. According to the researchers behind the study, a dose of 50 milligrams per day significantly reduced "after-eating" blood sugar from 12.47 to 11.16 mmol/L (224.5 to 200.9 mg/dL), while doses ranging from 100 to 300 milligrams per day significantly lowered fasting blood glucose from 8.64 to 7.54 mmol/L (155.5 to 135.7 mg/dL).

(Mmol/L stands for millimoles per liter, the global standard unit of measure for blood glucose.)

♦ *Relieving diabetic retinopathy*: Italian researchers investigated the effects of Pycnogenol on damage to the tiny blood vessels in the retina of the eye that can lead to vision loss and blindness.[2] They enlisted 20 people for this double-blind study, all of them suffering from retinopathy related to diabetes, as well as elevated blood pressure and clogged arteries. The volunteers were randomly assigned to receive either 150 milligrams of Pycnogenol or a placebo every day for 2 months. Then came a second phase of the study, in which an additional 20 volunteers were given 150 milligrams of Pycnogenol daily for 2 months. Between the two phases of the study, 30 people took Pycnogenol and 10 a placebo. The researchers used various tools to assess the volunteers' visual acuity, field of vision, and general eye health. The results were positive. In the placebo group, retinopathy progressively worsened, and visual acuity declined significantly. But in the Pycnogenol group, retinal function did not deteriorate, and visual acuity improved significantly. Fifty-three percent of those taking Pycnogenol had a "very good" or "good" response to treatment, while the remaining 47 percent showed a "moderate response." Among those taking the placebo, only 30 percent had a "good" response, and 10 percent showed no improvement at all. The researchers speculated that Pycnogenol may work by "sealing" leaky blood vessels in the eye.

♦ *Reducing blood pressure*: For a double-blind, placebo-controlled study published in *Life Sciences* in 2004, a team of Chinese and German researchers studied the effects of Pycnogenol in 58 adults with elevated blood pressure.[3] The volunteers were randomly assigned to receive either 100 milligrams of Pycnogenol or a placebo every day for 12 weeks. Everyone also took 20 milligrams of the standard blood pressure medication nifedipine. The goal was to see if Pycnogenol would help lower blood pressure and allow patients to reduce their dosage of the medicine. The results were positive. While the average dose of nifedipine needed by the placebo group to control blood pressure rose to 21.5 milligrams daily, in the Pycnogenol group it fell to an average of 15 milligrams per day. The researchers suggested that "Pycnogenol offers a broad spectrum of protection for the patient with hypertension."

Other studies have shown that Pycnogenol can reduce the formation of unnecessary blood clots (platelet aggregation), improve antioxidant capacity in the blood, increase "good" HDL cholesterol, and otherwise help strengthen cardiovascular health. All of these are important to diabetics, who often suffer from cardiovascular complications.

Summing Up the Evidence for Pycnogenol

Although Pycnogenol is not a cure for diabetes, a fair number of studies indicate that it can help control blood sugar and protect against several diabetes-related problems (such as diabetic retinopathy and cardiovascular disease). Therefore, it is fair to say that Pycnogenol is a four-star treatment for diabetes backed by strong evidence.

Available Forms

Pycnogenol is available in oral and topical supplement form.

How Much Pycnogenol Is Typically Used

There is no standard dose of Pycnogenol for diabetes. Based on the results of several studies, it appears that 100 to 200 milligrams per day is an effective dose range.

Possible Side Effects and Interactions

Pycnogenol may aggravate the symptoms of multiple sclerosis, rheumatoid arthritis, and other autoimmune diseases because of its immune-stimulating effects. For the same reason, it may interact with immunosuppressant drugs such as cyclosporine (Sandimmune), which help prevent rejection of transplanted organs. Pycnogenol's immune-stimulating actions also may interfere with the actions of immunosuppressant medications such as azathioprine (Imuran). If you're taking any medication, be sure to consult your doctor before adding Pycnogenol to your self-care regimen.

Alpha-Lipoic Acid

Rating: ☆☆☆ = Intriguing Evidence

A powerful free radical fighter that resides inside the mitochondria—the "energy factory" of a cell—alpha-lipoic acid (ALA) supports certain energy-producing reactions. ALA also helps recycle antioxidants such as vitamins C and E, "regenerating" them so that they can continue to exert their antioxidant effects.

In Germany, ALA—also known as thioctic acid—is used as a drug to treat diabetic neuropathy and certain liver ailments.[4] Several studies have looked into ALA's ability to help control blood sugar. Among them:

♦ In 1995 a team of German researchers published the results of their study examining whether ALA would improve insulin sensitivity and the hormone's ability to clear blood sugar from the bloodstreams in people with type 2 diabetes.[5] Thirteen people with type 2 were given a one-time-only injection of either 1,000 milligrams of ALA (brand name Thioctacid) or a placebo. The ALA improved insulin's ability to dispose of blood sugar. The placebo did not produce any significant change. As the researchers noted, "This is the first clinical study to show that alpha-lipoic acid increases insulin-stimulated glucose disposal" in people with type 2 diabetes.

♦ A team of German and American researchers examined the effects of ALA on glucose in their study of 20 people with type 2 diabetes.[6] All of the volunteers had well-controlled diabetes; that is, they were not suffering from any infections or other diabetes complications. All 20 received injections of 500 milligrams of ALA (Thioctacid) every day for 10 days. The ability of their own insulin to properly handle blood sugar was measured before and after the ALA treatments. The results were positive, showing that ALA improved the ability of insulin to dispose of glucose by some 30 percent. The researchers noted that 10 days of treatment with ALA "enhances insulin-stimulated whole body glucose disposal."

The positive results of these small trials encouraged the researchers to assess ALA in a larger study:

♦ For this multicenter study, 74 people with type 2 diabetes were randomly divided into four groups and given oral daily doses of 600, 1,200, or 1,800 milligrams of ALA, or a placebo.[7] All three dosages of ALA (Thioctacid) were found to be superior to placebo in increasing insulin sensitivity and the rate of clearance of blood glucose. The researchers concluded that "oral administration of alpha-lipoic acid can improve insulin sensitivity in patients with type 2 diabetes."

Another line of research inquiry focused on whether ALA can help with the nerve damage (neuropathy) often seen in diabetes:

♦ A meta-analysis appearing in *Diabetic Medicine* in 2004 summed up the current research into ALA's effect on diabetic polyneuropathy, or damage to many nerves due to diabetes.[8] This meta-analysis statistically merged the results of four clinical trials—all randomized, double-blind, and placebo-controlled, and involving a total of 1,258 people. In all of these trials, the volunteers were given intravenous infusions of 600 milligrams of ALA per day for 3 weeks. The researchers concluded that "treatment with alpha-lipoic acid (600 milligrams per day i.v.) over 3 weeks is superior to placebo in ameliorating both neuropathic symptoms and deficits" in patients with diabetic polyneuropathy.

Summing Up the Evidence for Alpha-Lipoic Acid

Given the fairly robust research findings on the use of alpha-lipoic acid for diabetes, it is fair to say that alpha-lipoic acid is a three-star treatment for diabetes backed by intriguing evidence.

Available Forms

ALA is found in foods such as liver and yeast. It also is available in supplement form.

How Much Alpha-Lipoic Acid Is Typically Used

There is no standard dose of ALA. Supplemental doses may range from 600 to 3,000 milligrams per day.

Possible Side Effects and Interactions

ALA may cause allergic skin conditions and upset stomach, and trigger low blood sugar (hypoglycemia). It also can bind with minerals, contributing to deficiencies of these nutrients in the body.

ALA may interact with diabetes drugs such as glipizide (Glucotrol), causing blood sugar to drop too low. If you're taking any medication, be sure to consult your doctor before adding ALA to your self-care regimen.

Blond Psyllium

Rating: ☆☆☆ = Intriguing Evidence

Perhaps best known as the active ingredient in the laxative Metamucil, blond psyllium is a common treatment for constipation and diarrhea, as well as for elevated blood pressure, elevated cholesterol, and other ailments. Its seeds and husk are coated with mucilage, a gummy substance that forms a thick gel when exposed to liquid in the intestines. Of all the species of psyllium, blond psyllium (*Plantago ovata*) contains the most mucilage.

In diabetes, mucilage helps control blood glucose by slowing the digestion and absorption of nutrients, which in turn slows the passage of glucose into the bloodstream. Psyllium also impairs the absorption of dietary fats and binds up bile acids, both of which help to lower blood cholesterol.

Several small studies have found that psyllium can improve blood sugar in people with type 2 diabetes, while helping to reduce elevated cholesterol and blood fat levels:

♦ A 1998 paper that appeared in the *Journal of Diabetes and Its Complications* reported the results of a double-blind study of 125 people suffering from type 2 diabetes.[9] The volunteers were divided into two groups. After receiving dietary counseling for 6 weeks, one group was given 15 grams of psyllium (Metamucil), and the other a placebo, every day for 6 weeks. Those taking the psyllium showed a significant reduction in blood sugar levels, total cholesterol, "bad" LDL cholesterol, and blood fats, plus an increase in "good" HDL cholesterol. The researchers concluded that psyllium "is useful as an adjunct to dietary therapy in patients with type 2 diabetes."

♦ The following year, a report published in the *American Journal of Clinical Nutrition* described the results of a double-blind study investigating the efficacy of psyllium in treating men who had type 2 diabetes and mild to moderate elevations in cholesterol and blood fat levels.[10] (Since diabetes is associated with an increased risk of developing heart disease, diabetics need to be careful to control their cholesterol and blood fats as well as blood glucose.) For this study, 34 men were randomly assigned to receive either 10.2 grams of psyllium (Metamucil) or a placebo daily. Their blood glucose, cholesterol, and blood fat levels were checked twice weekly. By the end of the 8-week study period, blood glucose levels were 19.2 percent lower after lunch and an average of 11 percent lower all day in the psyllium group than in the placebo group. The researchers reported that the psyllium was well tolerated and concluded that it improved blood glucose and blood fat control in men with type 2 diabetes plus elevated cholesterol and blood fats.

♦ These results were repeated in a 2002 study presented in the *European Journal of Clinical Nutrition*.[11] For this small-scale, 11-week study, 20 volunteers with type 2 diabetes were given 14 grams of psyllium fiber (brand name Plantaben) every day during weeks 2 through 7. At the end of weeks 1, 7, and 11, they also were given a breakfast meal containing specific amounts of sugar and other substances. Then their blood glucose, insulin, cholesterol, and other levels were measured to see how they responded to the test meal. The results were positive, with blood glucose, total cholesterol, and "bad" LDL cholesterol significantly declining after 6 weeks of psyllium treatment. The researchers concluded that psyllium had a "beneficial therapeutic effect" in controlling type 2 diabetes and in lowering the risk of coronary heart disease.

Summing Up the Evidence for Blond Psyllium

With a number of studies suggesting that blond psyllium can lower postprandial (after-meal) glucose and insulin levels in those with type 2 diabetes, and postprandial glucose levels in those with type 1 diabetes, it is fair to say that blond psyllium is a three-star treatment for diabetes backed by intriguing evidence.

Other Names

Blond psyllium is known to scientists as *Plantago ovata*, and in various parts of the world as Englishman's foot, Indian plantago, ispagol, psyllium, sand plantain, and spogel.

Available Forms

Blond psyllium is found in bulking laxatives such as Metamucil, as well as in some breads, cereals, and snack bars. It is also available as seeds, powder, tablets, and tincture.

How Much Blond Psyllium Is Typically Used

A standard dose of blond psyllium has not been set. For diabetes and elevated cholesterol, doses up to 15 grams per day have been used.

Possible Side Effects and Interactions

Taken orally, blond psyllium can cause abdominal pain, diarrhea, and constipation, among other side effects. Some people may experience an allergic reaction to it.

Blond psyllium may increase the risk of low blood sugar when combined with diabetes medications such as glipizide (Glucotrol). The fiber in blond psyllium may reduce the absorption of any drug taken orally. If you're taking any medication, be sure to consult your doctor before adding therapeutic amounts of blond psyllium to your self-care regimen.

Chromium

Rating: ☆☆☆ = Intriguing Evidence

The mineral chromium works with insulin to help cells take up fuel (glucose) from the bloodstream and release energy. Although the body contains only a small amount of chromium (about 6 milligrams), a shortfall of this mineral can diminish insulin's effectiveness as well as the body's ability to handle glucose. Low levels of chromium are characteristic of diabetes, although there is no proof that a lack of chromium actually causes the disease. Still, some people have used chromium to treat diabetes, as well as elevated cholesterol, heart disease, and obesity. It also is believed to improve athletic performance.

The idea that chromium might be helpful in the treatment of diabetes goes back at least 50 years, when researchers hypothesized that brewer's yeast contained a glucose tolerance factor (GTF) that prevented deliberately induced diabetes from taking root in laboratory animals. Several studies have shown that the mineral can indeed help improve glucose and insulin levels in diabetics. For example:

♦ Researchers from the US Department of Agriculture and Beijing Medical University studied the effects of chromium (in the form of chromium picolinate) on 180 men and women with type 2 diabetes. The volunteers were randomly assigned to one of three groups, receiving 1,000 micrograms of chromium, 200 micrograms of chromium, or a placebo.[12] (The supplements were supplied by Nutrition 21.) All of the volunteers continued with their regular diet, lifestyle habits, and medications during the study. When they were checked at 2 months and again 4 months later, the results were encouraging. After 2 months, the fasting insulin concentrations were significantly lower in both groups receiving chromium. At 2 and 4 months, the fasting and 2-hour "after-eating" glucose levels had fallen significantly in the group taking 1,000 micrograms of chromium, compared to those taking the placebo. At the 4-month mark, total cholesterol had fallen in those taking 1,000 micrograms of chromium. According to the researchers, the results "demonstrate that supplemental chromium had significant beneficial effects on . . . glucose, insulin, and cholesterol variables in subjects with type 2 diabetes."

♦ For a 2004 study published in the *International Journal of Vitamin and Nutrition Research*, Israeli researchers recruited 78 senior citizens, all with diabetes.[13] Thirty-nine of the volunteers were given 400 micrograms of chromium daily for 3 weeks, plus standard treatment, while the other 39 received only standard treatment. (The supplements were supplied by Solgar Vitamin and Herb.) Among those taking chromium, there was a significant drop in the fasting glucose level from 190 to 150 mg/dL, while total cholesterol fell from 235 to 213 mg/dL and triglycerides from 152 to 136 mg/dL. But there was no significant improvement in either fasting glucose or cholesterol levels among those taking the placebo. The researchers concluded that "dietary supplementation with chromium is beneficial in moderating glucose intolerance," and that the mineral appeared to lower cholesterol and fat in the blood.

♦ A study presented to the International Symposium on the Health Effects of Dietary Chromium in 1998 examined the link between chromium and gestational diabetes (pregnancy-related diabetes).[14] Thirty women between 20 and 24 weeks pregnant participated in this study. All of them were instructed to consume a diet designed to help keep their blood sugar under control. Then 10 were given the Recommended Dietary Allowance of chromium for pregnant women (4 micrograms per kilogram of body weight per day); another 10 received a "double dose" of chromium (8 micrograms per kilogram of body weight per day); and 10 took a placebo. Eight weeks later, the women who had taken either dose of chromium had lower blood sugar and insulin levels compared to baseline, and compared to the women taking the placebo. The researchers concluded that chromium supplementation "for gestational diabetic women improves glucose intolerance and lowers hyperinsulinemia" (elevated insulin levels).

♦ A recent paper published in *Diabetes Care* summed up the current research into chromium's effect on diabetes.[15] For this 2004 review, the two authors—one from the Harvard School of Public Health, the other from the Pennington Biomedical Research Center—gathered relevant chromium/diabetes studies. They concluded, "Growing evidence suggests that chromium supplementation, particularly at higher doses and in the form of [chromium picolinate], may improve insulin sensitivity and glucose metabolism in patients with glucose intolerance and type 1, type 2, gestational, and steroid-induced diabetes." The researchers went on to note that the studies supporting this conclusion have shortcomings, which call for more study.

Summing Up the Evidence for Chromium

A fair number of studies have shown that chromium is indeed helpful in controlling blood sugar levels in diabetics—although other studies have found the opposite. There are many reasons why some studies may say "yes" while others say "no," such as using different dosages or different forms of the mineral; focusing on different types of diabetes (type 1, type 2, gestational diabetes, and steroid-induced diabetes); and utilizing different tools to measure study results. At this point, it can be said that chromium is a three-star treatment for diabetes backed by intriguing evidence.

Available Forms

Chromium is found in foods such as broccoli, grape juice, English muffins, mashed potatoes, orange juice, bananas, and green beans. It is also available in supplement form.

How Much Chromium Is Typically Used

Chromium supplements come in several forms, including chromium picolinate and chromium chloride. The most important factor is how much elemental chromium the supplement contains. Be sure to check the label for the amount of elemental chromium before purchasing a supplement product. Supplemental doses may range from 200 to 1,000 micrograms per day.

Possible Side Effects and Interactions

The Food and Nutrition Board of the Institute of Medicine has not set a tolerable upper intake for chromium. However, some experts believe that taking more than 300 micrograms of the mineral every day for several months may be toxic to the liver, while others have suggested that long-term use may damage cellular DNA.

In supplement form, chromium can cause headaches, mood swings, and sleep disturbances. It also may interact with diabetes medications such as glyburide (DiaBeta), causing blood sugar to fall too low. If you're taking any medication, be sure to consult your doctor before adding chromium supplements to your self-care regimen.

Cinnamon

Rating: ☆☆ = Modest Evidence

The volatile oils in cinnamon bark are most likely the active ingredients in cinnamon, a spice that various cultures long have used as a treatment for poor appetite, infections, stomach upset, and diarrhea. It also appears as a flavoring in foods, beverages, mouthwash, and toothpaste, and as a fragrance in lotions, detergents, cosmetics, and other products.

Test-tube studies have shown that cinnamon can enhance the activity of insulin. This prompted Pakistani researchers to investigate whether the spice could improve blood sugar, cholesterol, and blood fat levels in people with type 2 diabetes:

+ Sixty men and women with type 2 diabetes were enrolled in this study, which was published in *Diabetes Care* in 2003.[16] The volunteers—average age 52—were randomly assigned to receive 1, 3, or 6 grams of cinnamon per day, or a placebo. Each volunteer took the prescribed dosage for 40 days. By the end of the study, all three dosages of cinnamon had reduced blood glucose levels significantly. The researchers concluded that cinnamon lowers blood sugar, blood fats, "bad" LDL cholesterol, and total cholesterol levels in people with type 2 diabetes, although the mechanisms involved remain a mystery. Figure 10-1 below shows how all three doses of cinnamon lowered fasting blood sugar over the course of 40 days. There was no change in blood sugar associated with the placebo.

Figure 10-1: Cinnamon Lowers Fasting Blood Sugar in People with Type 2 Diabetes

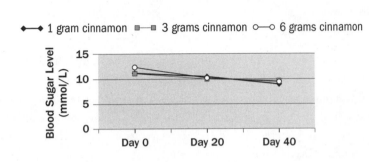

Summing Up the Evidence for Cinnamon

This single study on cinnamon for diabetes is intriguing but limited. At this point, it is reasonable to say that cinnamon is a two-star treatment for diabetes based on modest evidence.

Other Names

Known scientifically as *Cinnamomum verum*, cinnamon is referred to in various cultures as batavia cassia, cannelier de ceylan, Madagascar cinnamon, Panag cinnamon, and tvak.

Available Forms

Cinnamon is available as powder, tincture, extract, dried bark, leaves, oil, or tea.

How Much Cinnamon Is Typically Used

There is no standard dose of cinnamon. Supplemental doses may range from 125 to 250 milligrams per day.

Possible Side Effects and Interactions

Cinnamon is believed to be safe when taken orally in small amounts. It may interact with diabetes medications such as metformin (Glucophage), causing blood sugar to fall too low. If you're taking any medication, be sure to consult your doctor before adding therapeutic amounts of cinnamon to your self-care regimen.

Fenugreek

Rating: ☆☆ = Modest Evidence

Native to Northern Africa and India, fenugreek has a long history. Ancient Egyptians used it for incense and embalming; the Romans adopted it as an aid to women during labor; and Chinese doctors prescribed it for weakness and swelling of the legs and as a general tonic. Today, fenugreek serves as a treatment for diabetes as well as for constipation, elevated cholesterol and blood fats, kidney problems, and a number of other ailments. It also is an ingredient in spice blends, and a flavoring agent in various foods.

Although it isn't known exactly how fenugreek might lower blood sugar in people with diabetes, some studies suggest it may do just that:

♦ Indian researchers tested the effects of fenugreek in 25 people with mild to moderate type 2 diabetes for a 2001 double-blind study.[17] The participants were randomly assigned to receive 2 months of treatment with daily doses of either 1 gram of fenugreek seed extract or a placebo. Both groups continued with their standard care. Blood sugar and insulin levels were checked before and after treatment, with positive results. The researchers concluded that "adjunct use of fenugreek seeds improves glycemic control and decreases insulin resistance in mild type 2 diabetes patients."

♦ For a 1990 study published in the *European Journal of Clinical Research*, 10 volunteers with type 1 diabetes were randomly assisgned to one of two groups.[18] Group 1 followed a standardized diet that included 100 grams of defatted fenugreek seed powder, while group 2 followed the same diet without fenugreek. After 10 days, the groups switched treatments. Average fasting blood sugar levels fell from 15.1 to 10.9 mmol/L (271.8 to 196.2 mg/dL) on the fenugreek diet. "After-eating" glucose levels also declined, as did the level of sugar in the urine (a sign of diabetes) by 54 percent. The researchers concluded, "The fenugreek diet significantly reduced fasting blood sugar and improved the glucose tolerance test."

Summing Up the Evidence for Fenugreek

A small body of clinical studies—plus numerous case histories—supports the use of fenugreek as an adjunct treatment for diabetes. Thus, it is reasonable to say that fenugreek is a two-star treatment for diabetes backed by modest evidence.

Other Names

Fenugreek is known to scientists as *Trigonella foenum-graecum*, and in various parts of the world as bird's foot, bockshornsame, Greek clover, Greek hay seed, and hu lu ba, among other names.

Available Forms

Fenugreek is available in whole, powder, fluid extract, capsule, and tea form.

How Much Fenugreek Is Typically Used

There is no standard dose of fenugreek for diabetes. Some studies have used supplemental doses of up to 100 grams of fenugreek seed powder per day.

Possible Side Effects and Interactions

Fenugreek's side effects include diarrhea, flatulence, and allergic reactions such as hoarseness and wheezing. It may interact with diabetes drugs such as acarbose (Precose), causing blood sugar to fall too low. It also may raise the risk of liver damage when combined with pain relievers such as acetaminophen (Tylenol). If you're taking any medication, be sure to consult your doctor before adding fenugreek to your self-care regimen.

Glucomannan

Rating: ☆☆ = Modest Evidence

Glucomannan is a soluble dietary fiber derived from konjac flour, a substance with a long history in China and Japan as a folk remedy for various ailments. It remains popular in those countries as a general health remedy and as a thickening agent for food. In the United States, glucomannan supplements serve as a treatment for diabetes, elevated cholesterol, and constipation as well as a weight-loss aid.

♦ Researchers from the University of Toronto and the University of Milan reported on the results of their double-blind crossover gluco-mannan/diabetes study in *Diabetes Care* in 1999.[19] Eleven men and women with type 2 diabetes, as well as elevated blood pressure and cholesterol, were observed for 8 weeks. Then they were randomly assigned to eat biscuits containing glucomannan (brand name Dicoman) or containing wheat fiber (as a placebo) for 3 weeks. Next came a 2-week "washout" period, during which the participants did not eat biscuits. This was followed by another 3-week period in which the participants switched treatments—that is, those who had been eating the glucomannan-enriched biscuits received the placebo biscuits, and vice versa. Throughout the entire study, all of the participants followed a standard cholesterol-lowering diet and continued with their medications. The results were intriguing, with glucomannan reducing blood levels of fructosamine, a short-term marker of diabetes control. Glucomannan also reduced systolic blood pressure by 6.9 percent and the ratio of total cholesterol to HDL cholesterol by 2.3 percent. The researchers concluded that adding glucomannan-enriched biscuits to standard treatment "improved metabolic control beyond the effect of conventional treatment alone in high-risk individuals with type 2 diabetes."

♦ A similar study was conducted by researchers from Taiwan and published in the *Journal of the American College of Nutrition* in 2003.[20] Twenty-two people age 45 or older—all with type 2 diabetes and taking standard diabetes medicines—enrolled in this randomized, double-blind crossover study. The volunteers were assigned to receive 4 weeks of treatment with either glucomannan fiber (with the dosage increasing from 1.2 to 3.6 grams per day) or a placebo. Then each group crossed over and took the other treatment for an additional 4 weeks. Fasting blood glucose levels fell by 12.3 percent with glucomannan, but rose by 10.2 percent with the placebo. The effect on the 2-hour "after-eating" blood sugar levels was similar; they dropped by 12.2 percent with the glucomannan but rose by 12.6 percent with the placebo. In addition, glucomannan reduced total cholesterol and LDL cholesterol. The study's authors noted that glucomannan could be an adjunct treatment for people suffering from diabetes and elevated blood fat levels.[21]

Figure 10-2 below shows the 2-hour "after-eating" blood sugar levels, a key diabetes test. The average blood glucose levels were similar at the beginning of the study. They dropped when glucomannan was taken but rose when the placebo was taken.

Figure 10-2: 2-Hour "After-Eating" Blood Sugar Levels

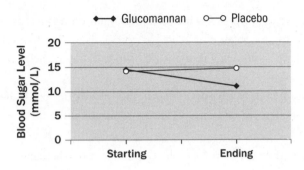

Summing Up the Evidence for Glucomannan

As suggested by the research available today, it is reasonable to say that glucomannan is a two-star treatment for diabetes based on modest evidence.

Available Forms

Glucomannan is available in powder and supplement form.

How Much Glucomannan Is Typically Used

There is no standard dose of glucomannan. Supplemental doses of up to 10 grams per day have been used.

Possible Side Effects and Interactions

Glucomannan may cause obstruction of the esophagus and/or gastrointestinal tract. If it's taken in combination with diabetes medications such as miglitol (Glyset), blood sugar levels may drop too low. Glucomannan also may hamper the absorption of drugs taken orally. If you're taking any medicine, be sure to consult your doctor before adding therapeutic amounts of glucomannan to your self-care regimen.

Guar Gum

Rating: ☆☆ = Modest Evidence

Guar gum is a soluble dietary fiber that comes from the seed of the guar plant, native to India. In manufacturing, it is used as a thickener, stabilizer, and/or binding agent in foods, beverages, lotions, and creams.

When mixed with liquid in the intestines, guar gum expands, giving more "heft" to feces and promoting bowel action. This makes it an effective remedy for constipation. Because it absorbs fluid, it may be helpful for treating diarrhea as well.

Some studies have investigated whether guar gum could help manage diabetes and elevated cholesterol. Here is a sampling:

♦ A team of researchers from the Department of Medicine of the University of Manchester in England conducted a double-blind, double-placebo, crossover study involving 19 people with type 2 diabetes who also were obese.[22] This 36-week study was divided into three periods of 12 weeks each. In random order, patients received 15 grams of guar gum (brand name Guarem) for 12 weeks, 1,500 milligrams of the diabetes drug metformin (Glucophage) for 12 weeks, and a placebo for 12 weeks. Both guar gum and metformin reduced the patients' fasting blood sugar levels and LDL cholesterol.

♦ In 1993 Finnish researchers reported on their study of guar gum in the *American Journal of Clinical Nutrition*.[23] The eight men and seven women in this study—all of whom had been suffering from type 2 diabetes for an average of 6 years—were given a placebo for 8 weeks, then 15 grams of guar gum every day for 32 weeks, then a placebo for another 8 weeks. The researchers tracked the patients' response to the guar gum and the placebo, finding that guar gum improved long-term control of blood sugar, "after-eating" clearance of blood sugar, and blood fat levels. They concluded that "guar gum has favorable long-term effects" on blood sugar and blood fat concentrations.

♦ For an intriguing study involving 14 people with type 2 diabetes, researchers from King's College and the University of Surrey in London gave breakfast to their study participants, then analyzed their blood.[24] The breakfast consisted of bread containing 7.6 grams of guar gum, or a "placebo" bread that did not contain guar gum. Blood samples were drawn before the volunteers ate and at 8 separate times after they had completed their meals. The results were positive, with guar gum significantly reducing the "after-eating" rise in blood sugar and insulin.

Summing Up the Evidence for Guar Gum

In addition to lowering blood sugar and sometimes insulin levels, guar gum reduces cholesterol levels—an important consideration for diabetics, who are at increased risk for clogged arteries and heart attacks. Guar gum has performed well, alone and in combination with other substances, in studies testing its effects on diabetes. It is reasonable to say that guar gum is a two-star treatment for diabetes based on modest evidence.

Other Names

Guar gum is known scientifically as *Cyamopsis tetragonoloba*, and in various cultures as aconite bean, Calcutta lucerne, guar, Indian cluster bean, Indian guar plant, and jaguar gum.

Available Forms

Guar gum is available in powder, tablet, and granule form.

How Much Guar Gum Is Typically Used

There is no standard dose of guar gum. Some successful studies used 15 grams of guar gum per day.

Possible Side Effects and Interactions

Among guar gum's possible side effects are nausea, diarrhea, dizziness, and sweating. If taken with inadequate amounts of fluid, it can cause obstruction of the esophagus and/or bowel. It may interact with diabetes drugs such as tolazamide (Tolinase), causing blood sugar to drop too low. It also may hamper the absorption of all drugs taken orally. If you're taking any medication, be sure to consult your doctor before adding therapeutic amounts of guar gum to your self-care regimen.

Vanadium

Rating: ☆☆ = Modest Evidence

Vanadium is a nonessential mineral found in various foods. It's considered nonessential because so far, nutrition researchers have not determined what vital role it may play in human health. The mineral does, however, seem to influence the way in which the body handles insulin and blood sugar. Some studies suggest that supplemental vanadium might helpful for those with diabetes:

+ Researchers tested the effects of vanadium in 10 people with diabetes (5 of whom were insulin-dependent, and five of whom were noninsulin-dependent).[25] The volunteers were given 125 milligrams of a form of vanadium called metavanadate every day for 2 weeks. The mineral triggered "a significant decrease in insulin requirements" in those with insulin-dependent diabetes. Total cholesterol levels also declined significantly in both groups of volunteers.
+ For a 1995 study published in the journal *Metabolism*, eight people with noninsulin-dependent diabetes were given 100 milligrams of vanadium (in the form of vanadyl sulfate) every day for 4 weeks.[26] Then six of the eight were given a placebo for another 4 weeks. The results were positive, with vanadyl sulfate producing "modest reductions" in fasting blood sugar levels.

Summing Up the Evidence for Vanadium

With support from a small number of clinical studies, it is fair to say that vanadium is a two-star treatment for diabetes backed by modest evidence.

Available Forms

Vanadium is available in supplement form.

How Much Vanadium Is Typically Used

There is no standard dose of vanadium for diabetes. Daily doses of 50 to 100 milligrams of vanadium, in the form of vanadyl sulfate, have been used in some studies.

Possible Side Effects and Interactions

In supplement form, vanadium can cause cramps and diarrhea. It also may interact with blood thinners such as aspirin and heparin (Hep-Lock) to increase the risk of bruising and bleeding, and with diabetes drugs such as glyburide (DiaBeta) to cause a significant drop in blood sugar. If you're taking any medication, be sure to consult your doctor before adding vanadium to your self-care regimen.

Bitter Melon

Rating: ☆ = Preliminary Evidence

A cousin to cantaloupe, casaba, and honeydew, bitter melon is eaten as a vegetable in India and parts of Asia, South America, and Africa. It has antibacterial properties and is a traditional remedy for psoriasis, ulcers, constipation, and other ailments.

Animal studies have suggested that bitter melon also can lower blood sugar levels. Now researchers are looking into whether it has the same benefit in humans. For example:

♦ A 2004 study looked at the effects of vanadium in 15 people with type 2 diabetes.[27] For this nonrandomized study, the volunteers were given standard diabetes medicines for 7 days, then half the dose of the standard medicines plus 400 milligrams of a bitter melon extract daily for another 7 days. The results were intriguing, with bitter melon plus a half-dose of the standard medicine lowering blood sugar further than a full dose of medicine. The researchers concluded that bitter melon extract works synergistically with standard diabetes medicines to improve their blood sugar–lowering ability.

♦ Researchers from Sher-e Bangal Medical College in Bangladesh tested the effects of bitter melon extract in 100 people with moderate type 2 diabetes.[28] This was not a study; instead, it was a series of individual patients undergoing treatment with the herb. The researchers reported that in 85 percent of the volunteers, the herbal extract led to significant reduction of fasting and "after-eating" blood sugar levels.

Summing Up the Evidence for Bitter Melon

Animal and laboratory studies, plus case histories and nonrandomized studies, have indicated that bitter melon can lower elevated blood sugar. However, the large-scale randomized, double-blind, controlled studies necessary to make a definitive statement about the herb's effects have not been performed. Based on what we know so far, it is reasonable to say that bitter melon is a one-star treatment for diabetes based on preliminary evidence.

Other Names

Bitter melon is known to scientists as *Momordica charantia*, and in various parts of the world as African cucumber, balsamo, bitter cucumber, carilla gourd, karela, pepino montero, and sushavi.

Available Forms

Bitter melon is available as a food, as well as in juice and capsule form.

How Much Bitter Melon Is Typically Used

There is no standard dose of bitter melon. One study used 400 milligrams of bitter melon extract per day.

Possible Side Effects and Interactions

Bitter melon's side effects are not known, but since it appears to potentiate diabetes medicines, it may cause blood sugar to dip too low. In addition, it may increase the risk of liver damage when combined with pain relievers such as acetaminophen (Tylenol) or with cholesterol-lowering drugs such as atorvastatin (Lipitor). If you're taking any medication, be sure to consult your doctor before adding therapeutic amounts of bitter melon to your self-care regimen.

Gymnema sylvestre

Rating: ☆ = Preliminary Evidence

Gymnema sylvestre comes from a plant grown in India. It is said that the plant was given the Hindu name of *gurmar*, meaning "sugar destroyer," because chewing the leaves takes away the ability to taste sweetness.

Ayurvedic physicians use the herb to treat diabetes, malaria, and constipation.

♦ Researchers from the University of Madras in India published the results of their study of *Gymnema sylvestre* in the *Journal of Ethnopharmacology* in 1990.[29] All of the 22 volunteers in this nonrandomized study had type 2 diabetes, and all were taking standard medicines for blood sugar control. They were given 400 milligrams of *Gymnema sylvestre* extract per day for 18 to 20 months in addition to their regular diabetes medications. While taking the herbal extract, "the patients showed a significant reduction in blood glucose," and were able to use less of their standard medicines. Figure 10-3 below shows the decline in blood sugar levels for each patient from the beginning to the end of the study.

Figure 10-3: Blood Sugar Falls with *Gymnema sylvestre* Treatment

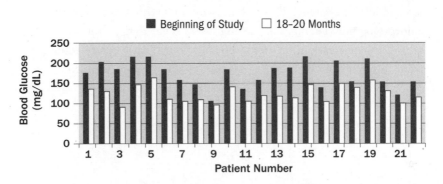

♦ Some of the same researchers who conducted the above study collaborated on a similar one, also published in the *Journal of Ethnopharmacology* in 1990.[30] For this nonrandomized study, 64 people with type 1 diabetes who were taking insulin were divided into two groups. The first group was given 400 milligrams of *Gymnema sylvestre* extract per day in addition to their insulin for periods ranging from 2 to 30 months. The second group took insulin only. Blood insulin requirements and fasting blood sugar levels dropped in the *Gymnema sylvestre* group. The researchers concluded that the *Gymnema sylvestre* extract "appears to enhance endogenous insulin"—that is, insulin produced by the body rather than injected as a medicine—possibly by revitalizing the liver cells that produce insulin.

Summing Up the Evidence for *Gymnena sylvestre*

Without data from quality randomized human trials to draw on, it is best to say that *Gymnema sylvestre* is a one-star treatment for diabetes based on preliminary evidence.

Available Forms

Gymnema sylvestre is available in extract form.

How Much *Gymnema sylvestre* Is Typically Used

There is no standard dose of *Gymnema sylvestre* for diabetes. Studies involving the herbal extract generally used about 400 milligrams per day.

Possible Side Effects and Interactions

Gymnema sylvestre can impair the ability to taste sweetness and cause nausea and loss of appetite. The herb may interact with diabetes drugs such as chlorpropamide (Diabinese), causing blood sugar to drop too low. If you're taking any medication, be sure to consult your doctor before adding therapeutic amounts of *Gymnema sylvestre* to your self-care regimen.

ALTERNATIVE APPROACHES TO

DIARRHEA

Blond psyllium	☆☆☆☆
Probiotics	☆☆☆☆
Lactobacillus	☆☆☆☆/☆☆☆
Bovine colostrum	☆☆☆
Saccharomyces boulardii	☆☆☆
Zinc	☆☆☆
Guar gum	☆☆
Homeopathy	☆☆

Diarrhea is the passing of loose, watery stool, which may be accompanied by an increase in the volume of stool or the frequency of bowel movements. Normal stool is between 60 and 90 percent water; in cases of diarrhea, the water content can exceed 90 percent.

The main symptom of diarrhea is a stool consistency that can range from soft and poorly formed to completely liquid. Other symptoms include gas, intestinal cramps, and a feeling of urgency to defecate. Nausea and vomiting also may occur, especially if the diarrhea is due to an intestinal infection or exposure to toxins. Uncontrolled diarrhea can lead to dehydration, low blood levels of electrolytes (sodium, potassium, chloride, and magnesium), malnutrition, low blood pressure, fainting, arrhythmias, and even kidney failure.

CAUSES

Generally, anything that speeds the transit of stool through the large intestine can cause diarrhea. This includes certain drugs (laxatives, antibiotics, and prostaglandins) and food substances (caffeine and magnesium); bacterial and viral infections; parasites; certain medical conditions (hyperthyroidism and pancreatic or duodenal tumors); and certain medical procedures (intestinal bypass, surgical removal of part of the digestive system, or surgical cutting of the vagus nerve to reduce acid secretion in the stomach). Sometimes inflammatory conditions affecting the area near the colon—such as diverticulitis, appendicitis, hemorrhagic ovarian cysts, and pelvic inflammatory disease—are to blame. Diarrhea also may be due to malabsorption, the result of insufficient digestive enzymes, or conditions such as celiac disease that destroy villi, the fingerlike projections that line the intestinal walls and are responsible for nutrient absorption.

In a general sense, we can speak of two types of diarrhea: *acute*, which lasts less than 2 weeks, and *chronic*, which lasts longer than 2 weeks.

The cause of acute diarrhea, or *gastroenteritis*, is almost always infectious—that is, exposure to bacteria such as *Campylobacter*, salmonella, and *Escherichia coli*; viruses such as rotavirus and cytomegalovirus; and parasites such as *Cryptosporidium paruum* and *Giardia lamblia*. Acute diarrhea also can occur with intestinal diseases, food intolerances, and medication reactions.

Chronic diarrhea is often the result of a long-standing infection (salmonella causes a particularly persistent one). Other potential causes include inflammatory bowel disease, tumors, malabsorption, or any disorder that speeds the transit of food through the intestines.

STANDARD TREATMENTS

The first-line treatment for diarrhea—whether acute or chronic—involves replacing fluids and electrolytes, pinpointing the cause of the diarrhea, and, if possible, putting a stop to it. For example, if you're lactose-intolerant, you can relieve diarrhea by avoiding lactose-containing foods or taking a lactase supplement. (Lactase is the enzyme that helps digest lactose, the primary sugar in milk.)

Cramping and inflammation of the intestines may be treated with antispasmodic drugs. Diarrhea that's triggered by toxins, chemicals, or infectious organisms may respond to medicines such as kaolin-pectin, which bind up the offending substances and also increase the firmness of stool. In more serious cases of diarrhea, antibiotic medications may be necessary.

As you read through the following discussion of diarrhea remedies, you'll notice some overlap between *Lactobacillus, Saccharomyces boulardii,* and probiotics. This is because some of the studies focused on several probiotics at once, so *Lactobacillus* and/or *Saccharomyces boulardii* may appear in multiple trials. We thought that each of the individual entries was important enough to stand on its own and that trying to combine them into one entry on probiotics would be confusing. Thus, we present them as three separate entries.

RATING POPULAR ALTERNATIVE TREATMENTS FOR DIARRHEA

Blond Psyllium

Rating: ☆☆☆☆ = Strong Evidence

Blond psyllium—the active ingredient found in the laxative Metamucil—is well-known as a constipation remedy. But it's also surprisingly effective in treating diarrhea. Its seeds are coated with mucilage, a gummy substance that absorbs water in the intestines and forms a thick, gooey gel. Because it attracts water in the intestines, blond psyllium can make the contents of the intestines more solid and slow the transit time of the stool—which is exactly what's needed in cases of diarrhea.

Some interesting studies of the effects of blond psyllium on diarrhea include the following:

+ A 2001 study published in *Nursing Research* tested the effects of psyllium on 39 nonhospitalized adults with fecal incontinence, the inability to control loose or liquid stools.[1] The participants were randomly assigned to take 7.1 grams of blond psyllium (Metamucil), 25 grams of gum arabic, or a placebo every day for 31 days. They also recorded their food intake and the characteristics of their stool and produced a stool sample for analysis before and after the 31-day treatment period. Both psyllium and gum arabic were helpful in relieving diarrhea, reducing the proportion of incontinent stools by more than half compared to the placebo.

The researchers concluded that both psyllium and gum arabic were "associated with a decrease in the percentage of incontinent stools and an improvement in stool consistency."

♦ Canadian researchers examined the effects of psyllium on cancer patients undergoing radiation therapy, which can trigger gastrointestinal side effects such as diarrhea.[2] This was a pilot study designed to collect information and set the stage for further research, rather than an experimental study. Sixty patients undergoing radiation therapy to the pelvis were randomly assigned to two groups. One group took blond psyllium (Metamucil) while the other did not. Those taking the psyllium showed a significant drop in the incidence and severity of diarrhea. They also were able to cut back on their usage of antidiarrheal medicine, although the reduction was not statistically significant.

♦ Patients who are tube-fed are at higher than average risk for developing diarrhea. In 1991 researchers from the Portland Veterans Affairs Medical Center randomly assigned 49 tube-fed patients to two groups.[3] One group received 3 teaspoons of blond psyllium (Hydrocil) per day for 6 days; the other did not. The researchers found that the use of blond psyllium firmed the stools and reduced diarrhea in tube-fed patients.

Summing Up the Evidence for Blond Psyllium

Several studies of blond psyllium as a treatment for diarrhea have produced positive results, leading to the conclusion that blond psyllium is a four-star treatment for diarrhea backed by strong evidence.

Other Names

Blond psyllium is known to scientists as *Plantago ovata* and in various parts of the world as Englishman's foot, Indian plantago, ispaghula, ispagol, psyllium, sand plantain, and spogel.

Available Forms

Blond psyllium is found in bulking laxatives such as Metamucil, as well as in some breads, cereals, and snack bars. It is also available as seeds and in supplement form as powder, tablets, and tincture.

How Much Blond Psyllium Is Typically Used

A standard dose of blond psyllium has not been set. Supplemental doses range up to 20 grams per day.

Possible Side Effects and Interactions

In therapeutic amounts, blond psyllium can cause abdominal pain and constipation, among other side effects. Some people may experience allergic reactions to it.

Blond psyllium may increase the risk of low blood sugar when combined with antidiabetes drugs such as glipizide (Glucotrol). If you're taking any medication, be sure to consult your doctor before adding blond psyllium to your self-care regimen.

Probiotics

Rating: ☆☆☆☆ = Strong Evidence

It may seem odd to think that bacteria can be good for you. Yet the intestinal tract is filled with beneficial bacteria that help break down food and certain drugs, support nutrient absorption and immune function, and prevent other, harmful bacteria from gaining a foothold.

Probiotics are living microscopic organisms that promote the growth of the beneficial bacteria, yeasts, and other substances that coexist in the gut with disease-causing bacteria. However, the delicate balance between the good and bad microorganisms can be upset by infections, antibiotics, radiation, or abdominal surgery, among other things—destroying the good bacteria and allowing the overgrowth of the bad.

That's when the intestines need to be "re-seeded" with beneficial microorganisms—most notably members of the *Lactobacillus* and *Bifidobacterium* species, along with certain yeasts. Among the probiotics are *L. acidophilus, L. delbrueckii, L. casei, L. reuteri, B. bifidum, B. lactis, Streptococcus salivarius, S. thermophilus,* and *Saccharomyces boulardii.*

Various studies, including those that follow, have shown that probiotics can help prevent diarrhea in children. Diarrhea is a common problem among children in the United States, prompting well over 100,000 hospitalizations and a couple of million doctor visits each year. This makes children particularly useful and accessible group to study.

♦ A 1994 study published in the journal *Lancet* looked at the effects of *B. bifidum* plus *S. thermophilus* on acute diarrhea in infants.[4] This double-blind, placebo-controlled trial investigated whether diarrhea could be prevented in infants who had been admitted to a chronic care hospital for other reasons. The 55 infants, ranging in age from 5 months to 24 months, were observed for a total of 4,447 patient-days. Some of the youngsters were given a standard infant formula, while others were given the same formula with added *B. bifidum* and *S. thermophilus* (supplied by Carnation Nutritional Products). Over the course of the study, only 7 percent of those taking the probiotics developed diarrhea, compared to 31 percent of those receiving the standard formula. The researchers concluded that "supplementation of infant formula with *B. bifidum* and *S. thermophilus* can reduce the incidence of acute diarrhea and rotavirus shedding in infants admitted to [the] hospital."

♦ A similar study published in 2004 examined whether probiotics could prevent the development of diarrhea in healthy children.[5] The 90 children participating in this double-blind, placebo-controlled study were randomly assigned to receive either infant formula or infant formula plus *B. lactis*. Of those receiving the probiotic, 28.3 percent developed diarrhea, compared to 38.7 percent of those who did not receive the probiotic. In addition, the infants drinking *B. lactis* had diarrhea for an average of 1.2 days, compared to an average of 2.3 days in those drinking the plain formula.

The results were equally positive when the studies of probiotics for diarrhea were statistically combined.

♦ Antibiotics can trigger diarrhea and other gastrointestinal problems by killing off *Lactobacillus* and other friendly bacteria in the gastrointestinal tract. A group of British researchers published their meta-analysis of the efficacy of probiotics as a treatment for antibiotic-associated diarrhea in the *British Medical Journal* in 2002.[6] The researchers used statistical methods to merge nine randomized, double-blind, placebo-controlled studies looking at antibiotic-associated diarrhea. The treatment periods ranged from 5 to 49 days. The authors noted that their results were limited because they included only a small number of studies in the meta-analysis. However, they concluded that probiotics "may be useful in preventing antibiotic associated diarrhea." The results of the individual studies used in the meta-analysis are listed in Table 11-1 on the opposite page.

Table 11-1: Results of Studies Used in *British Medical Journal* 2002 Meta-analysis[7]

STUDY	PROBIOTIC USED	PERCENT OF PATIENTS WITH DIARRHEA AT END OF STUDY	
		Probiotics Group	Placebo Group
Adam et al.[8]	*Saccharomyces boulardii*	4	17
Goetz et al.[9]	*Lactobacillus acidophilus* and *Lactobacillus bulgaricus*	0	14
Surawicz et al.[10]	*Saccharomyces boulardii*	9	22
Wunderlich et al.[11]	*Enterococcus faecium SF68*	9	27
Tankanow et al.[12]	*Lactobacillus acidophilus* and *Lactobacillus bulgaricus*	66	69
Orrhage et al.[13]	*Lactobacillus acidophilus* and *Bifidobacterium longum*	20	70
McFarland et al.[14]	*Saccharomyces boulardii*	7	15
Lewis et al.[15]	*Saccharomyces boulardii*	21	17
Vanderhoof et al.[16]	*Lactobacillus GG*	7	26

♦ Italian researchers also focused on antibiotic-associated diarrhea in their 2002 meta-analysis of probiotics.[17] When they statistically merged seven placebo-controlled studies involving 881 patients, they were able to conclude that the evidence suggests a "strong benefit" for probiotics in preventing or treating antibiotic-associated diarrhea.

Summing Up the Evidence for Probiotics

Although there have been disappointing results from some studies, there are enough successful randomized, double-blind, placebo-controlled studies to allow us to say that probiotics are a four-star treatment for diarrhea backed by strong evidence.

Available Forms

Probiotics may be found in certain brands of yogurt and other foods. They're also available in capsule, tablet, and powder form.

Amounts of Probiotics Typically Used

There is no standard dose of probiotics, which are measured in viable organisms rather than milligrams or milliliters. Typical supplemental doses may range from 5 billion to 30 billion viable organisms per day.

Possible Side Effects and Interactions

The more common side effects of probiotics include constipation and gas. The risk of interactions with medicines depends on the probiotic. See the possible interactions for *Lactobacillus* and *Saccharomyces boulardii* in this chapter. As with all supplements and drugs, be sure to read the label directions carefully before adding probiotics to your self-care regimen.

Lactobacillus

Rating for Rotaviral Diarrhea: ☆☆☆☆ = Strong Evidence

Rating for Traveler's Diarrhea, Antibiotic-Associated Diarrhea, and Non-Rotaviral Diarrhea: ☆☆☆ = Intriguing Evidence

Lactobacillus is a group of lactic-acid-producing bacteria found in the human gastrointestinal and genitourinary tracts. It helps increase the availability of minerals, stabilize the mucosal barrier of the gastrointestinal tract, and ward off the harmful actions of certain bacteria. Members of this group include *L. acidophilus*, *L. rhamnosus*, and *L. bulgaricus*.

Lactobacillus and Acute Diarrhea in Children

As far back as the 1950s, researchers were speculating that *Lactobacillus* and other friendly bacteria might help prevent or cure diarrhea in children. A few of the more interesting studies follow:

- In 2002 Danish researchers presented the results of their study of 69 children hospitalized due to acute diarrhea.[18] The youngsters were randomly assigned to receive two daily doses of either 10 billion colony-forming units of *Lactobacillus*—a blend of *L. rhamnosus* and *L. reuteri*—or a placebo. (The *Lactobacillus* strains were provided by Chr. Hansen A/S.) At the end of the 5-day treatment period, only 10 percent of those receiving *Lactobacillus* still had loose stools, compared to 33 percent of those taking the placebo. *Lactobacillus* also reduced the duration of diarrhea by 20 percent. The researchers concluded that these two strains of *Lactobacillus* helped ease acute diarrhea in hospitalized children.

Figure 11-1 below compares how long diarrhea and watery diarrhea continued in the *Lactobacillus* and control groups. These results are derived from children who entered the study within 60 hours after the onset of diarrhea.

Figure 11-1: *Lactobacillus* Reduces Duration of Diarrhea

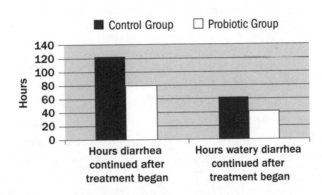

♦ A randomized study released in 2002 looked at the effects of two strains of *Lactobacillus* among children recruited from daycare centers who were suffering from acute diarrhea.[19] The children were assigned to receive either 20 billion colony-forming units of *Lactobacillus* (a mixture of *L. rhamnosus* plus *L. reuteri*, supplied by Chr. Hansen A/S) or a placebo every day for 5 days. The average duration of diarrhea was 76 hours in the *Lactobacillus* group, compared to 116 hours in the placebo group. The positive effects were even more pronounced in the children who received the treatment soon after the diarrhea began. The researchers remarked that this combination of probiotics "was effective in reducing the duration of diarrhea."

♦ A group of Finnish researchers published the results of their study in the *Journal of Pediatric Gastroenterology and Nutrition* in 1997.[20] Forty youngsters ranging in age from 6 months to 3 years who had been hospitalized with acute diarrhea were enrolled in the study. Three-quarters of them had rotavirus, a very common cause of severe diarrhea. The children were randomly assigned to receive from 10 billion to 100 billion colony-forming units of *L. reuteri* per day or a placebo for up to 5 days. By the second day of treatment, only 26 percent of those taking *L. reuteri* were experiencing watery diarrhea, compared to 81 percent of those receiving the placebo. The researchers concluded that "*L. reuteri* is effective as a therapeutic agent in acute rotavirus diarrhea in children."

A number of articles have summarized what we know about *Lactobacillus* and other probiotics for treating acute infectious diarrhea in children.

♦ One of these articles, which appeared in the *Journal of Pediatric Gastroenterology and Nutrition* in 2001,[21] reviewed the published randomized, double-blind, placebo-controlled studies of *Lactobacillus* and other probiotics for diarrhea in children. The researchers concluded that probiotics can be significantly beneficial and that *Lactobacillus* GG (a strain of *L. rhamnosus*) "showed the most consistent effect."

♦ A meta-analysis performed in 2002 by researchers from the University of Washington and Sea Mar Community Health Center in Seattle statistically merged nine existing randomized, double-blind, placebo-controlled studies of the effects of *Lactobacillus* on acute infectious diarrhea in children.[22] This produced a single larger, more powerful study that could provide a more definitive answer than could any of the individual trials. The authors concluded that "*Lactobacillus* is safe and effective as a treatment for children with acute infectious diarrhea." (The results of eight of the nine individual studies included in the meta-analysis are shown in the Table 11-2 on the following page.)

Table 11-2: *Lactobacillus* versus Placebo in the Treatment of Infectious Diarrhea in Children—Results from Individual Studies Used for Meta-analysis[23]

STUDY	NUMBER OF PARTICIPANTS	AVERAGE NUMBER OF DAYS DIARRHEA LASTED	
		Lactobacillus Group	Placebo Group
Simakachorn et al. 2000[24]	73	1.8	2.4
Guandalini et al. 2000[25]	260	2.4	3.0
Shornikova et al. 1997[26]	40	1.7	2.9
Shornikova et al. 1997[27]	46	1.5	2.5
Shornikova et al. 1997[28]	123	2.7	3.8
Kaila et al. 1992[29]	39	1.1	2.5
Pearce et al. 1974[30]	94	2.7	2.1
Chicoine et al. 1973[31]	54	2.5	2.8

Lactobacillus and Prevention of Acute Diarrhea in Adults

Of course, children aren't the only ones who develop diarrhea. Adults also can suffer.

♦ For one study, Israeli researchers tested the efficacy of *Lactobacillus* as a diarrhea preventive in 502 healthy young male military recruits. The men were randomly assigned to receive either 100 milliliters of yogurt containing *L. casei* or a "plain" yogurt without *Lactobacillus* 6 days a week for 8 weeks.[32] The researchers kept track of the incidence and duration of diarrhea for each study participant, and stool samples were checked for bacteria and parasites. The results were mildly positive, with 12.2 percent of the *Lactobacillus* group developing diarrhea, compared to 16.1 percent of the control group. The results were encouraging but not statistically significant.

Lactobacillus and Other Forms of Diarrhea

Lactobacillus also has been tested in people with diarrhea other than the acute infectious type.

♦ *Mild diarrhea*: Italian researchers randomly assigned 100 children brought to physicians for mild diarrhea to receive one of two treatments:

either drinking lots of fluid (a standard treatment) or drinking lots of fluid and taking *L. casei GG*.[33] Sixty-one of the children were infected with rotavirus, 39 were not. The average duration of diarrhea dropped from 6 to 3 days among those taking the *Lactobacillus*, whether or not they were infected with rotavirus. The researchers concluded that "oral administration of *Lactobacillus GG* is effective in rotavirus-positive and rotavirus-negative ambulatory children with diarrhea."

♦ *Antibiotic-associated diarrhea*: Researchers from the Department of Pediatrics at the University of Nebraska tested the effects of *Lactobacillus* in 188 children suffering from antibiotic-associated diarrhea.[34] The children, ranging in age from 6 months to 10 years, were randomly assigned to take daily doses of 10 billion to 20 billion *Lactobacillus GG* colony-forming units (supplied by CAG Functional Foods) or a placebo. The children also received their prescribed antibiotics. This was a double-blind trial, so the researchers, the patients, and their caregivers were unaware of who was receiving which treatment until the end of the study. *Lactobacillus GG* not only significantly reduced the number of bowel movements per day but also gave a firmer consistency to the stool. The researchers concluded that "*Lactobacillus GG* reduces the incidence of antibiotic-associated diarrhea in children treated with oral antibiotics for common childhood infections."

♦ *Antibiotic-associated diarrhea*: Finnish researchers tracked 16 healthy men who voluntarily took the antibiotic erythromycin for 7 days.[35] Half of the men, who ranged in age from 18 to 24, were randomly assigned to receive 250 milliliters of yogurt containing *Lactobacillus GG* per day. The rest received a pasteurized yogurt containing no live bacteria, which served as the placebo. Those taking the *Lactobacillus* developed antibiotic-induced diarrhea for 2 days, on average, compared to 8 days for those taking the placebo. The *Lactobacillus* group also had less antibiotic-related stomach pain and flatulence. The researchers suggested that taking *Lactobacillus GG* orally could help replenish intestinal colonies of helpful bacteria that are destroyed by antibiotics.

♦ *Persistent diarrhea*: For this double-blind, placebo-controlled study published in 2003, 89 children age 6 months to 2 years with persistent diarrhea were randomly assigned to receive pasteurized cow's milk in one of three forms: plain; containing *L. casei* and *L. acidophilus*; or containing the probiotic *S. boulardii*.[36] The children were treated for 5 days. Both *Lactobacillus* and *S. boulardii* significantly reduced the frequency of bowel movements and the duration of diarrhea, leading the researchers to conclude that these probiotics were "useful in the management of persistent diarrhea in children."

Summing Up the Evidence for *Lactobacillus*

Numerous researchers have investigated the effects of *Lactobacillus* on various types of diarrhea in children and adults. Some studies have produced positive results; others, negative results. The confusion is likely due to differences in the causes of diarrhea, the ages and stress levels of the patients, the types and dosages of *Lactobacillus*, and the designs of the studies. Despite these limitations, it's fair to say that:

- For rotaviral diarrhea, *Lactobacillus* is a four-star treatment backed by strong evidence.
- For traveler's diarrhea, antibiotic-associated diarrhea, and nonrotaviral diarrhea, *Lactobacillus* is a three-star treatment backed by intriguing evidence.

Available Forms

Lactobacillus is found in yogurt and other fermented milk products. It also is available in supplement form.

How Much *Lactobacillus* Is Typically Used

There is no standard dose of *Lactobacillus*, which is measured in viable organisms rather than milligrams or milliliters. Typical supplemental doses may range from 5 billion to 30 billion viable organisms per day.

Possible Side Effects and Interactions

Lactobacillus can cause flatulence and increase the risk of infection when taken with drugs that suppress the immune system, such as cyclosporine (Sandimmune). If you're taking any medication, be sure to consult your doctor before adding therapeutic amounts of *Lactobacillus* to your self-care regimen.

Bovine Colostrum

Rating: ☆ ☆ ☆ = Intriguing Evidence

Bovine colostrum is a substance produced by a cow during the first several days after giving birth to a calf. This "early milk" is rich in immune-boosting agents, growth factors, nutrients, and other substances that the newborn calf needs to survive and thrive. After a short while, the cow's colostrum gives way to "mature milk," which has a different composition. In humans, bovine colostrum has been used to strengthen the immune system, repair damage to the nervous system, and slow the aging process.

As far back as the 1950s, researchers theorized that bovine colostrum might be able to fend off infectious diarrhea by transferring "passive immunity" to humans. That is, something in the colostrum could do what patients were unable to do for themselves: destroy the organism that was causing the diarrhea.

A number of studies have tested the theory that bovine colostrum can prevent or treat diarrhea. These studies used either bovine colostrum or hyperimmune bovine colostrum (HBC), which is obtained by immunizing cows with one or more pathogens in order to get antibodies to those pathogens. Some interesting studies include the following:

♦ A 1988 double-blind study published in the *New England Journal of Medicine* looked at the effect of bovine colostrum on diarrhea.[37] Twenty volunteers were divided into two groups. One group was given an HBC preparation containing large amounts of antibodies against *Escherichia coli*, while the other was given a similar bovine colostrum preparation without these antibodies (the placebo). Both groups received treatment for 7 days. On the third day, the researchers deliberately exposed the volunteers to *E. coli*, a bacteria known to cause traveler's diarrhea. While 9 of the 10 taking the placebo preparation developed diarrhea, none of the 10 taking the HBC preparation did. The researchers concluded that hyperimmune bovine colostrum "may be an effective prophylaxis against traveler's diarrhea."

♦ A paper published in the *Journal of Infectious Diseases* in 1998 described what happened when 25 healthy adults participated in a study designed to see whether a hyperimmune bovine colostrum preparation could protect against a deliberate attempt to induce diarrhea.[38] For this randomized, double-blind study, 15 of the participants received HBC, while 10 received a placebo preparation. On the third day of treatment, all of the volunteers were exposed to *E. coli*. Seven of the 10 who were taking the placebo developed diarrhea, compared to only 1 of the 15 who were taking hyperimmune bovine colostrum.

♦ For a randomized, double-blind study published in the *Pediatric Infectious Disease Journal*, Bangladeshi researchers enlisted 80 children suffering from diarrhea caused by rotavirus.[39] The children were assigned to receive either 10 grams of hyperimmune bovine colostrum containing antibodies to rotavirus or a placebo every day for 4 days. Compared to those taking the placebo, those taking the HBC preparation had "significantly less daily and total stool output and stool frequency" and needed less oral rehydration. The researchers concluded that "treatment with antirotavirus immunoglobulin of bovine colostral origin is effective in the management of children with acute rotavirus diarrhea."

Several other studies of AIDS-related diarrhea[40,41,42] and diarrhea caused by rotavirus, *E. coli*, and other infectious microorganisms[43,44,45,46] have produced similar positive results.

Summing Up the Evidence for Bovine Colostrum

Although the research backing bovine colostrum for diarrhea is a little confusing, as several different preparations have been tested on various types of diarrhea, it is fair to say that bovine colostrum is a three-star treatment for diarrhea backed by intriguing evidence.

Available Forms

Bovine colostrum is available in powder and pill form. It has not been standardized, so the composition of various brands may differ significantly, depending on when it was gathered from the cow, what the cow had been eating, whether the cow was exposed to certain illnesses and developed antibodies to them, how the product was processed, and other factors.

How Much Bovine Colostrum Is Typically Used

There is no standard dose of bovine colostrum. Studies have used dosages ranging up to 10 grams per day.

Possible Side Effects and Interactions

Bovine colostrum can cause nausea and vomiting and trigger allergic reactions. It is not known to interact with medicines in a significant manner. As with all supplements and drugs, be sure to read the product label carefully before trying bovine colostrum.

Saccharomyces boulardii

Rating: ☆☆☆ = Intriguing Evidence

Saccharomyces boulardii—often referred to as *S. boulardii*—is a type of yeast widely used in Europe, South America, and other parts of the world as a treatment for diarrhea. *S. boulardii* was originally thought to be a unique yeast species but is now believed to be a strain of baker's yeast (*S. cerevisiae*).

A probiotic agent, *S. boulardii* helps repopulate the gastrointestinal tract with friendly bacteria and aid in the elimination of harmful intestinal organisms. In addition to diarrhea, *S. boulardii* has been used as a treatment for a number of ailments, including irritable bowel syndrome, ulcerative colitis, urinary tract infections, elevated cholesterol, Lyme disease, and fever blisters.

A number of studies have shown that *S. boulardii* can be helpful in preventing or treating different kinds of diarrhea:

- *Infectious diarrhea:* A study published in the *Journal of the American Medical Association* in 1994 tracked adults suffering from *Clostridium difficile*-associated disease.[47] (*C. difficile* is a kind of bacteria that can cause colitis and diarrhea, especially in those taking antibiotics that destroy beneficial bacteria in the intestinal tract.) For this double-blind study, 124 adults were randomly assigned to receive either 1 gram of *S. boulardii* or a placebo every day for 4 weeks, in addition to antibiotics. The recurrence rate of *C. difficile*-associated diarrhea was 34.6 percent in the *S. boulardii* group compared to 64.7 percent in the placebo group.
- *Antibiotic-associated diarrhea:* In 2005 Polish researchers published the results of a study involving 269 children, age 6 months to 14 years, who were undergoing antibiotic therapy.[48] In this double-blind study, the children were randomly assigned to receive either 500 milligrams of

S. boulardii or a placebo every day for as long as they were taking antibiotics. Those who received *S. boulardii* suffered from fewer bouts of diarrhea during antibiotic therapy and for up to 2 weeks afterward. The researchers noted that this was "the first randomized controlled trial evidence that *S. boulardii* effectively reduces the risk of antibiotic-associated diarrhea in children."

♦ *Antibiotic-associated diarrhea in hospitalized patients:* One hundred eighty hospitalized patients participated in a double-blind study testing the ability of *S. boulardii* to prevent antibiotic-associated diarrhea.[49] In addition to their prescribed antibiotics, the volunteers were randomly assigned to receive either 500 milligrams of *S. boulardii* or a placebo every day. Only 9.5 percent of those taking *S. boulardii* developed diarrhea, compared to 22 percent of those taking the placebo. The researchers concluded that "*S. boulardii* reduces the incidence of antibiotic-associated diarrhea in hospitalized patients."

♦ *Acute diarrhea:* Two hundred children suffering from sudden and severe (acute) diarrhea were randomly assigned to receive either 250 milligrams of *S. boulardii* a day or a placebo.[50] Following 5 days of treatment, those taking *S. boulardii* showed a significant drop in the frequency and overall duration of diarrhea. They also were able to leave the hospital sooner than those who were taking the placebo, with an average stay of 2.9 days for the *S. boulardii* group versus 3.9 days for the placebo group.

Summing Up the Evidence for *S. boulardii*

With several randomized, double-blind, placebo-controlled trials—including one published in the very mainstream *Journal of the American Medical Association*—finding that *S. boulardii* can be helpful in preventing or treating several types of diarrhea, it's fair to say that *S. boulardii* is a three-star treatment backed by intriguing evidence.

Other Names

Saccharomyces boulardii is also known as *S. boulardii* and saccharomyces.

Available Forms

S. boulardii is available in capsule form.

How Much S. boulardii Is Typically Used

There is no standard dose of *S. boulardii*. Supplemental doses may range up to 1 gram per day, taken as divided doses.

Possible Side Effects and Interactions

S. boulardii has side effects including flatulence and fungemia (fungi in the blood). It is not known to interact with drugs or increase their side effects in a significant manner. As with all supplements and drugs, be sure to read the product label carefully before trying *S. boulardii* supplements.

Zinc

Rating: ☆☆☆ = Intriguing Evidence

Zinc is an essential mineral that stimulates the activity of more than 100 enzymes in the body. It plays an important part in immune function, wound healing, taste and smell, DNA synthesis, and normal growth and development. Too little zinc can result in delayed sexual maturity, hair loss, poor appetite, diarrhea, impotence, and other problems.

In supplement form, zinc has been used to improve athletic performance and to treat colds, impaired fertility, and acne. A number of studies have locked out zinc's ability to help relieve diarrhea in children:

> ♦ For a 1995 study published in the *New England Journal of Medicine*, researchers from Johns Hopkins University and the All India Institute of Medical Sciences tested the effects of supplemental zinc on the severity and duration of acute diarrhea among children in New Delhi, India.[51] The 937 children participating in the randomized, double-blind, placebo-controlled study ranged in age from 6 months to 35 months and were suffering from acute diarrhea. All of the children received oral rehydration and nutritional supplements that did not contain zinc. In addition, some of the children were given 20 milligrams of elemental zinc. Among those taking the zinc, there was a 39 percent drop in the average number of watery stools per day and a 21 percent drop in the number of days with watery stools. The researchers concluded that "for infants and young children with acute diarrhea, zinc supplementation results in clinically important reductions in the duration and severity of diarrhea."

♦ A 2001 study published in the *British Medical Journal* looked at the effects of zinc supplementation in 685 rural African children.[52] The participants in this randomized, double-blind, placebo-controlled study ranged in age from 6 months to 31 months. For 6 days a week for 6 months, the children were assigned to receive either 12.5 milligrams of zinc sulphate or a placebo. Although the researchers were primarily interested in testing the effects of zinc on malaria and other diseases, they also kept track of episodes of diarrhea. They concluded that "zinc supplementation was significantly associated with a reduced prevalence of diarrhea."

♦ Looking for more definitive answers than any single study could provide, the Zinc Investigators' Collaborative Group prepared a meta-analysis that was published in the *American Journal of Clinical Nutrition* in 2000.[53] For this analysis, the researchers statistically merged seven randomized, controlled studies examining the effects of supplemental zinc on children under age 5 who lived in developing countries and suffered from acute or persistent diarrhea. They found that for acute diarrhea, those taking supplemental zinc had a "15 percent lower probability of continuing diarrhea on a given day." And for persistent diarrhea, those taking zinc had a "24 percent lower probability of continuing diarrhea . . . and a 42 percent lower rate of treatment failure or death." This led the researchers to conclude that taking oral zinc supplements "reduces the duration and severity of acute and persistent diarrhea."

Summing Up the Evidence for Zinc

We don't know exactly how zinc might prevent or treat diarrhea. We do know that even a mild zinc deficiency can weaken the immune system, perhaps allowing bacteria to settle in and cause diarrhea. And once diarrhea has begun, zinc can be lost in the stool, further depleting the body's stores of this vital mineral. If appetite is depleted, less zinc may be taken in from food, leading to a greater risk of deficiency.

Since much of the zinc–diarrhea research has been conducted in countries where many children are malnourished, we may not be able to apply the study results directly and uncritically to well-nourished children in developed countries. Yet given that many children in developed countries may already have marginal zinc deficiencies, and that diarrhea itself can deplete zinc stores even further, it is reasonable to conclude that supplementation with zinc may be helpful. Therefore, based on the available research, we can say that zinc is a three-star treatment for diarrhea backed by intriguing evidence.

Available Forms

Zinc is found in oysters, chicken leg, pork tenderloin, plain yogurt, pecans, cashews, and other foods. It's also available in supplement form.

How Much Zinc Is Typically Used

The Food and Nutrition Board has set the Recommended Dietary Allowances for zinc at 11 milligrams for adult men and 8 milligrams for adult women. Here are the board's recommendations for children:

Age	Daily Recommendation	Tolerable Upper Limit per Day
0–6 months	2 mg	4 mg
7–12 months	3 mg	5 mg
1–3 years	3 mg	7 mg
4–8 years	5 mg	12 mg
9–13 years	8 mg	23 mg
Boys 14–18	11 mg	34 mg
Girls 14–18	9 mg	34 mg
Adult males	11 mg	40 mg
Adult females	8 mg	40 mg

Some studies have produced good results using 20 milligrams of elemental zinc per day.

Possible Side Effects and Interactions

Taking excessive amounts of zinc can lower the levels of "good" HDL cholesterol and weaken the immune system. In addition, zinc may hamper the absorption of antibiotics such as ciprofloxacin (Cipro), reducing levels of the drug in the body. If you're taking any medication, be sure to consult your doctor before adding therapeutic amounts of zinc to your self-care regimen.

Guar Gum

Rating: ☆☆ = Modest Evidence

The guar bean, which grows primarily in India and Pakistan, contains a soluble dietary fiber in its seed called guar gum. When mixed with water, guar gum forms a gel. Used in food manufacturing as a stabilizer in ice cream, cheese, and other food products, guar gum has nearly eight times the thickening power of cornstarch. This property also may prove useful for treating diarrhea. Like blond psyllium, guar gum soaks up excess liquid in the intestines, helping to solidify the feces and slow transit time.

A small body of research suggests that guar gum may indeed be helpful for treating diarrhea:

♦ A 2005 study published in the *Archives of Disease in Childhood* looked at the effect of a particular brand of guar gum on persistent diarrhea in young children.[54] The 116 children, ranging in age from 5 months to 24 months, entered the hospital suffering from watery diarrhea that had lasted more than 2 weeks. They were randomly assigned to receive either a chicken diet plus guar gum (Benefiber) or a chicken diet without guar gum. Diarrhea was relieved in 84 percent of those who were receiving guar gum, compared to only 62 percent of those who were not receiving guar gum.

♦ Belgian researchers investigated the use of guar gum in patients with severe sepsis (an infection that enters the bloodstream, causing low blood pressure, organ failure, and other problems) or septic shock (low blood pressure and low bloodflow caused by an overwhelming infection).[55] Such patients are at risk for developing diarrhea, a risk made greater when they are tube-fed. For this double-blind, placebo-controlled study, 25 patients were randomly assigned to receive either a standard tube-feeding solution or the solution plus guar gum (Benefiber, 22 grams per liter of solution) for a minimum of 6 days. Compared to the placebo group, the guar gum group experienced significantly fewer days during which diarrhea occurred.

♦ Similar results were obtained by a team of Egyptian and Swiss researchers who published the results of their double-blind study in *Clinical Nutrition* in 2004.[56] The participants were 20 adult volunteers who were receiving tube feeding and who had persistent diarrhea. Some were randomly assigned to receive guar gum (Benefiber, 2 percent of the feeding solution) in addition to their tube feeding for 4 days. Among those receiving the guar gum, the number of liquid stools fell from two per day on the first day to one per day on the fourth day. But among those who did not get the guar gum, the number of liquid stools rose from 1.2 on the first day to 2.1 on the fourth day.

Summing Up the Evidence for Guar Gum

The positive results from the modest number of double-blind studies point to the conclusion that guar gum is a two-star treatment for diarrhea based on modest evidence.

Other Names

Guar gum is known scientifically as *Cyamopsis tetragonoloba* and in various cultures as aconite bean, Calcutta lucerne, guar, Indian cluster bean, Indian guar plant, and jaguar gum.

Available Forms

Guar gum is available in powder, tablet, and granule form.

How Much Guar Gum Is Typically Used

There is no standard dose of guar gum. Doses of up to 15 grams a day (5 grams three times a day) have been used.

Possible Side Effects and Interactions

Among guar gum's possible side effects are nausea, dizziness, and sweating. If taken with inadequate amounts of fluid, it can cause obstruction of the esophagus or bowel.

Guar gum may interact with diabetes drugs such as tolazamide (Tolinase), causing blood sugar to drop too low. It also may hamper the absorption of drugs taken orally. If you're taking any medication, be sure to consult your doctor before adding guar gum to your self-care regimen.

Homeopathy

Rating: ☆☆ = Modest Evidence

The core principle of homeopathy is "like cures like." A homeopathic remedy contains a miniscule amount of a substance that, in larger doses, would cause the very disease that it's intended to treat. For example, if a person has a rash, giving him or her a highly diluted solution of substances that would cause a rash in larger doses may strengthen the body's natural defenses and make the rash disappear. It's somewhat akin to a vaccine, which stimulates the immune system to mount a defense against a certain enemy by presenting it with a weakened or dead version of that enemy.

Homeopathic treatment is highly individualized and can vary considerably from person to person. That said, some studies have found the homeopathic approach to be effective against diarrhea:

♦ A 1994 study presented in *Pediatrics* examined the use of homeopathic remedies for acute childhood diarrhea.[57] For this double-blind trial, 81 children ranging in age from 6 months to 5 years were randomly divided into two groups. Each child was examined by a homeopathic physician, and the child's individual characteristics (i.e., the amount and characteristics of the stool, the presence of vomiting or abdominal pain, the child's appetite and thirst) were noted and entered into a computer program that selected a specific homeopathic medicine. All children received standard rehydration therapy; then some were randomly selected to receive a personalized homeopathic medicine, while others received a placebo medicine. Those in the homeopathy group showed a statistically significant decrease in the duration of diarrhea (the number of days it lasted) as well as a statistically significant drop in the number of stools per day after 72 hours of treatment. The researchers concluded that "homeopathic [remedies] may be beneficial in the treatment of acute childhood diarrhea."

♦ In 2000 several of the researchers from the University of Washington in Seattle who worked on the 1994 study attempted to duplicate their results among children in Kathmandu, Nepal.[58] These researchers enlisted 126 children, ranging in age from 6 months to 5 years, who had passed more than three unformed stools during the 24 hours prior to joining the study. The children were randomly assigned to receive an individually selected homeopathic medicine or a placebo, which they were to take after every episode of diarrhea for the next 5 days. One hundred sixteen children completed the study, during which all were rehydrated. The children taking the homeopathic medicine produced an average of 3.2 stools per day over the 5-day treatment period, compared to 4.5 per day among those receiving only the placebo. The researchers concluded that the results were consistent with those of the previous study and that "homeopathic treatment decreases the duration of diarrhea and the number of stools in children with acute childhood diarrhea."

♦ Several members of the team that conducted the two previous studies joined forces to prepare a meta-analysis examining the effects of homeopathy on acute childhood diarrhea.[59] Three double-blind studies previously conducted were statistically merged to produce a single larger, more powerful study. This study looked at 242 children with acute diarrhea, ranging in age from 6 months to 5 years. All of the children received rehydration and were randomly assigned to receive either individualized homeopathic treatment or a placebo. The children in the homeopathy group experienced 3.3 days of diarrhea, on average, compared to 4.1 days for those in the placebo group. The researchers concluded that "individualized homeopathic treatment decreases the duration of acute childhood diarrhea."

Summing Up the Evidence for Homeopathy

Evaluating the effectiveness of homeopathic treatment is difficult because the treatment is, by design, very individualized. It's virtually impossible to say that a particular homeopathic medicine works or doesn't work, or that one homeopathic medicine is superior to another. In this case, the circumstances are further complicated by the fact that the same three researchers participated in both studies as well as in the meta-analysis. A body of evidence collected by disparate teams of researchers with different backgrounds and inclinations is considered superior to a body of evidence collected by the same group of people working together again and again.

With these caveats in mind, it is fair to say that homeopathy is a two-star treatment for diarrhea based on modest evidence.

Finding a Homeopathic Physician

For more information on homeopathy, or to find a qualified homeopathic practitioner, visit the National Center for Homeopathy Web site: www.homeopathic.org.

ALTERNATIVE APPROACHES TO

FIBROMYALGIA

Acupuncture ☆☆☆☆
Baths ☆☆
Physical manipulation ☆☆

Fibromyalgia literally means pain in the body's fibrous tissues—the muscles, tendons, and ligaments. It involves a cluster of symptoms (which is why it's sometimes referred to as fibromyalgia syndrome), the most notable of which is a severe aching and stiffness in the muscles that is often worse in the morning. The pain settles in at least 11 of 18 specific points on the body, called tender points.

Another symptom is fatigue; up to 90 percent of those with fibromyalgia experience a bone-deep fatigue that leaves them totally drained of energy. Unfortunately, the sleep that they so desperately need tends to elude them, as sleep disturbances afflict almost all fibromyalgia sufferers.

Not surprisingly, many who have fibromyalgia find themselves depressed, with 25 percent hit hard enough to be diagnosed as clinically depressed and in need of psychological care. Another distressing symptom of fibromyalgia is "fibro fog"—a combination of mental confusion, memory lapses, poor concentration, and word mix-ups. Other symptoms that can affect those with fibromyalgia include anxiety, constipation, diarrhea, chronic headaches, numbness and tingling in the arms and legs, restless leg syndrome, and temporomandibular disorder.

Although fibromyalgia is a chronic condition, its symptoms tend to come and go. Flare-ups can be aggravated by allergies, hormonal fluctuations, infections, stress, anxiety, depression, lack of sleep, cold environments, and weather changes.

CAUSES

Perhaps the most frustrating aspect of fibromyalgia is that no one knows what causes it. Many researchers believe that fibromyalgia is the result of some abnormality in physiology that's set off by exposure to a triggering event such as a viral or bacterial infection, an injury, or the onset of another disease such as lupus or rheumatoid arthritis. The underlying physiological abnormality could be a faulty immune system, hormonal irregularities, changes in the levels of substances that transmit pain signals, or the body's response to stress.

STANDARD TREATMENTS

The standard treatments for fibromyalgia syndrome include medicines to quell the pain (such as analgesics and nonsteroidal anti-inflammatory drugs) as well as medications to improve sleep and ease depression, anxiety, and other symptoms as they arise. For more severe pain, local anesthetics or cortisone injections may be prescribed. While all of these medicines help to a certain degree, they don't correct the underlying problem(s) and must be taken indefinitely. Cognitive behavioral therapy and other forms of counseling may be used to ease psychological symptoms and to help patients go on with their day-to-day routines.

RATING POPULAR ALTERNATIVE TREATMENTS FOR FIBROMYALGIA

Acupuncture
Rating: ☆ ☆ ☆ ☆ = Strong Evidence

Acupuncture is an ancient Chinese discipline that treats disease by balancing the flow of energy in the body. It's based on the idea that everyone is born with a certain amount of energy, which moves through the body along tiny invisible channels called meridians. If any of these meridians becomes blocked, the flow of energy slows or stops and the body becomes ill. In acupuncture, needles unblock the meridians and let the energy move freely again, allowing the body to heal itself.

A small number of studies have indicated that acupuncture can be helpful in relieving symptoms of fibromyalgia. For example:

♦ For a double-blind study published in the *British Medical Journal* in 1992, 70 patients with fibromyalgia were randomly assigned to receive either six sessions of electroacupuncture (stimulation of traditional acupuncture points with a mild electrical current) or six sham procedures (serving as the control treatment) over the course of 3 weeks.[1] The researchers tracked eight factors—such as changes in pain threshold, quality of sleep, and the number of pain pills taken—to see if the treatment was helping. Among those receiving electroacupuncture, there was "a significant improvement" in seven of eight measures compared to zero of eight among those receiving sham acupuncture. The researchers concluded that "electroacupuncture is effective in relieving symptoms of fibromyalgia."

♦ For their 2000 open study, Swiss researchers used acupuncture to treat 20 fibromyalgia patients, with the treatments being tailored to each patient's needs.[2] The average number of tender points fell from 16.1 to 13.8, and the patients were better able to tolerate pain in 10 of 12 of their tender points. The researchers concluded that "acupuncture is a useful method to treat patients with fibromyalgia."

♦ A 1998 study discussed in *Rheumatology International* tested the effects of acupuncture in 29 men and women—average age 48, all suffering from fibromyalgia.[3] Pain levels and positive tender points were tracked using the visual analogue scale (VAS). The average VAS score, which was 64.0 at the beginning of the study, fell to 34.5 after acupuncture treatment.

Summing Up the Evidence for Acupuncture

Although these and many other acupuncture/fibromyalgia studies have produced positive results, a large number of studies have produced equivocal or negative results. And many of the studies have been criticized for looking at small numbers of participants and for weaknesses in the study protocols.

In its 1997 consensus statement on acupuncture, the National Institutes of Health took note of these limitations but concluded that "acupuncture may be useful as an adjunct treatment or an acceptable alternative to be included in a comprehensive management program" for fibromyalgia. In addition, the World Health Organization has noted that acupuncture has a therapeutic effect on symptoms of fibromyalgia, although it cautions that further proof is necessary.[4]

The debate over the efficacy of acupuncture will undoubtedly continue for many years. Nevertheless, because of the recommendation from the World Health Organization, it is fair to say that acupuncture is a four-star treatment for fibromyalgia based on strong evidence.

Possible Side Effects

When properly administered, acupuncture usually produces no side effects. In rare cases, there may be slight bruising or a small amount of bleeding where the needles are inserted, or some dizziness.

Finding an Acupuncturist

For more information about acupuncture, or for help in finding a certified acupuncturist, visit the Web site for the National Certification Commission for Acupuncture and Oriental Medicine (NCCAOM): www.ncaom.org. The commission is the acupuncture profession's equivalent of the American Medical Association.

Baths

Rating: ☆☆ = Modest Evidence

Balneotherapy is a fancy word for bath therapy—that is, the use of hot water or mineral water baths to relieve symptoms of various ailments. Herbs and essential oils may be added to the bathwater to enhance its therapeutic effects. Although popular in Europe and Japan, balneotherapy has not received much attention from the medical community in the United States.

Most people with fibromyalgia love the idea of soaking in a nice hot bath, with good reason. Some studies suggest that bath therapy can reduce pain while enhancing the sense of well-being. Here is one example:

♦ For a study presented in the journal *Rheumatology International*, volunteers between ages 30 and 55 and suffering from fibromyalgia were randomly assigned to either engage in 3 weeks of mineral bath therapy or continue with their normal daily activities.[5] Those in the bath therapy group soaked for 20 minutes five times a week under the direction of a physiotherapist. At the end of the 3 weeks, these people showed a statistically significant drop in the number of tender points and depression. And here is the really interesting part: Six months after treatment, they still showed improvement in the number of tender points as well as a reduction in the negative impact of fibromyalgia on their lives. The researchers concluded that bath therapy "is effective and may be an alternative method in treating fibromyalgia patients."

Summing Up the Evidence for Baths

It's not clear why hot-water or mineral-water baths help relieve fibromyalgia symptoms. It may be that immersion in hot water itself is beneficial, aiding in relaxation and the relief of stress and tension. It may have something to do with the magnesium, calcium, and potassium typically used for mineral baths. Perhaps the herbs and essential oils that are sometimes added to the bathwater have an aromatherapeutic effect. Or it may simply be a powerful placebo effect.

Whatever the reason, bath therapy does seem to relieve some fibromyalgia symptoms. It is reasonable to conclude that baths are a two-star treatment for fibromyalgia based on modest evidence.

Finding a Balneotherapist

The best way to find a qualified balneotherapist is to ask your physician for a recommendation to a health professional with expertise and experience in bath therapy.

Physical Manipulation

Rating: ☆☆ = Modest Evidence

Physical manipulation—therapies such as chiropractic and osteopathic manipulation—have been proposed as a means of reducing some fibromyalgia symptoms.

Chiropractic is based on the principle that a properly aligned spine is the key to good health. The spine connects the brain to the body, and major nerves run along the spinal column. Any upset in the spine will automatically harm the body. By using chiropractic techniques to manipulate the spine, it should return to its proper position, allowing the body to heal itself.

The basic idea behind osteopathic manipulation, or osteopathy, is that physical or emotional stress results in misalignment not only of the spine but also of the muscles and bones. This misalignment interferes with blood circulation and nerve pathways, causing pain. The solution, according to osteopaths, is to realign both bones and muscles, which allows the body to heal itself. Doctors of Osteopathy (DOs) undergo training that is almost identical to that of medical doctors (MDs), and they are licensed to perform surgery and write prescriptions. However, DOs are taught to place more emphasis on the body's innate healing capacity.

Some studies suggest that both chiropractic and osteopathic manipulation can help with fibromyalgia symptoms. For example:

♦ For a randomized, crossover study published in the *Journal of Manipulative and Physiological Therapeutics* in 1997, researchers tested the effects of manipulative therapies in 21 fibromyalgia patients, ranging in age from 25 to 70.[6] The patients were divided into two groups, and all continued taking their medicines for the duration of the study. For the first 4-week period, some of the patients were assigned to receive chiropractic spinal manipulation, soft tissue therapy, and passive stretching. The rest received no manipulative therapies during this time and served as controls. During the second 4-week period, the control patients also received manipulative therapy. The chiropractic treatment improved the range of motion in the patients' backs and lowered their pain levels. According to the researchers, their study showed that chiropractic spinal manipulation "may be beneficial in the treatment of fibromyalgia patients, specifically in improving their range of motion, general flexibility, and reported pain levels."

♦ A 2000 study presented in the *Journal of Manipulative and Physiological Therapeutics* looked at the effects of chiropractic treatment on fibromyalgia.[7] Fifteen women, with an average age of 51, received a course of 30 treatments, each session including pressure on tender points and spinal manipulative therapy. Sixty percent of the women responded well, experiencing reductions in both pain intensity and fatigue, plus an improvement in sleep quality. Among those who responded to treatment, pain intensity scores fell by an average of 77.2 percent, sleep quality scores improved by 63.5 percent, and the fatigue level score dropped by 74.8 percent. The benefits of chiropractic manipulation were still apparent 1 month after the conclusion of treatment.

♦ Osteopathic manipulation was used in a 2002 study of 24 women suffering from fibromyalgia.[8] The volunteers were randomly assigned to receive one of four treatments: (1) individualized osteopathic manipulation; (2) individualized osteopathic manipulation plus education about self-treatment of tender points; (3) moist heat; or (4) no treatment. All of the volunteers continued to take their standard medicines. Those receiving osteopathic manipulation (with or without education) demonstrated superior results on "measures of pain threshold, perceived pain, . . . activities of daily living, and perceived functional ability."

Summing Up the Evidence for Physical Manipulation

With only a relatively small body of published evidence to draw upon, it is reasonable to say that physical manipulation is a two-star treatment for fibromyalgia based on modest evidence.

Finding a Practitioner

To learn more about chiropractic or to find a qualified chiropractor, visit the Web site for the American Chiropractic Association at www.amerchiro.org. The Web site for the American Osteopathic Association, www.osteopathic. org, also has a feature that allows you to search for DOs in your area.

13

ALTERNATIVE APPROACHES TO
HIGH BLOOD PRESSURE

Calcium	☆☆☆☆
Coenzyme Q_{10}	☆☆☆☆
Garlic	☆☆☆☆
Magnesium	☆☆☆☆
Omega-3 fatty acids	☆☆☆☆
Acupuncture	☆☆
Olive oil	☆☆

Hypertension is another word for high blood pressure, or a dangerous amount of force exerted by blood against the insides of arteries. The arteries carry blood away from the heart, bearing the brunt of the pressure exerted by the blood with each heartbeat. The arteries have tough, muscular, elastic walls that relax and widen as the blood pulses through, then become slightly narrower between heartbeats. Blood pressure is determined by the force of the blood as the heart pumps, multiplied by the amount of resistance that the arteries provide.

Blood pressure can rise for one of two reasons. Either the heart is working hard, causing an increase in the strength or rate of its pumping action and a corresponding increase in blood pressure, or the walls of the arteries have become narrow, stiff, or clogged with plaque, so the heart must pump hard to force blood through.

Hypertension is a serious condition that erodes artery linings, encouraging the build-up of plaque (a condition called *atherosclerosis*), and makes the arteries less resilient. Left untreated, hypertension can lead to heart disease, heart failure, aneurysm, stroke, kidney damage, retinal damage, and a shortened life expectancy.

SYMPTOMS

Hypertension affects some 50 million people in the United States, although fewer than 14 million have it under control. This is probably because hypertension is so easy to ignore: It has no obvious symptoms, at least in its early stages. As it becomes more severe, it may cause headaches, blurred vision, dizziness, blackouts, and nosebleeds, among other symptoms.

CAUSES

No one knows what brings on most cases of hypertension, although genetics are a likely contributor. Certain factors can hasten development of the condition or make it worse. They include overweight, lack of exercise, poor diet, stress, smoking, alcohol abuse, various hormones, and certain drugs. A small percentage of hypertension cases are the result of other conditions such as kidney disease, vascular tumors, thyroid disease, narrowing of the aorta, sleep apnea, or hyperparathyroidism.

STANDARD TREATMENTS

Since hypertension cannot be cured, the standard treatments are designed to keep it under control. First-line approaches include losing weight, lowering sodium intake, engaging in moderate aerobic exercise, refraining

UNDERSTANDING THE BLOOD PRESSURE NUMBERS

The only way to know for sure if you have hypertension is through a blood pressure screening. The reading consists of two numbers. The first or top number, called *systolic pressure*, measures the pressure inside your arteries as your heart is contracting. The second or bottom number, *diastolic pressure*, reflects the pressure inside your arteries when your heart is at rest.

According to the latest guidelines, normal blood pressure should be less than 120/80 mm Hg (millimeters of mercury). You have pre-hypertension if your systolic pressure is between 120 and 139, or your diastolic pressure is 80 between 89. You have significant hypertension if your systolic pressure is above 139 or your diastolic is above 89.

from smoking, and reducing excessive alcohol consumption. If blood pressure remains elevated, antihypertensive medications may be prescribed. Among these are diuretics and ACE inhibitors, which reduce blood volume; alpha-1 blockers, which reduce arterial resistance; beta-blockers, which slow the heart rate; and calcium-channel blockers, which relax arterial walls.

RATING POPULAR ALTERNATIVE TREATMENTS FOR HYPERTENSION

Calcium

Rating: ☆ ☆ ☆ ☆ = Strong Evidence

Although best known for building strong bones, the mineral calcium has many important functions in the body. It assists in wound healing, blood clotting, cellular metabolism, and muscle contraction. For these reasons, the body must maintain a certain amount of calcium in the blood and will withdraw calcium from bones to make up any deficit if blood levels begin to drop. A lack of dietary calcium can cause thinning of the bones, pain, and spastic muscle contractions.

A number of studies have examined whether calcium could help lower blood pressure. For example:

◆ For one study, researchers used data from the Tromsø Study to explore a possible link between calcium intake from dairy products and blood pressure.[1] This large-scale population study tracked the health and habits of thousands of men and women living in Tromsø, Norway. Analysis of the questionnaires and blood pressure readings revealed "a significant linear decrease in systolic and diastolic blood pressure with increasing dairy calcium intake in both sexes." In other words, the more calcium in the diet, the lower the blood pressure. Although the calcium-driven drop in blood pressure was small (only 1 to 3 mm Hg), the researchers noted that "calcium could have a significant effect on primary prevention of cardiovascular disease."

◆ A 1998 study published in the *American Journal of Clinical Nutrition* looked at the effects of supplemental calcium in African-American adolescents.[2] One hundred sixteen boys and girls, with an average age of 15.8 years, were randomly assigned to receive either 1,500 milligrams of elemental calcium or a placebo every day for 8 weeks. This double-blind, placebo-controlled trial had a crossover design, so those who took the calcium switched to the placebo for an additional 8 weeks, and vice versa. The results were positive, with calcium supplementation reducing diastolic blood pressure by an average of 1.9 mm Hg. The reduction was greatest in those who had begun the study with the lowest dietary calcium intakes. Although the magnitude of the blood pressure reduction was modest, the researchers concluded that "calcium supplementation may lower diastolic blood pressure in African-American adolescents with low dietary intakes of calcium."

◆ Chinese researchers looked at the effects of calcium supplements among a population in which dietary calcium intake is often low.[3] Ninety-eight adults, ranging in age from 30 to 64, participated in this double-blind study. They were randomly assigned to receive either 800 milligrams of calcium or a placebo daily for 5 weeks. Among those taking calcium, systolic pressure fell by an average of 4.7 mm Hg, and diastolic pressure by 2.7 mm Hg. The researchers concluded that calcium supplementation could be beneficial in areas where sodium intake is high, calcium intake is low, and hypertension is common.

◆ Several review studies and meta-analyses have concluded that calcium can help lower elevated blood pressure. To cite one example, a 1999 meta-analysis published in the *American Journal of Hypertension* pooled the results of 42 randomized clinical trials to find that calcium supplementation could reduce systolic blood pressure by 1.44 mm Hg and diastolic pressure by 0.84 mm Hg.[4] The researchers concluded that "calcium supplementation leads to a small reduction in systolic and diastolic blood pressure."

Summing Up the Evidence for Calcium

The weight of scientific evidence suggests that calcium can produce a small drop in elevated blood pressure, especially in those who are calcium deficient. It is fair to conclude that calcium is a four-star treatment for elevated blood pressure backed by strong evidence.

Available Forms

Among the food sources of calcium are dairy products, canned salmon or sardines (with bones), dried figs, smoked oysters, spinach, tofu, broccoli, almonds, and papaya.

Calcium is also available in supplements, often in the form of calcium carbonate or calcium citrate. Calcium carbonate costs less than calcium citrate, and it concentrates more calcium per pill. However, calcium citrate is less constipating than calcium carbonate, and according to some studies, it is better absorbed.

How Much Calcium Is Typically Used

There is no set dosage of calcium for treating hypertension. Studies have used dosages of up to 2,000 milligrams per day.

Possible Side Effects and Interactions

The Food and Nutrition Board of the Institute of Medicine has set a tolerable upper intake for calcium of 2,500 milligrams per day for adults. Taking more than this can lead to kidney damage. Calcium supplements also may cause belching, gastrointestinal irritation, and constipation.

It's interesting to note that calcium may interfere with the actions of medicines to control elevated blood pressure and angina, such as nisoldipine (Sular) and diltiazem (Cardizem). It also may reduce the effectiveness of aspirin and other pain relievers. If you're taking any medication, be sure to consult your doctor before adding therapeutic amounts of calcium to your self-care regimen.

Coenzyme Q_{10}

Rating: ☆☆☆☆ = Strong Evidence

Coenzyme Q_{10} is an enzyme that's found throughout the body as well as in many foods. Called CoQ_{10} for short, it helps lower total cholesterol and "bad" LDL cholesterol, inhibit the conversion of LDL to its more dangerous oxidized form, improve the flow of oxygen to the heart muscle, and assist the body in generating energy. It also may help keep blood pressure at normal levels, which is vitally important since elevated blood pressure is a major risk factor for cardiovascular disease. In Europe and Japan, CoQ_{10} is given to millions of people as a treatment for high blood pressure, angina, and congestive heart failure, among other ailments.

A fair number of studies have tested the effects of CoQ_{10} on blood pressure. For example:

♦ A 2001 study published in the *Southern Medical Journal* looked at the effects of CoQ_{10} on elevated blood pressure in adults.[5] Eighty men and women, most of whom had systolic hypertension, participated in this double-blind study. The volunteers were randomly assigned to receive either 120 milligrams of CoQ_{10} (brand name Q-Gel) per day or a placebo. Among those taking CoQ_{10}, systolic pressure fell by an average of 17.8 mm Hg. Diastolic blood pressure was not affected. The researchers concluded that CoQ_{10} "may be safely offered to hypertensive patients as an alternative treatment option."

♦ Another study of the effects of CoQ_{10} on hypertension was published in the *Journal of Human Hypertension* in 1999.[6] The 59 adult volunteers in this double-blind study had been taking medicines for elevated blood pressure for more than a year and also were suffering from coronary artery disease. They were randomly divided into two groups, one of which took 120 milligrams of CoQ_{10} (Q-Gel) per day, the other a B-complex vitamin daily. Everyone continued with their standard medication for the duration of the study. In the CoQ_{10} group, the average systolic pressure fell from 168 to 152 mm Hg and the average diastolic pressure from 106 to 97 mm Hg. Compared to the placebo group, blood sugar and blood fat levels fell significantly in the CoQ_{10} group, while "good" HDL cholesterol rose significantly. The researchers concluded that treating people who have elevated blood pressure and coronary artery disease with 120 milligrams of CoQ_{10} per day "may be associated with a significant reduction in systolic and diastolic blood pressure."

♦ Seventy-four people with type 2 diabetes participated in a double-blind, placebo-controlled study published in the *European Journal of Clinical Nutrition* in 2002.[7] The volunteers were randomly assigned to one of four groups for 12 weeks of daily treatment. The groups received 200 milligrams of CoQ_{10} (brand name CoQ); the cholesterol and blood-fat-lowering drug fenofibrate (Lofibra); both; or neither. The CoQ_{10} regimen significantly lowered systolic pressure by 6.1 mm Hg and diastolic pressure by 2.9 mm Hg. The researchers concluded that supplementation with CoQ_{10} "may improve blood pressure" in people with type 2 diabetes.

♦ Researchers from the Institute for Biomedical Research at the University of Texas, Austin, studied 109 people with hypertension. All the participants were given an average daily dose of 225 milligrams of CoQ_{10}, while they continued taking their medicines. The researchers noted a "definite and gradual improvement" during the first 6 months of the study, with many patients able to reduce the amount of drug therapy they needed. After the initial 6-month period, blood pressure and drug requirements stabilized, with the patients enjoying "significantly improved systolic and diastolic blood pressure." Notably, 51 percent of patients were able to stop using up to three of their standard antihypertensive drugs after 4½ months on CoQ_{10}.

♦ Australian researchers examined the medical literature for their 2003 review, published in *Biofactors*.[8] In the eight studies that qualified for review, systolic pressure fell by an average of 16 mm Hg and diastolic pressure by 10 mm Hg. The researchers concluded that "being devoid of significant side effects, CoQ_{10} may have a role as an adjunct or alternative to conventional agents in the treatment of hypertension."

Summing Up the Evidence for Coenzyme Q_{10}

In general, studies show that a dose of 100 to 225 milligrams of CoQ_{10} per day triggers a significant and consistent reduction in blood pressure, with systolic pressure falling by an average of 15 points and diastolic pressure by an average of 10 points. People with hypertension who, at the outset, have the lowest levels of CoQ_{10} in the bloodstream seem to respond best when taking this supplement. It is worth noting that CoQ_{10} often works so well that about half of those who take it can reduce or even eliminate their blood pressure medications.

CoQ_{10} has been used to relieve the main symptom of angina—chest pain that is caused by narrowing of the coronary arteries, which places a strain on the heart. When volunteers were given either CoQ_{10} or a placebo for a month, those who took the CoQ_{10} had 53 percent fewer episodes of angina and were able to exercise longer on a treadmill.

CoQ_{10} has been studied extensively in this country and abroad. It is fair to say that CoQ_{10} is a four-star treatment for elevated blood pressure backed by strong evidence.

Available Forms

The body manufactures its own CoQ_{10}. You can get additional amounts of this heart-healthy enzyme from supplements as well as from a variety of foods, including beef, chicken, trout, salmon, oranges, and broccoli. Unfortunately, levels of CoQ_{10} may run low in those who take Lipitor or other statin drugs to combat elevated blood fats and cholesterol, since these drugs interfere with the body's production of the enzyme.

How Much Coenzyme Q_{10} Is Typically Used

There is no standard dose of CoQ_{10}. Supplemental doses for hypertension may range from 60 to 300 milligrams per day.

Possible Side Effects and Interactions

In various studies, people have taken dosages of CoQ_{10} from 300 milligrams per day for a year to 100 milligrams per day for up to 6 years, with no serious adverse effects other than an occasional case of stomach upset.

Because CoQ_{10} can lower blood pressure, it may adversely interact with blood pressure medicines such as atenolol (Tenormin). If you're taking any medication, be sure to consult your doctor before adding CoQ_{10} to your self-care regimen.

Garlic

Rating: ☆☆☆☆ = Strong Evidence

Garlic, the off-white bulb with the papery skin that is also known as the "stinking rose," has been used for thousands of years as a food and a medicine. Studies have shown that garlic not only has powerful antibiotic properties but also can help treat high cholesterol and blood fats, arthritis, diarrhea, and colds, among many other ailments.

Garlic's therapeutic benefits may even extend to blood pressure, as the following studies suggest.

+ German researchers enlisted 47 men with mild hypertension for their double-blind study, which was published in 1990.[9] All of the volunteers had systolic blood pressure ranging from 95 to 104 mm Hg. They were randomly assigned to receive either 600 milligrams of garlic powder (Kwai) or a placebo every day for 12 weeks. The results were positive, as shown by comparisons of before and after supine (lying down) blood pressure readings. The average diastolic pressure fell by 13 percent and the average systolic pressure by 11 percent among those taking garlic, compared to 4 percent and 5 percent among those taking the placebo. The researchers concluded that this garlic preparation produced "statistically significant reductions in blood pressure."

+ Forty-one men with moderately elevated cholesterol participated in a double-blind, crossover study comparing the effects of aged garlic extract to placebo.[10] The volunteers were randomly assigned to receive either 7.2 grams of aged garlic extract (Kyolic AGE) or a placebo every day for 6 months. Then they switched to the other treatment for an additional 4 months. The garlic extract produced a 5.5 percent reduction in systolic blood pressure, leading the researchers to conclude that "blood pressure is beneficially affected by garlic administration."

Summing Up the Evidence for Garlic

Although there are negative studies, there are enough positive studies to have convinced Germany's Commission E to approve the use of garlic as a treatment for elevated blood pressure. Thus, it is fair to say that garlic is a four-star treatment for elevated blood pressure backed by strong evidence.

Available Forms

You can find garlic in supermarkets as raw cloves, bottled chopped garlic, or garlic powder. A single raw clove equals about 3 grams of garlic. It is also available in capsule, extract, oil, and syrup form.

How Much Garlic Is Typically Used

There is no standard dose of garlic for hypertension. Typical supplemental doses may range from 600 to 1,200 milligrams of extract or 300 milligrams of powder per day.

Possible Side Effects and Interactions

Therapeutic amounts of garlic may cause dizziness, headache, irritation of the gastrointestinal tract, thinning of the blood, and prolonged bleeding time. When combined with blood pressure medications such as benazepril (Lotensin), garlic may cause blood pressure to drop too low. It also may interact with antidiabetes drugs such as glipizide (Glucotrol), raising the risk of low blood sugar. If you're taking any medication, be sure to consult your doctor before adding therapeutic amounts of garlic to your self-care regimen.

Magnesium

Rating: ☆☆☆☆ = Strong Evidence

The fourth most abundant mineral in the body, magnesium plays a role in more than 300 biochemical reactions. This essential mineral is necessary to maintain a normal heart rhythm, manufacture fats and proteins, build and maintain strong bones and teeth, produce energy, and ensure the proper function of nerves and muscles.

Magnesium also appears to be important in regulating blood pressure. A number of observational studies have linked a diet rich in magnesium, potassium, and other minerals to a reduced risk of developing hypertension. Some researchers have zeroed in on the effects of magnesium supplementation in people with elevated blood pressure. Among the relevant studies:

- Swedish researchers conducted a double-blind, crossover study involving 17 patients with elevated diastolic blood pressure.[11] Each day for 9 weeks, the volunteers took magnesium (brand name Emgesan) in doses starting at 15 mmol (375 milligrams) and increasing to 40 mmol (600 milligrams), or a placebo. The results were positive, with magnesium producing a significant decrease in average systolic pressure from 154 mm Hg to 146 mm Hg and in average diastolic pressure from 100 mm Hg to 92 mm Hg.
- A 1996 study published in the *International Journal of Cardiology* examined the effects of magnesium on 15 men and women ranging in age from 36 to 65.[12] All of the volunteers in this randomized, double-blind, crossover study had been diagnosed with mild to moderate hypertension. They were given either 600 milligrams of magnesium or a placebo every day for 6 weeks. Magnesium supplementation reduced average systolic

pressure by 7.6 mm Hg and average diastolic pressure by 3.8 mm Hg. The researchers noted that while the mineral worked well for some patients, it did not help others.

♦ A 1999 report published in the *Annals of Epidemiology* looked at the effects of magnesium on 7,731 men and women, ages 46 to 64, who did not have hypertension at the start of this observational study.[13] The researchers tracked the participants' health and habits for 6 years, then divided them into four groups according to the amount of magnesium in their blood. They found that the higher the blood level of magnesium, the lower the risk of hypertension. Among the women in the study, those with the highest levels of magnesium were 30 percent less likely to develop hypertension than those with the lowest levels. Similarly, the men with the highest levels of magnesium were 18 percent less likely to develop hypertension. The researchers concluded that low blood levels of magnesium "may play a modest role in the development of hypertension."

♦ Korean researchers searched through the scientific literature to find 20 randomized studies, involving a total of 1,200 people, that examined the effects of magnesium on hypertension.[14] Fourteen of these studies involved people who already had elevated blood pressure, while six looked at people with normal blood pressure. After statistically merging the individual studies to create a single large study, the researchers concluded that magnesium supplementation can lead to a small reduction in blood pressure.

Summing Up the Evidence for Magnesium

There is little doubt that ample amounts of various nutrients, including magnesium, are necessary to keep blood pressure within healthful limits. It's also clear that supplemental magnesium can sometimes help prevent and/or reduce elevated blood pressure. However, we don't yet know who will benefit from supplemental magnesium and whether the drop in pressure will be enough to stave off the consequences of hypertension. For now, it is fair to say that magnesium is a four-star treatment for elevated blood pressure backed by strong evidence.

Available Forms

Among the food sources of magnesium are Florida avocados, toasted wheat germ, pumpkin seeds, cooked soybeans, spinach, dry roasted almonds, peanuts, and cashews. Supplemental magnesium takes many forms, including magnesium oxide, magnesium citrate, magnesium gluconate, magnesium chloride, and magnesium taurate. Magnesium taurate is more expensive than other forms but may have some ability to lower blood pressure on its own.

How Much Magnesium Is Typically Used

The Food and Nutrition Board has set the Recommended Dietary Allowances for magnesium at 400 milligrams for men ages 19 to 30; 420 milligrams for men 31 and older; 310 milligrams for women 19 to 30; and 320 milligrams for women 31 and older. There is no set dose of magnesium for treating hypertension, though typical therapeutic doses may range from 200 to 800 milligrams of elemental magnesium per day. (Read the label carefully to see how much elemental magnesium a supplement product contains.)

Possible Side Effects and Interactions

The Food and Nutrition Board of the Institute of Medicine has set a tolerable upper intake for magnesium at 350 milligrams per day for adults. Taking too much supplemental magnesium can cause diarrhea, lethargy, and weakness. In addition, magnesium may interact with aminoglycoside antibiotics such as streptomycin to trigger neuromuscular weakness, and it may reduce the absorption of quinolone antibiotics such as ciprofloxacin (Cipro). If you're taking any medication, be sure to consult your doctor before adding therapeutic amounts of magnesium to your self-care regimen.

Omega-3 Fatty Acids
Rating: ☆☆☆☆ = Strong Evidence

The omega-3 fatty acids are beneficial fats found primarily in cold-water fish that can help prevent heart disease in humans. They work by lowering the risk of clot formation within the blood vessels and reducing inflammation. Omega-3s are essential fatty acids, meaning they cannot be synthesized by the body and must be obtained from the diet. Thebest known of the omega-3s are eicosapentaenoic acid (EPA) and docosahexaenoic (DHA) acid.

Numerous studies have indicated that the omega-3 fatty acids can reduce elevated blood pressure. For example:

◆ Norwegian researchers presented the results of their study of omega-3 fatty acids in the *New England Journal of Medicine* in 1990.[15] The 156 men and women participating in the study, all of whom had mild hypertension, were randomly assigned to receive 10 weeks of daily treatment with either 6 grams of omega-3 fatty acids (85 percent of which was EPA and DHA combined) or placebo. In the omega-3 fatty acid group, average systolic pressure fell by 4.6 mm Hg and average diastolic pressure by 3.0. There was no significant improvement in the placebo group. The researchers concluded that EPA and DHA "may reduce blood pressure in essential hypertension." (Essential hypertension, the most common form, is elevated blood pressure for which no obvious cause can be found.)

◆ A study published in *Hypertension* in 1998 tracked 63 men and women with elevated blood pressure who had been taking antihypertension medication for at least 3 months.[16] The volunteers were randomly assigned to eat a daily fish meal supplying 3.6 grams of omega-3 fatty acids; to lose weight; to do both; or to do neither. After 16 weeks, both eating the omega-3-rich fish and losing weight had significantly lowered 24-hour ambulatory blood pressure levels (the continuous reading of blood pressure as a patient goes through 24 hours of regular activities). The researchers concluded that "incorporation of fish into a weight-reducing diet has additive effects in reducing ambulatory [blood pressure], as well as beneficial effects on heart rate, in overweight hypertensives taking antihypertensive medication."

◆ Seventy-eight people with uncontrolled hypertension participated in a 1995 double-blind study published in the *Annals of Internal Medicine*.[17] The volunteers were randomly assigned to receive either 4 grams of omega-3 fatty acids (EPA plus DHA) or a placebo every day for 16 weeks. The omega-3's lowered systolic blood pressure by an average of 3.8 mm Hg and diastolic pressure by an average of 2.0 mm Hg, compared to placebo.

Several studies have reviewed the current state of knowledge regarding omega-3 fatty acids and elevated blood pressure.

◆ The Agency for Healthcare Research and Quality, part of the US Department of Health and Human Services, published one such review in 2004.[18] According to the conclusions of this review, the evidence suggests that fish oil has a very small but beneficial effect on elevated blood pressure.

♦ A meta-analysis that appeared in the prestigious medical journal *Circulation* combined the results of 31 placebo-controlled studies of fish oil and hypertension, involving 1,356 people.[19] The authors of this study concluded that "there is a dose-response hypotensive effect of fish oil in hypertensive patients." In other words, fish oil does indeed reduce blood pressure in people with mild hypertension, and the effects become more pronounced as the dosage increases.

Summing Up the Evidence for Omega-3 Fatty Acids

Given the large number of studies indicating that omega-3 fatty acids from food or supplements can be helpful for reducing high blood pressure, plus the favorable review from the Agency for Healthcare Research and Quality, it is safe to conclude that the omega-3 fatty acids are a four-star treatment for elevated blood pressure backed by strong evidence.

Available Forms

The best sources of omega-3 fatty acids are cold-water fatty fish such as mackerel, salmon, herring, anchovies, and tuna. As a general rule, the fattier the fish is, the more omega-3s it contains. The human body can manufacture omega-3s from alpha-linolenic acid (ALA), which is found in walnuts, flaxseed, and various other plant foods. Omega-3 fatty acids also are available in supplement form, labeled as fish oil, omega-3, EPA, DHA, or some combination of these.

Amounts of Omega-3 Fatty Acids Typically Used

There is no standard dosage of omega-3 fatty acids for lowering elevated blood pressure. Many of the studies examining omega-3s as a treatment for hypertension have used dosages of up to 6 grams per day.

Possible Side Effects and Interactions

The omega-3 fatty acids are found in common foods and have been granted Generally Regarded as Safe (GRAS) status by the US government. Among their possible side effects is prolonged bleeding time, which may be a problem for those who have bleeding disorders, those who are taking medicines to thin the blood, or those who will be undergoing surgery.

Along the same line, the omega-3 fatty acids may raise the risk of bruising and bleeding when taken with drugs that thin the blood, such as aspirin and heparin (Hep-Lock). They also may interact with blood pressure medications such as atenolol (Tenormin), causing blood pressure to fall too low. If you're taking any medication, be sure to consult your doctor before adding therapeutic amounts of omega-3s to your self-care regimen.

Acupuncture

Rating: ☆☆ = Modest Evidence

A traditional Chinese healing discipline, acupuncture involves the use of needles to free energy, which moves through the body via tiny invisible channels called meridians. When the meridians become blocked, energy flow slows or stops, and illness can result.

While acupuncture has a long history as a treatment for pain, a number of studies have found it to be helpful for reducing high blood pressure as well.

♦ An early study, published in 1975 in the *American Journal of Chinese Medicine*, tested the effects of acupuncture in people with hypertension.[20] The 28 volunteers, average age 57, were given between 10 and 40 acupuncture treatments, depending on their individual needs. As shown in Figure 13-1, 16 of the participants had an "excellent" response to treatment, 8 had a "moderate" response, and only 4 showed no improvement at all.

Figure 13-1: Change in Systolic Blood Pressure Following Acupuncture Treatment

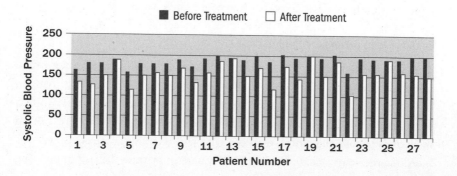

♦ For a 2003 study published in the *Journal of Traditional Chinese Medicine*, 87 people with a variety of health concerns—including 24 with elevated blood pressure—were treated with acupuncture.[21] Their blood pressure was monitored over the course of their treatment sessions. Even though they were receiving acupuncture for various reasons, and not necessarily for elevated blood pressure, systolic pressure fell in all 87 volunteers, most markedly in those with hypertension. The drop was considered statistically significant.

♦ A team of researchers from Taiwan and San Francisco enlisted 50 people suffering from untreated hypertension to test the effects of acupuncture on blood pressure and on the internal secretion of renin, an enzyme involved in the regulation of blood pressure.[22] After the volunteers' blood pressure was checked, they were given acupuncture; then their blood pressure was rechecked 30 minutes later. Systolic pressure fell from 169 mm Hg to 151 mm Hg, while diastolic pressure fell from 107 mm Hg to 96 mm Hg. The activity of renin in the bloodstream also dropped. The researchers concluded that "acupuncture decreases blood pressure in hypertensive patients and . . . that the decrease results, at least in part, from a decrease in renin secretion."

Summing Up the Evidence for Acupuncture

These and other studies are intriguing but are limited by the fact that they tend to involve small numbers of patients, run for short periods of time, lack randomization, and lack a placebo control in the form of "sham" acupuncture or something similar. Further, while many studies have produced positive results, a large number of studies have produced equivocal or negative results. The debate over the efficacy of acupuncture undoubtedly will continue for many years, until large-scale, double-blind studies using "sham" acupuncture or some other acceptable placebo control are performed. Based on what we know today, it is fair to say that acupuncture is a two-star treatment for elevated blood pressure backed by modest evidence.

Possible Side Effects

When properly administered, acupuncture usually produces no side effects. In rare cases patients have reported slight bruising or a small amount of bleeding where the needles are inserted, as well as some dizziness.

Finding an Acupuncturist

For more information about acupuncture, or to locate a certified acupuncturist, visit the National Certification Commission for Acupuncture and Oriental Medicine (NCCAOM) Web site: www.nccaom.org. The commission is the acupuncture profession's equivalent of the American Medical Association.

Olive Oil

Rating: ☆☆ = Modest Evidence

For thousands of years, olive oil—the "liquid gold" that comes from the fruit of the olive tree (*Olea europaea*)—has been prized for its nutritional, medicinal, and symbolic significance. It contains large amounts of monounsaturated fatty acids and antioxidants and is a major component of the Mediterranean diet, which has long been associated with heart health.

Known for its effectiveness at lowering blood cholesterol, olive oil also has been linked to reductions in blood pressure in a number of population and clinical studies. For example:

♦ Italian researchers compared the effects of extra-virgin olive oil to placebo for a study published in the *Archives of Internal Medicine* in 2000.[23] For this double-blind, crossover study, 23 people with hypertension were randomly assigned to consume diets containing either extra-virgin olive oil or sunflower oil (placebo) for 6 months. Then the groups switched diets. The researchers looked for several indications of improvement, including changes in blood pressure readings and the amount of blood pressure medication the participants needed to take. They found that compared to the placebo diet, the olive oil diet significantly lowered resting blood pressure—both systolic and diastolic. In addition, the olive oil diet reduced the need for blood pressure medicines by 48 percent, compared to 4 percent with the placebo diet. The researchers concluded that "a slight reduction in saturated fat intake, along with the use of extra-virgin olive oil, markedly lowers [the] daily antihypertensive dosage requirement."

♦ A similar study, presented in *Clinical Nutrition* in 2004, was performed with elderly patients.[24] For this study, 31 people who were undergoing treatment for hypertension and another 31 who had normal blood pressure were randomly assigned to consume diets enriched with either virgin olive oil or sunflower oil (placebo). The groups then switched diets. The results were positive, as the olive oil diet "normalized systolic pressure" among those with hypertension. The researchers concluded that dietary virgin olive oil "proved to be helpful in reducing the systolic pressure" of elderly patients being treated for hypertension.

♦ The Spanish SUN (Seguimiento Universidad de Navarra) Project tracks the health and habits of university graduates. For an article published in the journal *Lipids* in 2004, researchers used data collected from 6,863 study participants, all of whom had been followed for at least 2 years, comparing olive oil consumption to the incidence of hypertension.[25] The researchers found that for men, the risk of developing hypertension fell as consumption of olive oil rose. Interestingly, this correlation did not hold true for women.

♦ The EPIC (European Prospective Investigation into Cancer and Nutrition) Study is a large-scale trial looking into the causes of cancer and other ailments.[26] Greek researchers used data collected from 20,343 Greek study participants who did not have elevated blood pressure to see if olive oil consumption was linked to reductions in hypertension. After analyzing the participants' health and habits, the researchers concluded that the intake of olive oil "is inversely associated with both systolic and diastolic blood pressure." This means that the more olive oil the study participants consumed, the lower their systolic and diastolic blood pressure readings were.

Summing Up the Evidence for Olive Oil

These studies of olive oil are enticing because they seem to corroborate the heart-healthy effects of the Mediterranean diet. However, we still don't have results from large-scale, double-blind clinical studies specifically examining the relationship between olive oil and blood pressure that would allow us to make a definitive determination. Given what we know to date, it is reasonable to say that olive oil is a two-star treatment for elevated blood pressure backed by modest evidence.

How Much Olive Oil Is Typically Used

There is no standard dose of olive oil. Typical supplemental doses may range from 30 to 40 grams (2 to 4 tablespoons) per day.

Possible Side Effects and Interactions

In therapeutic amounts, olive oil may trigger biliary colic in those with gallstones. It also may interact with diabetes medications such as glimepiride (Amaryl), causing blood sugar to drop too low. If you're taking any medication, be sure to consult your doctor before adding therapeutic amounts of olive oil to your self-care regimen.

ALTERNATIVE APPROACHES TO

HIGH CHOLESTEROL

Blond psyllium	☆☆☆☆☆
Oats	☆☆☆☆☆
Omega-3 fatty acids	☆☆☆☆☆
Plant sterols/stanols	☆☆☆☆☆
Soy	☆☆☆☆☆
Nuts	☆☆☆☆
Policosanol	☆☆☆

Cholesterol is a waxy, fatty substance that the body uses to insulate nerves and produce cell membranes. It also plays an important role in the manufacture of bile acids, the sex hormones estrogen and testosterone, and vitamin D. But excess amounts of cholesterol floating through the bloodstream can clog arteries, leading to heart attacks and strokes.

The most common cholesterol measurements are:

♦ Total cholesterol—all of the different kinds of cholesterol in the bloodstream combined into one measurement.
♦ LDL cholesterol—primarily carries cholesterol to organs and tissues. When oxidized, LDL tends to leave deposits on the walls of arteries, which is why it's referred to as the "bad" cholesterol.
♦ HDL cholesterol—primarily carries cholesterol away from artery walls and to the liver for excretion, thus lowering total cholesterol levels. This is why it's referred to as the "good" cholesterol.

It's recommended that total cholesterol be kept between 130 mg/dL (milligrams per deciliter of blood) and 199 mg/dL, as levels above 200 mg/dL reflect an increased risk of heart disease. LDL levels should be below 100 mg/dL, and HDL levels above 40 mg/dL.

Elevated blood fats (triglycerides) are also considered a risk factor for coronary heart disease and so are routinely measured. It's recommended that triglycerides be kept below 150 mg/dL.

SYMPTOMS

Unhealthy cholesterol levels don't cause pain or any other symptoms. Over time, however, they can cause atherosclerosis, a build-up of plaque in the arteries that can lead to heart disease, heart attack, and stroke. Chest pain most likely won't occur until the blood vessels are about 75 percent blocked—and it may not occur at all. Generally, the only way you'll know if your cholesterol levels are too high (or too low, in the case of HDL) is to have your blood analyzed by a lab.

CAUSES

High total cholesterol and high LDL have been linked to a diet high in fat (particularly saturated fat and trans fats) or cholesterol; obesity, particularly abdominal obesity; smoking; and a lack of exercise. Low HDL is usually the result of too little exercise, obesity, or smoking.

STANDARD TREATMENTS

The primary treatment for elevated total cholesterol or LDL or low HDL is a diet low in cholesterol and fat (especially saturated fat and trans fats) and high in complex carbohydrates, fruits and vegetables, and fiber. Some people may need to lose weight, increase their physical activity, and quit smoking. If these lifestyle measures don't improve the cholesterol numbers enough, a cholesterol-lowering medication—perhaps one of the statin drugs, such as Lipitor or Crestor—may be prescribed.

RATING POPULAR ALTERNATIVE TREATMENTS FOR HIGH CHOLESTEROL

Blond Psyllium

Rating: ☆☆☆☆☆ = Convincing Evidence

A soluble fiber, blond psyllium has been used by various cultures to treat constipation, diarrhea, elevated blood pressure, elevated cholesterol, and diabetes, among other ailments. It's found in the laxative Metamucil and in some frozen foods, where it's used as a stabilizer or thickener. Its active ingredient is mucilage, a clear, colorless gelling agent contained in the husk of the psyllium seed. When ingested, mucilage swells and forms a thick, gooey mass in the intestines. This mass helps increase stool size and weight and gently stimulates production of a bowel movement. Although there are many species of psyllium, blond psyllium (*Plantago ovata*) is the one with the highest mucilage content.

Since soluble fiber is known to lower cholesterol when combined with a low-fat diet, blond psyllium has been investigated as a possible treatment for elevated cholesterol. Studies such as the following suggest that it can be effective.

♦ Two hundred eighty-six people with mildly to moderately elevated cholesterol participated in a 1998 study comparing the effects of blond psyllium to placebo.[1] The volunteers—whose LDL cholesterol levels ranged from 130 to 220 mg/dL—were randomly assigned to receive blond psyllium via a variety of cereals, snack bars, and breads in one of the following amounts: 3.4 grams per day for the low-dose group; 6.8 grams for the medium-dose group; 10.2 grams for the high-dose group; and no blond psyllium for the placebo group. The volunteers consumed foods providing the specified amount of blond psyllium every day for 24 weeks. The results of this double-blind study were positive, with LDL levels in the high-dose group averaging 5.3 percent lower than those in the placebo group at the 24-week mark. The researchers noted that while the 5.3 percent drop was modest, the LDL cholesterol in the high-dose psyllium group "remained lower throughout the 24-week treatment period, indicating the potential for long-term benefit."

♦ A double-blind study published in the *American Journal of Clinical Nutrition* in 2000 compared the effects of psyllium to placebo in men and women with elevated cholesterol.[2] Two hundred forty-eight volunteers were randomly assigned to receive either 10.2 grams of psyllium (Metamucil) or a placebo every day for 26 weeks. All of the study participants also followed a standard cholesterol-lowering diet. The results were positive, with those in the psyllium group showing a 4.7 percent drop in total cholesterol and a 6.7 percent reduction in LDL cholesterol, compared to those in the placebo group. The researchers concluded,

"Psyllium therapy is an effective adjunct to diet therapy and may provide an alternative to drug therapy for some patients."

♦ For a 2005 study published in the *Archives of Internal Medicine*, researchers pitted psyllium (Metamucil) against the standard drug simvastatin (Zocor).[3] The 68 participants in this double-blind study were randomly assigned to one of three groups:

◊ Moderate-dose medicine—10 milligrams of simvastatin plus a placebo daily

◊ Moderate-dose medicine plus psyllium—10 milligrams of simvastatin plus 15 grams of blond psyllium (Metamucil) daily

◊ High-dose medicine—20 milligrams of simvastatin plus a placebo daily

After 8 weeks, those taking the moderate-dose medicine plus placebo had lowered their LDL cholesterol by an average of 55 mg/dL. By comparison, LDL cholesterol fell by 63 points among those taking the high-dose medicine plus placebo, as well as those taking the moderate-dose medicine plus psyllium. The researchers concluded that the mix of psyllium and moderate-dose medicine was as effective as high-dose medicine for lowering LDL cholesterol. Table 14-1 below summarizes the results of this study.

Table 14-1: Psyllium Performs Well Compared to Statin Drug

	CHANGES AFTER 8 WEEKS OF TREATMENT		
	10 mg simvastatin	20 mg simvastatin	Psyllium plus 10 mg simvastatin
Total cholesterol mg/dL	-57	-61	-66
LDL cholesterol mg/dL	-55	-63	-63
Blood fats (triglycerides) mg/dL	-23	-8	-17
HDL cholesterol mg/dL	+2	+4	-3

♦ A 1997 meta-analysis published in the *Journal of Nutrition* looked at 11 published and unpublished randomized, controlled studies.[4] The studies lasted from 14 to 56 days and involved the volunteers eating cereal enriched with blond psyllium. After statistically merging the results of the individual studies, the researchers found that eating psyllium-enriched cereal as part of a low-fat diet triggers reductions in total cholesterol and LDL cholesterol "over that which can be achieved with a low-fat diet alone."

♦ A 2000 meta-analysis published in the *American Journal of Clinical Nutrition* looked at eight blond psyllium/high cholesterol studies involving more than 600 people.[5] The authors of this analysis concluded, "Psyllium supplementation significantly lowered serum total and LDL cholesterol concentrations in subjects consuming a low-fat diet."

Summing Up the Evidence for Blond Psyllium

Both theory and clinical studies support the idea that blond psyllium, combined with a low-fat diet, can reduce total cholesterol and LDL cholesterol. In recognition of this finding, the United States Food and Drug Administration has allowed food manufacturers to make a health claim for products containing blond psyllium, saying that as part of a diet low in cholesterol and saturated fat, soluble fiber from blond psyllium "may reduce the risk of heart disease." In addition, Germany's Commission E has approved the use of blond psyllium (*Plantago ovata*) as a treatment for elevated cholesterol levels. Given the solid research and the thumbs-up from the FDA, it is safe to say that blond psyllium is a five-star treatment for elevated cholesterol backed by convincing evidence.

Other Names

Blond psyllium is known to scientists as *Plantago ovata* and in various parts of the world by other names, including Englishman's foot, Indian plantago, ispagol, psyllium, sand plantain, and spogel.

Available Forms

Blond psyllium is found in bulking laxatives such as Metamucil, supplements, and some breads, cereals, and snack bars. It is also available in the form of seeds, powder, tablets, and tincture.

How Much Blond Psyllium Is Typically Used

A standard dose of blond psyllium has not been set. Successful studies have used dosages of about 10 to 15 grams per day.

Possible Side Effects and Interactions

Taken orally, blond psyllium can cause abdominal pain, diarrhea, constipation, and other side effects. Some people may experience allergic reactions to it.

Blond psyllium may increase the risk of low blood sugar when combined with diabetes medications such as glipizide (Glucotrol). If you're taking any medication, be sure to consult your doctor before adding blond psyllium to your self-care regimen.

Oats

Rating: ☆☆☆☆☆ = Convincing Evidence

A kind of grain consumed for centuries by animals and humans alike, oats have been used by various cultures to treat numerous ailments, including elevated cholesterol, constipation, and diabetes. When applied as a poultice, oats also can help relieve the itchiness of eczema, dermatitis, chicken pox, and other skin conditions.

Oats contain soluble fiber, the kind that dissolves in water. Among the soluble fibers is one known as beta-glucan, which is believed to be responsible for the cholesterol-lowering effect of oats. The studies of oats' ability to lower cholesterol include the following:

♦ A 1991 study published in the *American Journal of Clinical Nutrition* involved 20 men with elevated cholesterol.[6] The men were randomly placed on a standard American diet with either 110 grams of oat bran (supplied by the Quaker Oats Company) or 40 grams of wheat bran every day for 3 weeks. The oat bran "significantly decreased total cholesterol by 12.8 [percent and] low-density lipoprotein [LDL] cholesterol by 12.1 [percent]." The wheat bran had no significant positive effect.

♦ A 1998 study, published in the *Journal of the American College of Nutrition*, put both oat bran and psyllium (another source of soluble fiber) to the test.[7] Sixty-six men, with cholesterol levels that ranged from normal to elevated, participated in the 8-week trial. They were randomly assigned to eat 100 grams of cookies daily. The cookies supplied 2.8 grams of soluble fiber from oat bran, 1.7 grams of soluble fiber from psyllium, or 0.6 gram of soluble fiber from wheat bran. The cookies containing the wheat bran served as the control because wheat bran is not known to lower cholesterol. The cookies made with oat bran reduced LDL cholesterol by an average of 26 percent, and the cookies made with psyllium lowered it by 22.6 percent. By comparison, the cookies made with wheat bran did not have any significant positive effect.

♦ A study published in the *Journal of the American Dietetic Association* in 2001 examined the effects of oats and soy on cholesterol levels.[8] For this study, 127 postmenopausal women with moderately elevated cholesterol levels were placed on a standard cholesterol-lowering diet for 3 weeks. As expected, their total cholesterol, LDL cholesterol, and blood fat levels dropped. Then they were randomly assigned to follow one of four dietary treatments: oats/milk powder, oats/soy protein powder, wheat/milk powder, or wheat/soy protein powder. In both oat groups, the women ate either two servings of cooked oatmeal (Quaker Oats) or a ready-to-eat oat bran cereal (Quaker Oats) every day. After the women had been on these new diets for 6 weeks, those in the oats/milk and oats/soy groups saw their total cholesterol drop by an additional 3 percent and their LDL cholesterol by more than 5 percent. Those in the wheat/milk and wheat/soy groups did not see positive changes.

♦ A meta-analysis, published in the *Journal of the American Medical Association* in 1992, examined published and unpublished studies of oats and cholesterol.[9] The researchers found 10 randomized, controlled trials meeting their quality criteria and statistically merged them to produce a meta-analysis. According to the researchers, their meta-analysis "supports the hypothesis that incorporating oat products into the diet causes a modest reduction in blood cholesterol level."

Summing Up the Evidence for Oats

A large body of scientific evidence supports the hypothesis that oats can reduce cholesterol. The United States Food and Drug Administration acknowledged this evidence in 1997 by allowing manufacturers to place the following claim on oat products: "A diet high in soluble fiber from whole oats (oat bran, oatmeal, and oat flour) and low in saturated fat and cholesterol may reduce the risk of heart disease." Given the solid research and the thumbs-up from the FDA, it is safe to say that oats are a five-star treatment for elevated cholesterol backed by convincing evidence.

Amount of Oats Typically Used

There is no standard dose of oats for elevated cholesterol. Typical dosages may range from 50 to 150 grams of whole oats per day supplying between 2.5 and 7.5 grams of soluble fiber.

Possible Side Effects and Interactions

Among oats' possible side effects are increased frequency of bowel movements, flatulence, and anal irritation. Oats may hamper the absorption of certain cholesterol-lowering drugs, such as atorvastatin (Lipitor). They also may reduce the effectiveness of morphine sulfate (MS Contin) and similar medications. If you are taking any medication, be sure to consult your doctor before adding oats to your self-care regimen.

Omega-3 Fatty Acids

Rating: ☆☆☆☆☆ = Convincing Evidence

Clinical trials and large population studies have shown that omega-3 fatty acids—which are found primarily in cold-water fatty fish—can reduce the incidence of heart disease. Although they don't appear to lower total cholesterol or LDL cholesterol, the omega-3s have demonstrated an ability to reduce high triglycerides, an important predictor of heart disease.

♦ The effects of omega-3 fatty acids were compared to those of corn oil for a 2003 randomized, double-blind study published in the *American Journal of Clinical Nutrition*.[10] Twenty-four obese men with elevated cholesterol and triglycerides and 10 lean men with normal cholesterol and triglycerides were assigned to receive either 4 grams of fish oil containing EPA and DHA (brand name Omacor) or a placebo every day for 6 weeks. The results were positive, with fish oil supplementation significantly lowering triglycerides by 18 percent.

♦ A double-blind study involving 57 men and women with low HDL cholesterol was published in the *Journal of the American College of Nutrition* in 2005.[11] The volunteers were randomly assigned to receive either 1.52 grams of the omega-3 fatty acid DHA (provided by Martek Biosciences Inc.) or a placebo every day for 6 weeks. The omega-3 fatty acids produced a statistically significant improvement in triglycerides, lowering them by 21 percent compared to 7 percent in the placebo group.

The researchers concluded that fish oil has "favorable effects on triglycerides," but noted that LDL cholesterol levels rose.

♦ In 2002 the American Heart Association published an "AHA Scientific Statement" in the journal *Circulation*.[12] This paper reviewed the evidence from population studies and randomized, controlled trials regarding omega-3 fatty acids and cardiovascular disease. Although the authors' focus was on cardiovascular disease as a whole, they did review the omega-3 fatty acid/blood fat studies and noted that the ability of omega-3 fatty acids from fish oil to lower triglycerides was "well established." The AHA paper cited a review, published in the *American Journal of Clinical Nutrition* in 1997, in which evidence from a significant body of studies showed that fish oil reduces blood fat levels by 25 to 30 percent.[13]

♦ In 2004, the Agency for Healthcare Research and Quality—part of the US Department of Health and Human Services—published an Evidence Report looking at the effects of omega-3 fatty acids on cardiovascular disease risk factors.[14] The agency noted that there is "strong evidence" that fish oils "have a strong beneficial effect" on triglycerides.

Summing Up the Evidence for Omega-3 Fatty Acids

Given the positive reviews in the American Heart Association Scientific Statement and the Agency for Healthcare Research and Quality Evidence Report, it is fair to say that omega-3 fatty acids are a five-star treatment for elevated cholesterol backed by convincing evidence.

Available Forms

The best sources of omega-3 fatty acids are cold-water fatty fish such as mackerel, herring, anchovies, salmon, tuna, bluefish, and swordfish. As a general rule, the fattier a fish is, the more omega-3s it contains. The human body also can manufacture omega-3s from alpha-linolenic acid, which is found in walnuts and flaxseed. Omega-3 fatty acids are available in supplement form, labeled as fish oil, omega-3, EPA, DHA, or some combination of these.

Dosage of Omega-3 Fatty Acids Typically Used

There is no standard dosage of omega-3 fatty acids. The American Heart Association offers these suggestions:

- If you don't have heart disease, eat at least two servings of a variety of fish per week—preferably the fatty kinds like salmon, which contain omega-3 fatty acids.
- If you have heart disease, take in at least 1 gram of DHA or EPA per day. You can get these omega-3s from foods or supplements.
- If you need to lower your triglycerides, take 2 to 4 grams of EPA and DHA per day, under your physician's care.

Possible Side Effects and Interactions

The omega-3 fatty acids are found in common foods and have been granted Generally Regarded as Safe (GRAS) status by the US government. Among their possible side effects are belching, heartburn, and nausea. The omega-3s also can prolong bleeding time, which may be a problem for those who have bleeding disorders, those who are taking medicines to thin the blood, or those who will be undergoing surgery soon.

Along the same line, the omega-3 fatty acids may interact with aspirin, heparin, and other drugs that thin the blood, increasing the risk of bleeding. If you're taking any medication, be sure to consult your doctor before adding omega-3 supplements to your self-care regimen.

Plant Sterols/Stanols

Rating: ☆☆☆☆☆ = Convincing Evidence

Soy, pine tree, and other plants contain substances called sterols, which structurally resemble cholesterol. Way back in the 1950s, researchers noted that such plant-derived sterols could lower cholesterol levels by interfering with the absorption of cholesterol in the intestines. As the focus of most research shifted toward emerging cholesterol-lowering drugs, the sterols were pushed to the scientific back burner. But in the past decade or so, interest in these substances has been revived, with studies investigating the therapeutic properties of individual sterols, different "versions" of the sterols, and the sterols as a group.

The most common sterols found in plants are *sitosterol*, *campesterol*, and *stigmasterol*. Sterols may be chemically modified, or esterified, so that more of them can be incorporated into fatty foods. Stanols are sterols that have been saturated and given new names. For example, saturated sitosterol becomes *sitostanol*. (Although we tend to think of "saturated" as a nutritional dirty word, in this case conversion to the saturated form has some benefits.)

A significant body of research has linked plant sterol/stanols to lower cholesterol levels. For example:

♦ Researchers from England's Oxford University and other scientific centers tested the effects of plant sterols on cholesterol for a 2001 study published in the journal *Atherosclerosis*.[15] Sixty-two people with familial hypercholesterolemia (an inherited disorder that causes elevated cholesterol levels) volunteered to participate. Thirty of the volunteers were taking statin drugs to control their elevated cholesterol, while the other 32 were not. For this double-blind trial, the volunteers were randomly assigned to receive either 25 grams of a fat spread containing 2.5 grams of plant sterols (supplied by Van den Bergh Foods) or a placebo spread every day. (The spread could be put on bread or otherwise added to the diet.) After 8 weeks, the groups switched to the other spread for 8 weeks. The researchers concluded that a fat spread "enriched with vegetable oil sterols reduced LDL cholesterol by 10 to 15 percent" and that the sterol-fortified spread was of equal benefit to those taking statin drugs and those not taking the medicines.

♦ Researchers from the Mayo Clinic looked at the effects of various formulations of stanols for a double-blind study published in *Mayo Clinic Proceedings* in 1999.[16] For the 8-week study period, 318 people with mildly elevated cholesterol levels were randomly assigned to receive one of three possible doses of a margarine-like spread containing 2 to 3 grams of stanols (supplied by McNeil CPC) or a placebo spread. All of the doses of stanols were effective, with the largest dose lowering total cholesterol by 6.4 percent and LDL cholesterol by 10.1 percent. The researchers concluded that their study "has shown the efficacy of stanol ester in lowering [total cholesterol] and [LDL cholesterol] levels in a population of mildly hypercholesterolemic men and women consuming a prudent US diet without significant adverse effects."

♦ Canadian researchers enlisted 16 people with elevated cholesterol levels for their 2002 randomized, double-blind, crossover study comparing the effects of sterols and stanols to placebo.[17] There were four dietary treatments: diet with plant sterols (primarily sitosterol, campesterol, and stigmasterol); diet with plant stanols (sitostanol and campestanol); diet with mixed sterols and stanols; and diet with placebo cornstarch. Each of the dietary treatments lasted 21 days, and each of the volunteers followed each of the diets in random order. The results were positive. Compared to the placebo diet, the diet with sterols produced total cholesterol that was 7.8 percent lower and LDL cholesterol that was 11.3 percent lower. The results were even better for the diet with stanols, as total cholesterol was 11.9 percent lower and LDL cholesterol was 13.4 percent lower. On the diet of mixed sterols plus stanols, total cholesterol was 13.1 percent lower and LDL was 16.0 percent lower than on the placebo diet.

♦ Seventy men and women, average age 58, participated in a randomized, double-blind, placebo-controlled study testing the effects of sterols on mildly elevated cholesterol.[18] The volunteers were encouraged to follow a standard fat-lowering diet; then they were assigned to 4 weeks of daily treatment with either three servings of chocolate containing 1.8 grams of a sterol/stanol mixture or just chocolate. The sterol/stanol mixture (provided by Forbes Medi-Tech) contained sitosterol, campesterol, sitostanol, and campestanol. The results were positive, with the sterol/stanol mixture producing a statistically significant reduction in total and LDL cholesterol. Table 14-2 below compares the effects of the sterol/stanol mixture to placebo.

Table 14-2: Sterols/Stanols Added to Chocolate Reduce Total and LDL Cholesterol[19]

	PERCENTAGE DECREASE IN TOTAL AND LDL CHOLESTEROL	
	Total Cholesterol	LDL Cholesterol
Phytosterol group	-6.4%	-10.3%
Placebo group	0.0%	+0.8%

♦ Several reviews and meta-analyses have investigated the effectiveness of plant sterols/stanols for lowering cholesterol. One of the most recent of these, a 2005 meta-analysis published in the journal *Pharmacotherapy*, combined data from 23 individual studies that had lasted from 4 to 52 weeks to determine the effects of certain natural therapies on LDL cholesterol.[20] According to the meta-analysis results, consuming 3.4 grams of plant sterol and stanol esters per day lowered LDL cholesterol by 11 percent.

♦ A 2002 critical review published in the *Journal of Nutrition* looked at the effects of plant sterols and stanols on cholesterol, concluding that "the efficacy of plant sterols and stanols as cholesterol-lowering agents has been well established."[21]

Summing Up the Evidence for Plant Sterols/Stanols

Research into plant sterols/stanols continues, with lively scientific debate centering around questions such as the right mix of sterols/stanols, the best source, the optimal dosage, whether sterols or stanols are preferable for long-term treatment, and which "delivery vehicle" is best—margarine-like spreads, milk, orange juice, or something else. Although many questions have yet to be answered, the United States Food and Drug Administration is satisfied that there is enough positive research to allow food manufacturers to make a health claim for products containing plant sterol/stanol esters. Specifically, manufacturers may say that as part of a diet low in cholesterol and saturated fat, plant sterol/stanol esters "may reduce the risk of heart disease." This endorsement from the FDA, combined with the substantial body of positive research, indicates that plant sterols/stanols are a five-star treatment for elevated cholesterol backed by convincing evidence.

Available Forms

Various combinations of plant sterol/stanols are available in supplement form and in foods such as salad dressing, mayonnaise, and margarine. Look for products such as Benecol and Take Control margarines, Rice Dream Heartwise rice milk, and Minute Maid HeartWise orange juice. Be sure to check labels before making a purchase, because formulations can change over time.

Amount of Plant Sterols/Stanols Typically Used

There is no standard dose of plant sterols/stanols for elevated cholesterol. Supplemental doses may range from 2 to 4 grams per day.

Possible Side Effects and Interactions

The side effects of sterols and stanols vary with the individual supplements. Sitostanol, for example, may trigger diarrhea and excessive fat in the stool.

As with all supplements and drugs, be sure to read the label directions carefully before trying plant sterols/stanols.

Soy

Rating: ☆☆☆☆☆ = Convincing Evidence

Soy, a kind of bean that is found worldwide, has been used medicinally in China for thousands of years. Containing isoflavones and other health-promoting substances, soy has a long history as a treatment for fever, headache, lack of appetite, various kinds of liver disease, and "female complaints." Over the past several decades, its effectiveness as a possible treatment for elevated cholesterol—as well as cancer, hot flashes, osteoporosis, and other ailments—has made it the subject of numerous scientific studies. Among them:

♦ Researchers from Wake Forest University School of Medicine enlisted 51 women, ages 45 to 55, to test the effects of soy protein supplementation on cholesterol levels, blood pressure, and menopausal symptoms.[22] For this double-blind, crossover study, the women were given three different treatments, each for 6 weeks: 20 grams of soy protein once daily, 10 grams of soy protein twice daily, or 20 grams of complex carbohydrates serving as a placebo. (The soy protein supplements were provided by Protein Technologies International.) The women took the treatments in random order, not knowing which they were using at any given time. The researchers concluded that soy protein could lower cholesterol, with "significant declines in total cholesterol (6 percent lower) and [LDL] cholesterol (7 percent lower)," when taken either once or twice daily. Table 14-3 below summarizes the key results from the study.

Table 14-3: Two Different Doses of Soy Reduce Cholesterol and Blood Fats[23]

	LEVEL AT END OF STUDY		
	Soy Once Daily	Soy Twice Daily	Placebo
Total cholesterol	198.6 mg/dL	195.7 mg/dL	208.1 mg/dL
LDL cholesterol	119.4 mg/dL	116.8 mg/dL	125.4 mg/dL
HDL cholesterol	52.2 mg/dL	52.2 mg/dL	53.3 mg/dL
Blood fats (triglycerides)	128.5 mg/dL	140.9 mg/dL	156.3 mg/dL

♦ Italian researchers compared the effects of soy milk to cow's milk in people with severely elevated cholesterol levels who either could not take or did not respond well to the statin drugs often prescribed for this condition.[24] The 21 volunteers were randomly assigned to consume either a high-protein soy milk drink or a cow's milk drink (the placebo) for 4 weeks. Then they switched and consumed the other drink for an additional 4 weeks. The high-protein soy milk drink produced statistically significant drops of 6.5 to 7.4 percent in total cholesterol, compared to small or not statistically significant reductions seen with the cow's milk.

♦ For a 1998 study published in the *American Journal of Clinical Nutrition*, 66 women with elevated cholesterol levels were given one of three treatments designed to test the effects of soy protein and isoflavones.[25] For this double-blind, randomized trial, the women were put on a standard cholesterol-lowering diet. They also were given 40 grams of soy protein with a moderate amount of isoflavones (brand name Supro 675), 40 grams of soy protein with a large amount of isoflavones (supplied by Protein Technologies International), or a placebo every day. Both doses of soy protein reduced cholesterol compared to the placebo, triggering approximately a 6 percent drop in total cholesterol.

Several experts have searched the medical literature in order to synthesize and refine current knowledge of soy's effect on cholesterol.

♦ For a 1995 meta-analysis published in the *New England Journal of Medicine*, researchers from the University of Kentucky statistically merged 38 controlled trials.[26] This "new look" at the data revealed that daily consumption of soy protein (averaging 47 grams per day) could lead to average decreases of 23.2 mg/dL in total cholesterol, 21.7 mg/dL in LDL cholesterol, and 13.3 mg/dL in blood fats (triglycerides). The authors of this meta-analysis concluded that "consumption of soy protein rather than animal protein significantly decreased serum concentrations of total cholesterol, LDL cholesterol, and triglycerides" without significantly raising or lowering HDL cholesterol. Table 14-4 on the next page summarizes the results of this meta-analysis.

Table 14-4: Meta-Analysis Combining Results of 38 Soy/Cholesterol Studies[27]

	Number of Studies	Number of Volunteers	Change in Value	Percentage Change
Total cholesterol	38	730	-23.2	-9.3%
LDL cholesterol	31	564	-21.7	-12.9%
Blood fats (triglycerides)	30	628	-13.3	-10.5%

♦ A meta-analysis prepared by researchers from the Chinese University of Hong Kong and published in the *American Journal of Clinical Nutrition* in 2005 also produced positive results.[28] This meta-analysis, which statistically combined 28 studies, found that soy protein with isoflavones could lower total cholesterol by 3.77 percent, LDL cholesterol by 5.25 percent, and blood fats (triglycerides) by 7.27 percent, while raising HDL cholesterol by 3.03 percent. Interestingly, this analysis found that men typically showed larger declines in total cholesterol and LDL cholesterol due to soy consumption than women did.

♦ In 2005 the Agency for Healthcare Research and Quality, part of the US Department of Health and Human Services, published an Evidence Report examining the effects of soy on various diseases.[29] The authors of this paper reviewed 61 studies of the effects of soy products on cholesterol, finding that total cholesterol levels fell approximately 5 mg/dL more in those taking soy than in those in control groups. A meta-analysis of 52 studies showed that consumption of soy triggered a statistically significant 3 percent decline in LDL cholesterol.

Summing Up the Evidence for Soy

More than 30 clinical trials have found that soy protein can reduce total cholesterol, LDL cholesterol, and blood fat levels, with some even suggesting that it can raise levels of protective HDL cholesterol. In addition, the United States Food and Drug Administration allows food manufacturers to attach the following health claim to products containing soy: "25 grams of soy protein a day, as part of a diet low in saturated fat and cholesterol, may reduce the risk of heart disease." Thus, it is fair to say that soy is a five-star treatment for elevated cholesterol backed by convincing evidence.

Available Forms

Soy comes in the form of soybeans, soy flour, soy milk, soy oil, tofu, miso, tempeh, natto, and other foods. Soy isoflavones also come in extract form.

How Much Soy Is Typically Used

There is no standard dose of soy, although supplemental doses may range as high as 50 grams of soy protein per day. The US Food and Drug Administration says that 25 grams per day, as part of a diet low in cholesterol and saturated fat, is an adequate amount.

Possible Side Effects and Interactions

Soy can cause constipation, nausea, and insomnia. It also can trigger allergic reactions in some people.

Those with breast cancer or a family history of breast cancer should be very cautious about using soy products, as there is conflicting evidence about whether soy has a positive or negative effect on the disease. The use of soy isoflavone extract is not recommended, as too many soy chemicals may interfere with mineral absorption, thyroid function, and/or mental function.

Soy may interact with and reduce the effectiveness of medications for cancer, such as tamoxifen (Nolvadex), and may inhibit the absorption of thyroid medications such as levothyroxine (Synthroid). If you're taking any medication, be sure to consult your doctor before adding therapeutic amounts of soy to your self-care regimen.

Nuts

Rating: ☆☆☆☆ = Strong Evidence

Nuts—which technically are single-seeded fruits with dry, tough fruit layers—are good sources of fiber, B vitamins, and magnesium. Although they typically are high in fat, the kind of fat they contain is mostly monounsaturated or polyunsaturated, which can help keep cholesterol levels under control. Nuts also help manage blood sugar and contain estrogen-like properties that may help relieve certain menopausal symptoms.

Although they are high in calories, nuts don't necessarily contribute to obesity. One study of more than 26,000 people found that those who ate the largest amounts of nuts were actually less likely to be obese. This is probably due to the fact that nuts are filling and satisfying.

Several population studies have linked the increased consumption of nuts to lower levels of cholesterol and a reduced risk of heart disease. The idea that adding nuts to the diet might lower cholesterol was tested in studies such as these:

♦ For a single-blind, controlled study published in the *New England Journal of Medicine* in 1993, 18 men with cholesterol levels between 137 and 250 mg/dL were randomly placed on one of two diets.[30] The diets were identical except that one contained walnuts. After 4 weeks of following these diets, those eating more walnuts had total cholesterol levels that were 12.4 percent lower and LDL cholesterol levels that were 16.3 percent lower than those who followed the control diet.

♦ A team of Canadian and American researchers tested the effects of almonds on elevated triglycerides and other heart disease risk factors for a 2002 study published in *Circulation*.[31] For this controlled, crossover study, 27 men and women with elevated triglycerides were randomly assigned to receive daily doses of one of the following:

◊ A full dose of almonds (73 grams of whole, raw, unblanched almonds)
◊ A full dose of low-saturated-fat, whole-wheat muffins (147-gram muffins)
◊ A half-dose of almonds plus a half-dose of muffins (37 grams of almonds plus 75 grams of muffin)

Each of the participants took each of the three supplements for one month apiece. The results were positive, with researchers noting that supplementing a healthful diet with almonds could reduce the risk of heart disease. Specifically, 37 grams of almonds a day—which the researchers described as "a handful"—lowered LDL cholesterol by 4.4 percent, while 73 grams a day reduced LDL cholesterol by 9.4 percent.

♦ Spanish researchers tested the effects of walnuts in 21 men and women with elevated cholesterol levels for a 2004 study published in *Circulation*.[32] The volunteers in this randomized, crossover trial adopted either a Mediterranean-type diet designed to lower cholesterol or the same diet with walnuts partially replacing olive oil, avocados, and other selected foods. The participants followed one of the diets for 4 weeks, then switched to the other for 4 weeks. The results were positive, with the walnut diet producing statistically significant reductions of 4.4 percent in total cholesterol and 6.4 percent in LDL cholesterol.

A number of review studies examining the nut–cholesterol question have been published.

♦ Writing in the *Journal of Nutrition* in 2005, South African researchers looked at 23 studies involving nuts.[33] They observed that the participants in 3 almond studies (50 to 100 grams per day), 2 peanut studies (35 to 68 grams per day), 1 pecan nut study (72 grams per day), and 4 walnut studies (40 to 84 grams per day) showed decreases in total cholesterol between 2 and 16 percent and LDL cholesterol between 2 and 19 percent compared to the participants consuming control diets.

♦ A 2002 review paper published in the *Journal of Nutrition* focused on the health benefits of walnuts.[34] The author of this review examined five controlled, peer-reviewed, human clinical studies of walnuts and heart health, concluding that the evidence "consistently demonstrated walnuts as part of a heart-healthy diet [and] lower blood cholesterol concentrations." The author added that the results of these experimental trials were supported by data gathered in population studies but that the trials were of relatively short duration.

♦ In 1999 researchers from the Harvard School of Public Health noted that "several clinical studies have observed beneficial effects of diets high in nuts (including walnuts, peanuts, almonds, and other nuts) on blood lipids"—that is, on cholesterol and blood fats.[35]

Summing Up the Evidence for Nuts

With a substantial body of research to support them, nuts appear to have a place in the treatment of elevated cholesterol levels. However, many questions—including the best kinds and amounts of nuts—have yet to be addressed. With this in mind, it is fair to say that nuts are a four-star treatment for elevated cholesterol backed by strong evidence.

Amount of Nuts Typically Used

There is no standard dose of nuts. One study found good results when participants ate 5 ounces (about 1¼ cups) of nuts per week. Various types of nuts have been used in the studies, so we cannot yet say that one type of nut is better than others, overall, for most people.

Possible Side Effects and Interactions

Some people can experience a life-threatening allergic reaction when exposed to certain kinds of nuts, most commonly peanuts and walnuts. If this should happen to you, seek emergency medical care as quickly as possible.

Policosanol

Rating: ☆☆☆ = Intriguing Evidence

Policosanol, a natural substance derived from sugarcane, is called "nature's statin" because it appears to lower cholesterol via the same mechanism employed by the statin drugs—but it doesn't trigger some of the side effects seen with these medicines. Policosanol is believed to help reduce the risk of heart attack and related illnesses by lowering total cholesterol and LDL cholesterol; increasing HDL cholesterol; inhibiting the conversion of LDL to its more dangerous oxidized form; clearing away cholesterol deposits in the heart, liver, and fatty tissues; and inhibiting the formation of blood clots.

Several studies have shown that policosanol can help lower elevated cholesterol levels.

◆ In a study published in 2002, Cuban researchers enlisted 205 volunteers to test the effects of policosanol in people who had elevated cholesterol and were also taking beta-blockers, a type of blood pressure medication.[36] The volunteers, ages 60 to 80, were randomly assigned to receive either 5 milligrams of policosanol or placebo every day for 3 years. At study's end, the data showed that policosanol had lowered total cholesterol by 23.2 percent, LDL cholesterol by 34.3 percent, and blood fats by 21.2 percent and raised HDL by 12.3 percent compared to placebo.

◆ Policosanol was pitted head-to-head against the standard cholesterol-lowering drug lovastatin (Mevacor) in a randomized, double-blind study published in 2002.[37] The 36 volunteers for this study had elevated cholesterol levels as well as type 2 diabetes. After following a cholesterol-lowering diet for 4 weeks, they were randomly assigned to receive either 10 milligrams of policosanol or 20 milligrams of lovastatin every day for 8 weeks. Both policosanol and lovastatin produced statistically significant reductions in total cholesterol, LDL cholesterol, and blood fats, and increases in HDL cholesterol. (See Table 14-5 below.) The researchers noted that while policosanol and the drug produced similar reductions in these crucial heart disease risk factors, policosanol was "slightly more effective" in reducing two important heart disease risk factor ratios (LDL to HDL and total cholesterol to HDL), in increasing protective HDL levels, and in slowing the oxidation of LDL to its more dangerous form.

Table 14-5: Policosanol and Lovastatin Improve Cholesterol/Blood Fat Levels[38]

	Policosanol	Lovastatin
Total cholesterol	-21.1%	-18.0%
LDL cholesterol	-29.9%	-25.0%
Blood fats (triglycerides)	-13.6%	-10.9%
HDL cholesterol	+12.5%	+8.3%

♦ In one of the larger policosanol studies, 589 men and women with elevated cholesterol levels and elevated blood pressure were randomly assigned to receive either policosanol or a placebo every day for 1 year.[39] Those in the policosanol group began with 5 milligrams per day, doubling to 10 milligrams per day if the smaller dose did not lower their cholesterol levels sufficiently after 6 months. The final results were positive, with policosanol producing statistically significant reductions of 15.4 percent in total cholesterol, 20.5 percent in LDL cholesterol, and 11.9 percent in blood fats, along with an increase of 12.7 percent in HDL cholesterol compared to baseline levels. The researchers concluded that "policosanol administered long term is effective in lowering" total and LDL cholesterol levels and blood fats as well as in raising HDL cholesterol.

♦ A 2005 meta-analysis published in the journal *Pharmacotherapy* combined the data from 29 randomized, double-blind, placebo-controlled studies.[40] These studies involved more than 2,900 people, lasted from 4 to 104 weeks, and gave the volunteers policosanol doses averaging 12 milligrams per day. As Table 14-6 on the next page shows, policosanol therapy reduces total cholesterol, LDL cholesterol, and blood fats while increasing HDL cholesterol.

Table 14-6: Policosanol Outperforms Placebo in Meta-Analysis of 29 Cholesterol Studies[41]

	Change Triggered by Policosanol	Change Triggered by Placebo
Total cholesterol	-16.2%	-0.6%
LDL cholesterol	-23.7%	-0.1%
Blood fats (triglycerides)	-12.4%	+2.4%
HDL cholesterol	+10.6%	-3.3%

Summing Up the Evidence for Policosanol

Policosanol has performed well in numerous studies involving some 3,000 volunteers, with some of them taking the supplement for up to 2 years. However, the bulk of the studies were performed by the same group of researchers from the Surgical Medical Research Center in Havana, Cuba. Their methodology and techniques may be first-rate, but medical evidence produced primarily by a single researcher or group of researchers is considered inferior to the same amount of evidence generated by different researchers working with different population groups. With this in mind, it is fair to say that policosanol is a three-star treatment for elevated cholesterol backed by intriguing evidence.

Available Forms

Policosanol is available in supplement form.

How Much Policosanol Is Typically Used

There is no standard dose of policosanol. Supplemental doses may range from 5 to 20 milligrams per day.

Possible Side Effects and Interactions

Policosanol has been used in various long-term, large-scale studies and has been given to the elderly and to patients with diabetes or severe liver or kidney problems without triggering significant side effects. It may interact with drugs that thin the blood, such as ibuprofen (Advil) or heparin, which could increase the risk of bleeding and bruising. If you're taking any medication, be sure to consult your doctor before adding policosanol to your self-care regimen.

15

ALTERNATIVE APPROACHES TO

INSOMNIA

Acupuncture ☆☆☆☆
Melatonin ☆☆
Valerian ☆☆
Yoga ☆☆

Insomnia is prolonged or abnormal sleeplessness that can manifest in different ways. For example, if you have *sleep-onset insomnia*, you're not able fall asleep once you go to bed. You may count sheep, toss and turn, or turn on the lights and read, but sleep eludes you. If your problem is *sleep maintenance insomnia*, you have no trouble falling asleep. In the middle of the night, however, you suddenly find yourself wide awake and unable to nod off again.

Another version of insomnia involves waking up at least an hour earlier than necessary and staying awake. Or you may have no trouble falling asleep and staying asleep—but your sleep quality is poor, leaving you exhausted and unrefreshed when you wake up.

Insomnia is a common problem that affects about 70 million Americans, nearly 60 percent of whom have a chronic disorder.[1] The elderly are the most likely to have sleep problems, which affect more than half of those over age 65. But a surprising number of children—about 25 percent of kids ages 1 to 5—also suffer from sleep disturbances.

SYMPTOMS

The most obvious symptom of insomnia is an inability to fall asleep, stay asleep, or be refreshed by sleep. All of these result in next-day fatigue, irritability, anxiety, depression, and difficulty concentrating. Insomnia can be self-perpetuating because it tends to make people anxious about not sleeping enough. This anxiety, in turn, can make sleep even more elusive.

CAUSES

The causes of insomnia can run the gamut from something as simple as a poor sleep environment—one that is too hot, too cold, too noisy, or not dark enough or that has an uncomfortable mattress or pillow—to a medical condition. Some physical conditions that are known to disrupt sleep include changes in hormone levels; fluctuations in body temperature; low blood sugar; allergies, sleep apnea and other breathing problems; urinary problems; heartburn and other gastrointestinal problems; pain; and dementia. During menopause, women may have trouble sleeping due to hot flashes, night sweats, or bladder problems. Lifestyle factors such as lack of exercise, working irregular shifts, and jet lag can contribute to insomnia.

Anxiety and depression can make sleeping difficult, as can psychological conditions such as anorexia nervosa, mania, schizophrenia, and panic disorder. Certain mood-altering substances and medications also can interfere with sleep. They include alcohol, caffeine, cigarettes, and cocaine in the former category amphetamines, antidepressants, beta-blockers, decongestants, diet pills, and steroids in the latter.

STANDARD TREATMENTS

Standard treatments for insomnia begin with environmental and lifestyle changes and may progress to medications. Generally, it's important to establish good sleeping habits, to follow a bedtime routine, to create an environment that encourages sleep, to stay away from substances that can interfere with sleep, and to get plenty of exercise (but not too close to bedtime). Relaxation techniques such as meditation and hot baths (though again, not too close to bedtime) can be helpful in calming the body and the mind so that you can fall asleep and stay asleep.

For particularly stubborn sleep problems, some doctors may prescribe sleep aids in the form of sedatives, mild tranquilizers, or antianxiety drugs. Benzodiazepines, originally designed to treat anxiety, are the most common sleep aids currently prescribed.

RATING POPULAR ALTERNATIVE TREATMENTS FOR INSOMNIA

Acupuncture

Rating: ☆☆☆☆ = Strong Evidence

Acupuncture is an ancient Chinese discipline in which very fine needles are inserted at certain points on the body. These points are located along tiny invisible channels known as meridians. Energy moves through the body along these meridians. If energy becomes blocked, it can lead to illness. The purpose of acupuncture is to unblock this vital energy, so the body can heal itself.

Acupuncture is known for its extremely calming effect on the nervous system. It is thought to help correct imbalances in the body that may contribute to insomnia, as well as bring about a general sense of well-being.

◆ Canadian researchers looked at the effects of acupuncture on 18 adults suffering from anxiety and insomnia.[2] In this open study, published in 2004, twice-weekly acupuncture treatments for 5 weeks led to significant improvements in the amount of time the volunteers needed to fall asleep, their total sleep time, and other measures of sleep quality. There also was a significant increase in nighttime secretion of melatonin, which may be a factor in improved sleep.

◆ For a 2005 study reported in the journal *Acupuncture in Medicine*, 30 pregnant women suffering from insomnia were randomly assigned to either an acupuncture group or a control (no acupuncture) group.[3] Both groups were given instruction in sleep hygiene (good sleep habits). They rated the severity of their insomnia on a numeric scale from 0 to 10, with 0 indicating good sleep and 10 indicating severe insomnia. At the end of the 8-week treatment period, the rating in the acupuncture group had fallen by 5.1 points, which the researchers considered a large and statistically significant improvement. The rating in the control group, meanwhile, showed no improvement.

Summing Up the Evidence for Acupuncture

Although these and many other acupuncture/insomnia studies have produced positive results, a large number of studies have produced equivocal or negative results. And many of the studies have been criticized for looking at small numbers of participants and for weaknesses in the study protocols.

In its 1997 consensus statement on acupuncture, the National Institutes of Health (NIH) took note of these limitations but concluded that "acupuncture may be useful as an adjunct treatment or an acceptable alternative to be included in a comprehensive management program" for insomnia. In 2003 the World Health Organization stated that acupuncture can alleviate insomnia.[4]

The debate over the efficacy of acupuncture undoubtedly will continue for many years. Nevertheless, based on the NIH and World Health Organization statements, it is fair to say that acupuncture is a four-star treatment for insomnia backed by strong evidence.

Possible Side Effects

When properly administered, acupuncture usually produces no side effects. In rare cases, there may be slight bruising or a small amount of bleeding where the needles are inserted. Some people have reported dizziness after treatment.

Finding an Acupuncturist

For more information on acupuncture, or for help in finding a certified acupuncturist, visit the National Certification Commission for Acupuncture and Oriental Medicine (NCCAOM) Web site at www.nccaom.org. The commission is the acupuncture profession's equivalent of the American Medical Association.

Melatonin

Rating: ☆☆ = Modest Evidence

Melatonin is a natural hormone manufactured in the brain that plays a role in sleep and body rhythms. The body produces more melatonin at night to encourage sleepiness and less during the day to promote a more "awake" feeling. People with insomnia often have lower levels of melatonin than the general population, which may be a major contributing factor to their sleep troubles.

Several studies have indicated that melatonin may be a useful sleep aid in certain people, particularly older insomniacs. For example:

♦ Researchers from the Massachusetts Institute of Technology tested the effects of melatonin (supplied by Nestlé) on 30 insomniacs and normal sleepers over age 50.[5] For this double-blind, placebo-controlled study, the participants were given three varying doses of melatonin (0.1 milligram, 0.3 milligram, and 3.0 milligrams) and a placebo—each for a week, in random order. The doses were taken 30 minutes before bedtime. The middle dose, 0.3 milligram of melatonin, "restored sleep efficiency"—that is, it increased the amount of time spent asleep compared to the amount of time spent in bed. What's more, the melatonin levels did not remain high during daylight hours, which would contribute to daytime sleepiness.

♦ Israeli researchers studied the effects of melatonin on melatonin-deficient elderly insomniacs and published their findings in a 1995 edition of the journal *Sleep*.[6] The volunteers were given various doses of melatonin, both fast-release and sustained-release, for various periods of time. They also were given a placebo at specific times. The results were positive. One week of treatment with 2 milligrams of sustained-release melatonin improved sleep maintenance, while 1 week of treatment with 2 milligrams of fast-release melatonin improved the ability to initiate sleep. After the participants stopped taking melatonin, their sleep quality declined.

♦ For a randomized, double-blind, crossover study published in *Lancet* in 1995, 12 elderly volunteers complaining of insomnia were given 2 milligrams of controlled-release melatonin (brand name Circadin) every night for 3 weeks, then a placebo every night for the same amount of time.[7] The results were positive, with sleep efficiency being "significantly greater after melatonin than after placebo." The researchers concluded that "melatonin deficiency may have an important role in the high frequency of insomnia among elderly people. Controlled-release melatonin replacement therapy effectively improves sleep quality in this population."

Summing Up the Evidence for Melatonin

Although melatonin has performed well in several studies, it has not passed muster in others. This result is not surprising, given the numerous variables in the studies. They include the many causes and types of sleep disturbances; the different ages of the study participants; and other disparate characteristics of the participants—such as whether they were taking other medications, whether they had another medical condition such as depression or Alzheimer's, and whether they were at home or in the hospital during the study. Then there are the questions of their ability to produce their own melatonin and how their bodies use the hormone. Given the rather confusing, if hopeful, state of the research, it is fair to say that melatonin is a two-star treatment for insomnia backed by modest evidence.

Available Forms

Melatonin is available in tablet, capsule, lozenge, and tea form in health food and vitamin stores. Very small amounts of the hormone are found in rice, barley, oats, and certain other foods.

How Much Melatonin Is Typically Used

There is no standard dose of melatonin. Supplemental doses may range from 0.3 to 5 milligrams per day.

Possible Side Effects and Interactions

Among the more serious side effects of melatonin—typically seen with larger dosages—are depression, headache, lethargy, an increased risk of seizure, inhibition of ovulation, suppression of male sexual drive, and low sperm count. When combined with drugs or substances that depress the central nervous system, such as alcohol, melatonin may cause additional sedation. It also can stimulate immune function and may interfere with immunosuppressant drugs such as prednisone (Deltasone). If you're taking any medication, be sure to consult your doctor before adding melatonin to your self-care regimen.

Valerian

Rating: ☆☆ = Modest Evidence

Valerian, a flowering plant native to Europe and Asia, has been used since ancient Roman times to relax the central nervous system, relieve anxiety and stress, and induce sleep. Its medicinal compounds are found in the root; in fact, dried extracts of the root are ingredients in virtually all herbal sleep aids.

The use of valerian waned in the 1940s, when the pharmaceutical industry began to develop more-potent sleep aids. But interest in the herb revived in the 1970s with the advent of more natural approaches to maintaining good health. Since that time, valerian has been put to the test as a sleep aid in several studies. For example:

♦ One hundred twenty-eight people participated in a randomized, double-blind, placebo-controlled trial of the effects of valerian on sleep that was published in 1982.[8] All of the study volunteers received three doses of each of the following: 400 milligrams of a valerian extract; an over-the-counter product containing valerian plus hops (brand name Hova); and a placebo. The volunteers took one dose at a time on nonconsecutive nights and in random order, 1 hour before bedtime. The next day, they filled out a postsleep questionnaire. By the end of the study, the valerian—whether in extract form or in combination with hops—produced "a significant decrease in subjectively evaluated sleep latency scores and a significant improvement in sleep quality." Sleep quality in those who were habitually poor or irregular sleepers increased markedly with valerian but did not change in those who were habitually good sleepers.

♦ For a randomized, double-blind, controlled trial published in 2002, 202 people suffering from insomnia were given either 600 milligrams of a valerian extract (brand name Sedonium) or 10 milligrams of the standard medication oxazepam (Serax), which is sometimes prescribed for people who have trouble staying asleep.[9] The effects on sleep were measured by the Sleep Questionnaire B, the Clinical Global Impression Scale, and other tools, which found that the herb was as effective as the drug in improving sleep quality. The researchers concluded that during the 6-week study, the valerian extract demonstrated "comparable efficacy" to the drug. Both substances increased the duration of sleep and the sense of being refreshed after sleep, but valerian was less likely than oxazepam to produce a hangover effect the following day.

♦ A 2003 study performed by German researchers looked at the effects of both a single dose of valerian and a 2-week course of treatment with the herb.[10] Sixteen adults—all suffering from insomnia not associated with a medical condition or another underlying problem—participated in this randomized, double-blind crossover study. During one of two 2-week trial periods, the volunteers took 600 milligrams of valerian root extract (brand name Sedonium) 1 hour before bedtime each night. During the other 2-week trial period, they took a placebo. Valerian taken over the course of 2 weeks showed a positive effect on slow-wave sleep, a form of sleep that plays an important role in physical recovery. The herb also produced a "positive effect on sleep structure and sleep perception of insomnia patients." The single dose of valerian didn't appear to produce these results, which suggests that the herb must be taken over a longer period of time to be effective. The researchers recommended that valerian be used for the treatment of mild insomnia triggered by psychological/social factors, as opposed to underlying illness or another physical problem.

Summing Up the Evidence for Valerian

Although some studies have shown that valerian can be useful as a sleep aid, the results of other studies have muddied the waters, allowing some experts to claim the herb is effective while others say the evidence is inconclusive. At this point, it is best to say that valerian is a two-star treatment for insomnia backed by modest evidence.

Available Forms

Valerian is available in capsule, tincture, liquid, extract, crude herb, and tea form.

How Much Valerian Is Typically Used

There is no standard dose of valerian. Supplemental doses may range from 400 to 900 milligrams per day.

Possible Side Effects and Interactions

When taken for a long period of time (more than a month), valerian can cause uneasiness, restlessness, headache, irregular heartbeat, and insomnia. Though rare, there have been reports of gastrointestinal problems and contact allergies.

Valerian can interact with a large number of drugs—especially those with sedative effects, such as benzodiazepines (Valium) and barbiturates

(Seconal), possibly limiting their effectiveness or triggering side effects. If you're taking any medication, be sure to consult your doctor before adding valerian to your self-care regimen.

Yoga

Rating: ☆☆ = Modest Evidence

Yoga is the ancient practice of balancing mind, body, and spirit in an effort to achieve the highest form of good health. There are many kinds of yoga, all of which involve the use of various standing, sitting, or lying-down postures called *asanas*, which are held for a period of seconds or minutes and accompanied by deep breathing.

A relatively small amount of published research has examined yoga's effect on insomnia.

◆ A researcher from Brigham and Women's Hospital, Harvard Medical School, published the results of his study in *Applied Psychophysiology and Biofeedback* in 2004.[11] This study was based on the theory that chronic insomnia is affected by mental and physiological arousal and that soothing the arousal would aid in sleep. The 20 volunteers were given a 1-hour training session in which they learned the yoga exercises they would be using for the study. Then for the next 8 weeks, the volunteers performed these exercises each evening, just before bedtime. They kept daily sleep–wake diaries beginning 2 weeks before the yoga treatment and continuing throughout the 8 weeks of treatment. The results were positive, with yoga significantly improving sleep efficiency, total sleep time, sleep onset latency, and sleep quality—all of which are important subjective sleep measures.

◆ Researchers in India enlisted 69 residents of a senior citizens' home for their 2005 study of insomnia.[12] The participants were randomly assigned to practice yoga, take an Ayurvedic herbal formula, or receive no treatment over a period of 6 months. The yoga sessions—which were performed for 60 minutes, 6 days a week—included physical activity, yoga postures, relaxation, breathing techniques, and yoga philosophy. All of the participants filled out a daily sleep rating questionnaire. The results were positive, with those practicing yoga experiencing "a significant decrease in the time taken to fall asleep . . . an increase in the total number of hours asleep . . . and in the feeling of being rested in the morning."

Summing Up the Evidence for Yoga

Given that certain yoga practices can be mentally and psychologically sooth-ing, the idea that yoga can help relieve certain types of insomnia is plausible. However, the number of studies supporting its scientific validity as an insomnia remedy is small, and issues such as the most appropriate yoga styles or postures have not been addressed. Given the relative paucity of research and the many unanswered questions, it is reasonable to say that yoga is a two-star treatment for insomnia backed by modest evidence.

16

ALTERNATIVE APPROACHES TO

MENOPAUSAL HOT FLASHES

Black cohosh ☆☆☆☆
Soy ☆☆☆

Menopausal hot flashes are waves of heat that typically start in the chest or neck and spread upward to the face, increasing skin temperature by as much as 8 degrees. They significantly pump up heart and breathing rates and trigger drenching sweats. When they occur at night, hot flashes are referred to as night sweats; they can awaken a woman from a deep sleep to find herself and her nightclothes soaked with perspiration.

A hot flash is the body's way of cooling itself by allowing heat to escape through the skin, so as the skin heats up, the body's inner temperature may actually drop. Some women experience chills immediately after a hot flash, while others may have chills combined with a bout of drenching perspiration (a "cold sweat").

Hot flashes affect up to 85 percent of American women.[1] They usually begin as estrogen levels start to wane during perimenopause. Most women who experience hot flashes do so for about a year,[2] although some may have them for more than 5 years[3] and a few for up to 15 years.

SYMPTOMS

The most obvious symptom of a hot flash is a sudden feeling of heat that seems to come out of nowhere and spreads throughout the upper body and face. Hot flashes vary in intensity; while some generate a moderate sensation of warmth, others may be so intense that they feel like a fever. This sudden blast of heat is often followed by sweating, chills, and clamminess. Hot flashes may be accompanied by anxiety, dizziness, nausea, heart palpitations, and tingling in the fingers. Because they can disrupt sleep, hot flashes and accompanying night sweats often cause fatigue, irritability, and low energy the following day.

CAUSES

Hot flashes are the result of *vasomotor changes*—that is, changes in the action of the nerves and muscles that determine the width of blood vessels—linked to declining estrogen levels. Although no one knows for sure what causes these vasomotor changes, one theory holds that they have something to do with a confused hypothalamus. The hypothalamus is the part of the brain that regulates both the sex hormones and body temperature. When the body becomes too hot, the hypothalamus sends a message to the blood vessels just beneath the surface of the skin, instructing them to dilate so that heat from the blood can escape through the skin. But as estrogen levels begin to wane, the hypothalamus may start triggering the dilation of blood vessels even when it isn't necessary. So a blast of heat can suddenly spread throughout the upper body for no apparent reason.

STANDARD TREATMENTS

The most effective treatment for hot flashes is estrogen replacement therapy, which was the standard practice until 2002. That's when preliminary results from the Women's Health Initiative—a long-term study involving 16,000 women—showed that those who used hormone replacement therapy were at increased risk for breast cancer, blood clots, heart attacks, and strokes. Since then, physicians and their female patients have, for the most part, steered clear of hormone replacement as a treatment for hot flashes.

There are certain nonhormonal drugs that may help reduce the intensity of hot flashes—among them clonidine, a medication for high blood pressure, and the antidepressants paroxetine, sertraline, and venlafaxine. Nondrug treatments include avoiding hot beverages, caffeine, alcohol, and spicy foods; wearing clothing made from breathable fabrics and dressing in layers that can be removed and replaced according to body temperature; getting plenty of exercise; and losing excess weight.

RATING POPULAR ALTERNATIVE TREATMENTS FOR MENOPAUSAL HOT FLASHES

Black Cohosh

Rating: ☆ ☆ ☆ ☆ = Strong Evidence

Among Native Americans, black cohosh (*Cimicifuga racemosa*)—a member of the buttercup family—is a traditional remedy for "women's complaints" such as menstrual discomforts and the pain of childbirth. Since the 1700s, Western civilizations have been using the herb to treat menopausal symptoms. Up until the early 1900s, it was listed as a drug in the US Pharmacopoeia. Today it remains a popular remedy in Germany, where it is widely prescribed to treat menopausal complaints.

Black cohosh contains isoflavonoids, vitamin C, beta-carotene, selenium, and numerous other nutrients. In addition, the herb may exert estrogen-like effects in the body. A number of studies have indicated that black cohosh may be helpful in relieving hot flashes. Among them:

♦ A 2005 study published in *Obstetrics & Gynecology* looked at the effects of black cohosh extract on menopausal complaints.[4] For this double-blind study, 304 women were randomly assigned to receive either 20 milligrams of black cohosh (Remifemin) or a placebo twice daily for 12 weeks. The researchers used the Menopause Rating Scale 1 to track 10 menopausal complaints, including vaginal dryness, urinary tract symptoms, depression, and hot flashes. The herb worked best at alleviating hot flashes, causing a statistically significant drop in their frequency.

♦ A 2005 study published in *Gynecological Endocrinology* compared black cohosh to transdermal estradiol (a form of estrogen applied to the skin) in 64 postmenopausal women.[5] The volunteers were randomly assigned to use either 40 milligrams of black cohosh (Remifemin) or transdermal estradiol (Estraderm) every day for 3 months. Those given the estradiol also received a synthetic form of progesterone called dihydrogesterone during the last 12 days of the 3-month study period. Both the herb and the drug "reduced significantly the number of hot flushes per day," from approximately 10 to approximately 5. This finding led the researchers to conclude that black cohosh "may be considered a consistent and safe option to counteract specific symptoms in menopausal women."

♦ Researchers from Semmelweis University in Hungary enlisted slightly more than 2,000 women with "symptoms of menopause that were moderate in intensity" for their 2005 study of black cohosh.[6] The women—who either could not or would not use hormone replacement therapy—took 40 milligrams of black cohosh extract (Remifemin) per day for 12 weeks. The results were positive, with the weighted scores for hot flashes falling from 9.65 at the beginning of the study to 6.95 at week 4, 4.90 at week 8, and 3.33 at week 12. Figure 16-1 below shows the improvement in selected symptoms following treatment.

Figure 16-1: Drop in Symptom Scores Following Treatment with Black Cohosh

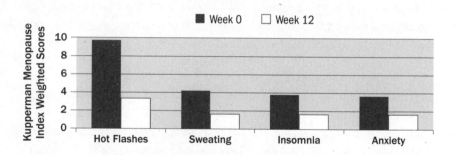

Summing Up the Evidence for Black Cohosh

The ending to the black cohosh story has yet to be written, for while many studies have shown it to be effective, others have not. Given the potentially significant differences in the black cohosh preparations and dosages, the severity of menopausal symptoms, and other variables in the various studies, the inconsistent results are not surprising. The weight of the evidence seems to suggest that black cohosh is helpful for many women experiencing hot flashes, leading to the conclusion that black cohosh is a four-star treatment for menopausal hot flashes backed by strong evidence.

Available Forms

Black cohosh is available as powdered rhizome, powdered and fluid extract, tincture, and capsules.

How Much Black Cohosh Is Typically Used

There is no standard dose of black cohosh, although some successful studies have used 40 milligrams of a standardized extract per day.

Possible Side Effects and Interactions

Black cohosh's side effects include lowered blood pressure, headache, and weight gain. In too-large doses, it may cause nausea, vomiting, sweating, and dizziness.

Black cohosh may interfere with the action of estrogens such as Premarin. It also may disrupt the absorption of ferrous fumarate (Femiron) and other medicines for iron-deficiency anemia. If you're taking any medication, be sure to consult your doctor before adding black cohosh to your self-care regimen.

Soy

Rating: ☆☆☆ = Intriguing Evidence

The soybean, which has been used medicinally in China for thousands of years, has become more and more popular in Western countries as a possible preventive or treatment for hot flashes during perimenopause and menopause. Scientists first got the idea that soy and soy products might help ease hot flashes, a common complaint among Western women, when they noticed that Japanese women almost never experienced them. One thing was strikingly different about the two populations: Japanese women ate several servings of soy each day, while Western women ate little or no soy. Could there be a connection?

The answer appears to be yes. Soy contains substances called isoflavones (e.g., genistin and diadzin), which exert weak estrogenic activity in the body. That is, these substances "plug into" estrogen receptors on cells and mimic the effects of the female hormone, but only to a small degree. In Japan, where dietary intake of soy is high (an average of 125 to 150 milligrams of soy isoflavones per day), only about 25 percent of women experience hot flashes—compared to 85 percent of North American women, who typically consume only about 1 milligram of soy isoflavones per day.[7]

Research into the effects of soy on hot flashes has produced some intriguing results. For example:

♦ A randomized study published in the journal *Menopause* in 2000 examined the effects of soy on 177 postmenopausal women suffering five or more hot flashes per day.[8] The women were randomly assigned to take either a soy isoflavone extract containing 50 milligrams total of genistin and diadzin or a placebo every day. After 12 weeks of treatment, the soy group showed a statistically significant drop in the frequency and severity of hot flashes. Those in the placebo group also improved, although not as much as the women taking the soy isoflavones. The researchers concluded that "soy isoflavone extracts provide an attractive addition to the choices available for relief of hot flashes."

♦ Italian researchers investigated the effects of soy protein on a total of 104 postmenopausal women.[9] For this randomized, double-blind, placebo-controlled trial, 51 women took 60 grams of soy protein (containing 76 milligrams of soy isoflavones, brand name Supro) per day. The other 53 women took a placebo. After 12 weeks of treatment, the women taking soy showed "a 45 [percent] reduction in their daily hot flushes versus a 30 [percent] reduction obtained with the placebo." The researchers concluded that adding soy protein to the diet "substantially reduced the frequency of hot flushes in climacteric women [women going through menopause]."

♦ For a randomized, double-blind study published in the journal *Menopause* in 2002, French researchers enlisted 75 volunteers who had undergone natural or surgical menopause and were experiencing seven or more hot flashes per day.[10] The participants were assigned to receive a soy isoflavone extract containing 70 milligrams total of genistin and diadzin (brand name Phytosoya) or a placebo every day for 4 months. Among those taking the soy extract, the average number of daily hot flashes dropped 38 percent by week 4, 51 percent by week 8, and 61 percent by week 16. This finding compared favorably to those taking the placebo, for whom the average number of daily hot flashes dropped only 21 percent. The researchers concluded, "Soy isoflavone extract may help to reduce the frequency of hot flushes in climacteric women and provides an attractive addition to the choices available for relief of hot flushes."

♦ In 2004, researchers from the University of Oklahoma Health Sciences Center examined the medical literature to produce a systematic review of menopause treatments.[11] They found soy protein to be among the complementary and alternative therapies "that have been shown to be safe and effective" for short-term relief of postmenopausal symptoms such as hot flashes.

Summing Up the Evidence for Soy

The soy picture is promising yet confusing because of its "dueling studies": Some say it does reduce the frequency and/or intensity of hot flashes, while others say it doesn't. This confusion is understandable because studies have used different forms and amounts of soy; have used different means of measuring changes in the frequency and intensity of hot flashes; have studied women who had experienced either natural or surgical menopause; and so on. In addition, most of the studies have been relatively short-term and therefore were unable to determine the effects of soy on hot flashes fter many months or years of use.

Until several large-scale, long-term studies have been conducted, we may not be able to explain why some women report good results with soy while others do not. In the meantime, it is fair to say that soy is a three-star treatment for menopausal hot flashes backed by intriguing evidence.

Available Forms

Soy is available as soybeans, soy flour, soy milk, soy oil, tofu, miso, tempeh, natto, and other foods. Soy isoflavones also come in extract form.

How Much Soy Is Typically Used

There is no standard dose of soy, although supplemental doses may be as high as 76 milligrams of soy isoflavones per day.

Possible Side Effects and Interactions

Soy's side effects include constipation, nausea, and insomnia. It may trigger an allergic reaction in some women.

Those with breast cancer or a family history of breast cancer should be very cautious about using soy products, as there is conflicting evidence about whether soy has a positive or negative effect on the disease. Although soy isoflavone extract has been used in some studies, it is not recommended because too many soy chemicals may interfere with mineral absorption, thyroid function, and/or cognitive function.

Soy may interact with and reduce the effectiveness of medicines for cancer, such as tamoxifen (Nolvadex). It also may interfere with the absorption of medicines for iron-deficiency anemia, such as ferrous fumarate (Femiron). If you're taking any medication, be sure to consult your doctor before adding therapeutic amounts of soy to your self-care regimen.

17

ALTERNATIVE APPROACHES TO

MIGRAINES

Acupuncture	☆☆☆
Magnesium	☆☆☆
Spinal manipulation	☆☆☆
Butterbur	☆☆
Feverfew	☆☆
Riboflavin	☆☆
Coenzyme Q_{10}	☆☆

Migraines are throbbing, pulsating, extremely painful headaches that settle in one side of the head. (The word *migraine* means "half a head.") More than 25 million Americans suffer from migraines, which can affect anyone at any age, though they typically begin during adolescence and young adulthood. In fact, 30 percent of those who experience migraines (known as *migraineurs*) are under age 10 when they suffer their first attacks.

Women are much more likely than men to have migraines, accounting for 70 percent of migraine patients.[1] Fortunately, both the number and the intensity of these headaches seem to decrease with age.

SYMPTOMS

Unlike other kinds of headaches, a migraine often progresses through five distinct stages. During stage one, sensitivity to light, noise, smell, or touch increases. There may be mood swings, speech or memory problems, cravings for sweets, or stiffness in the neck and shoulders—all signs of slight changes or upsets in brain activity.

In stage two, the migraineur may see a hazy light (an *aura*) surrounding an object, along with flashing or shimmering lights, sparkles, or zigzags.

During stage three, intense, throbbing pain settles in one side of the head, accompanied by nausea, vomiting, diarrhea, dizziness, weakness, and extreme sensitivity to light, noise, and smells. This stage can last for up to 3 days.

In stage four, the headache resolves itself, usually after plenty of rest and sleep—although the migraine may just disappear all of a sudden.

During stage five, once the headache has passed, the sufferer may feel achy, exhausted, or emotionally unstable for another day or two.

CAUSES

Migraines are the result of the narrowing and widening of blood vessels in the brain. The process begins when the blood vessels go into spasm and tighten up; then when they relax, they become unnaturally wide and leak plasma (the fluid part of blood) into nearby tissues. The immune system identifies the leaking plasma as the enemy, triggering an inflammatory response. This inflammation irritates the blood vessels and causes intense head pain as the blood pulses through them. The blood vessels may go through the process of clamping down and then widening excessively several times, keeping the painful migraine in play.

The constriction and dilation of the blood vessels can be set in motion by an array of factors, including alcohol consumption, cigarette smoke, certain foods, exercise, hormonal fluctuations, environmental factors, and chemical imbalances—particularly those involving serotonin, a brain chemical or neurotransmitter.

STANDARD TREATMENTS

The standard therapies for migraines fall into two categories: those that prevent the headaches and those that relieve the pain. Preventive treatments include identifying and eliminating migraine triggers like those described earlier, along with eating a healthful diet, getting regular exercise and plenty of sleep, and reducing or managing stress. Various medications may help prevent migraines, including botulinum toxin type A (Botox), antidepressants such as amitriptyline (Elavil), antiseizure medications such as divalproex sodium (Depakote), beta-blockers such as metoprolol (Lopressor), and calcium-channel blockers such as verapamil (Calan).

Pain-relieving treatments include rest and sleep, cool compresses, and avoiding light and noise. Also helpful are certain medications—among them beta-blockers such as propranolol (Inderal); ergot derivatives such as ergotamine (Cafergot); opioids such as oxycodone (OxyContin); nonsteroidal anti-inflammatory drugs such as aspirin; triptans such as almotriptan (Axert); and various combination drugs.

RATING POPULAR ALTERNATIVE TREATMENTS FOR MIGRAINES

Acupuncture

Rating: ☆☆☆ = Intriguing Evidence

The history of acupuncture as a treatment for pain dates back thousands of years. This traditional Chinese healing discipline builds on the principle that the body is brimming with energy or *qi* (pronounced "chee"), which travels around the body via a network of invisible channels called meridians. You might think of meridians as tiny rivers that wind their way throughout the body, occasionally coming close to the surface at various points called acupoints.

At times, the flow of qi can slow or become blocked, which practitioners of Traditional Chinese Medicine believe is the root of all disease. By inserting very fine needles into the appropriate acupoints, they can break up these blockages and restore the flow of qi, thus allowing the body to heal itself.

A number of studies have focused on the use of acupuncture as a treatment for migraines:

♦ Researchers from Memorial Sloan-Kettering Cancer Center randomly divided 401 volunteers with chronic headache disorder, primarily migraine, into two groups.[2] Over a period of 3 months, one group received standard care while the other group received standard care plus 12 acupuncture treatments. The researchers evaluated several indicators of headache status at the beginning of the study and again at 3 months and 12 months. They concluded that those who had received acupuncture "experienced the equivalent of 22 fewer days of headache per year." This group also "used 15 [percent] less medication . . . made 25 percent fewer visits to general practitioners . . . and took 15 percent fewer days off sick." As Figure 17-1 below shows, the Weekly Headache Score fell much more dramatically in the acupuncture group than in the standard care group. The weekly headache score is based on patients' ratings of the intensity of their migraines. The researchers concluded that "acupuncture leads to persisting, clinically relevant benefits for primary care patients with chronic headaches, particularly migraine."

Figure 17-1: Headache Score Falls in Acupuncture Group

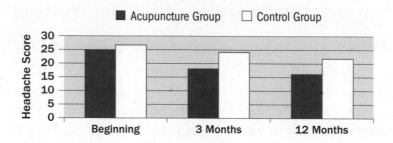

♦ A study conducted at the Center for Non-Conventional Medicines in Rome compared acupuncture to standard drug treatments for migraines.[3] One hundred twenty people suffering from migraine without aura were randomly assigned to either the acupuncture group or the standard treatment group. The researchers used a total score to measure the patients' frequency of migraines and other factors and to monitor their progress. The lower the total score, the better. Among those in the acupuncture group, the total score fell by 84 percent, compared to 64 percent in the standard treatment group.

♦ In an effort to see if acupuncture was as effective as the popular anti-migraine drug sumatriptan (Imitrex), a group of German and Swiss researchers divided 179 migraineurs into three groups.[4] When the volunteers noticed the first symptoms of a migraine, they were given traditional Chinese acupuncture, 6 milligrams of sumatriptan, or a placebo injection. The results were positive, with the acupuncture treatment preventing the development of a full-blown migraine in 35 percent of the patients who received it, compared to a 36 percent success rate with the drug and 18 percent with the placebo. Acupuncture was virtually as effective as the standard migraine medicine in aborting an impending migraine attack.

◆ For a 2002 study published in the journal *Headache*, 160 women suffering from migraine were randomly assigned to receive either acupuncture or the standard drug flunarizine (Sibelium).[5] Those in the acupuncture group received weekly treatment for the first 2 months, then monthly treatment for the next 4 months. Those in the drug group were given 10 milligrams of flunarizine daily for the first 2 months, followed by 10 milligrams for 20 days a month over the next 4 months. By the end of the 6-month study period, the number of migraine attacks and the need for medicines had dropped significantly in both groups. However, those receiving acupuncture showed significant reductions in pain intensity and side effects compared to the drug group. In short, acupuncture was as effective as the medicine in preventing migraines and was more effective at relieving pain in this group of women.

◆ The authors of a review study that appeared in the *Clinical Journal of Pain* in 2000 analyzed 27 clinical trials of acupuncture as a treatment for migraines and other types of headaches. According to the authors, 23 of the 27 trials found that "acupuncture offers benefits for the treatment of headaches."[6]

Summing Up the Evidence for Acupuncture

Although these and other acupuncture/migraine studies have produced positive results, many have been criticized for their small numbers of participants and weaknesses in their protocols. Also, a large number of studies have produced equivocal or negative results.

In its 1997 consensus statement regarding acupuncture and headaches, the National Institutes of Health took note of these limitations in concluding that "acupuncture may be useful as an adjunct treatment or an acceptable alternative to be included in a comprehensive management program" for headaches.

Based on what we know today, it is fair to say that acupuncture is a three-star treatment for migraines backed by intriguing evidence.

Possible Side Effects and Interactions

When properly administered, acupuncture usually produces no side effects. There have been a few cases of mild bruising or bleeding where the needles are inserted. Some people have reported dizziness after treatment, too.

Finding an Acupuncturist

To learn more about acupuncture, or to find a certified acupuncturist in your area, visit the Web site of the National Certification Commission for Acupuncture and Oriental Medicine (NCCAOM) at www.nccaom.com. The commission is the acupuncture profession's equivalent of the American Medical Association.

Magnesium

Rating: ☆☆☆ = Intriguing Evidence

Magnesium is an essential mineral that's necessary to convert fat, carbohydrates, and protein into energy and to regulate blood sugar, heartbeat, nerve impulses, the electrical balance within cells, and muscle contraction and relaxation. Magnesium also helps tone the blood vessels that feed the brain and keep them relaxed and open.

In some people, low blood levels of magnesium can cause the tiny muscles in the walls of the blood vessels to go into spasm. This clamping down on the blood vessels disrupts blood flow and may trigger a migraine. Low blood levels of magnesium—specifically serum ionized magnesium—have been associated with the onset of migraines in some people.

Several studies have indicated that magnesium can prevent and/or relieve migraines:

♦ In the mid-1990s, a team of physicians based at the New York Headache Center studied the effects of magnesium on migraines. Forty patients who were in the throes of a migraine headache were given intravenous infusions of magnesium sulphate.[7] Before they received the infusion, the volunteers rated the severity of their migraine pain on a scale of 1 to 10. Then they rated their pain twice more: 15 minutes after receiving the magnesium infusion and 24 hours later. The results of the study were positive: Within 15 minutes of receiving the magnesium sulphate, 9 of the

40 patients reported that their migraine pain had completely disappeared, while another 26 stated that their pain levels fell by half or more. Of this group of 35 responders, 21 were pain-free 24 hours later.

While intravenous magnesium sulphate appears to be effective for many, it certainly is not as practical as magnesium in tablet form. But can magnesium taken orally have the same pain-relieving effect? Some studies, including the following, suggest that it can:

♦ A team of German researchers randomly divided 81 men and women with migraine, ranging in age from 18 to 65, into two groups.[8] Every day for 12 weeks, one group received 600 milligrams of magnesium (trimagnesium dicitrate, brand name Magnesium Diasporal N 300) in tablet form, while the other group received a placebo. During this double-blind, placebo-controlled study, the researchers monitored the number of migraine attacks the participants experienced, the number of days they were migraine-free, and how often they used medicines to control their symptoms. During weeks 9 through 12, the number of migraine attacks dropped by 41.6 percent in the magnesium group compared to 15.8 percent in the placebo group. At the end of the study, the number of "migraine days" had fallen by 52.3 percent in the magnesium group, compared to 19.5 percent in the placebo group. The amount of medicine needed to control symptoms also fell significantly in the magnesium group. The researchers concluded that large doses of oral magnesium "appear to be effective in migraine prophylaxis."

♦ A 2000 study compared the effects of magnesium to two standard drugs and placebo.[9] Ninety-two men and women ranging in age from 20 to 54—all suffering from migraine, with or without aura—participated in this double-blind study. They were randomly assigned to receive 3 months of daily treatment with 1,830 milligrams of magnesium citrate, 10 milligrams of flunarizine (Sibelium), 10 milligrams of amitriptyline (Elavil), or placebo. As Table 17-1 on the next page shows, magnesium was about as effective as the two drugs in reducing the frequency and severity of migraines, and was superior to placebo. The researchers concluded that oral magnesium is effective for preventing migraines "and compares well to established drugs like flunarizine and amitriptyline both in effectiveness and occurrence of side effects."

Table 17-1: Magnesium Equal to Drugs and Superior to Placebo for Alleviating Migraine Symptoms[1]

	TREATMENT			
	Magnesium	Flunarizine	Amitriptyline	Placebo
Frequency of migraine attacks				
Beginning of study	4.2	4.1	4.3	4.3
End of 1st month	3.5	3.6	3.7	4.1
End of 2nd month	2.2	2.6	2.7	4.0
End of 3rd month	1.5	1.7	1.9	3.8
Severity of migraine attacks				
Beginning of study	2.7	2.9	2.7	2.7
End of 1st month	2.4	2.6	2.6	2.6
End of 2nd month	1.7	1.6	1.7	2.5
End of 3rd month	1.1	1.0	1.4	2.6

Magnesium has also been studied for its effect on menstrual migraines.

♦ A 1991 study published in the journal *Headache* involved 20 women suffering from menstrual migraines.[11] For this double-blind study, the women were randomly assigned to receive either 360 milligrams of magnesium pyrrolidone carboxylic acid (brand name MAG 2) or a placebo every day for 2 months. Although both treatments led to reductions in the Pain Total Index, magnesium produced better results, and only magnesium reduced the number of migraine days. The researchers concluded that magnesium supplementation could help prevent menstrual migraines.

Summing Up the Evidence for Magnesium

The idea that magnesium might prevent or relieve migraines is enticing, since for some people an intravenous injection of the mineral actually stops the headache in its tracks. Several studies of oral magnesium as a treatment for migraines suggest that the mineral is a three-star treatment for migraines backed by intriguing evidence.

Available Forms

Among the food sources of magnesium are Florida avocados, toasted wheat germ, pumpkin seeds, cooked soybeans, spinach, dry roasted almonds, peanuts, and cashews. The mineral also is available in supplement form.

How Much Magnesium Is Typically Used

There is no set dose of magnesium for treating migraines. Studies have used dosages ranging from 360 to 1,830 milligrams of magnesium per day.

Possible Side Effects and Interactions

The Food and Nutrition Board of the Institute of Medicine has set a tolerable upper intake for magnesium at 350 milligrams per day for adults. Taking too much supplemental magnesium can cause diarrhea, lethargy, and weakness. Supplemental magnesium can reduce the absorption of bisphosphonates such as alendronate (Fosamax) and tetracycline antibiotics such as demeclocycline (Declomycin). If you're taking any medication, be sure to consult your doctor before adding therapeutic amounts of magnesium to your self-care regimen.

Spinal Manipulation

Rating: ☆☆☆ = Intriguing Evidence

Both chiropractors and osteopathic doctors may use spinal manipulation to treat various health concerns.

Chiropractic treatment builds on the idea that disease results from the spinal vertebrae putting undue pressure on nearby nerves. This pressure affects the function of organs and tissues served by those nerves, damaging them and setting the stage for disease. Realigning the spine relieves the pressure on nerves, so the body can heal itself.

Several studies—some led by chiropractors, some by osteopaths—have investigated the effects of spinal manipulation on migraines:

◆ For a randomized, controlled study conducted by Australian researchers, researchers enlisted 127 migraineurs ranging in age from 10 to 70 and diagnosed according to guidelines set forth by the International Headache Society.[12] All experienced at least one migraine per month. Some of the participants received up to 16 sessions of chiropractic spinal manipulation over a 2-month period, while the rest (the control group) did not. All of the participants kept track of the frequency, intensity, and duration of their migraines, among other characteristics. Those receiving spinal manipulation showed a statistically significant reduction in migraine frequency (from 7.6 to 4.1 migraines per month). A significant number of volunteers also reported that "their medication use had reduced to zero" by the end of the study.

♦ Researchers from Northwestern College of Chiropractic in Minnesota compared spinal manipulation to the standard drug amitriptyline (Elavil) in their 1998 randomized trial.[13] The 218 migraineurs participating in this study were randomly assigned to receive spinal manipulation, amitriptyline, or both over the course of 8 weeks. Then they were observed for another 4 weeks to see if there were any "carry-over" effects. Throughout, the volunteers kept track of their headache symptoms, which were used to calculate a headache index score (with higher scores indicating more headache pain). By the end of the 8-week treatment period, headache index scores had fallen an average of 49 percent in those taking amitriptyline, 40 percent in those receiving spinal manipulation, and 41 percent in those receiving combined therapy. Four weeks later, those who had received spinal manipulation still showed a 42 percent reduction in their headache index scores, compared to a 24 percent drop among the amitriptyline group and a 25 percent drop in the combined therapy group. The researchers concluded that "spinal manipulation seemed to be as effective as a well-established and efficacious treatment (amitriptyline), and . . . should be considered a treatment option for patients with frequent migraine headaches."

♦ The Cochrane Library published a review of spinal manipulation studies in 2004.[14] The authors of the paper looked at 22 studies involving more than 2,600 patients, ranging in age from 12 to 78 and suffering from migraine and other types of headache. The authors concluded that "for the prophylactic treatment of migraine headaches, there is evidence that spinal manipulation may be an effective treatment option with a short-term effect similar to that of a commonly used, effective drug (amitriptyline)."

Summing Up the Evidence for Spinal Manipulation

There is a great deal of controversy regarding the effectiveness of spinal manipulation as a treatment for migraines. While there are studies and reviews that produced favorable results, there also are a number of studies and reviews in which spinal manipulation was found not to be helpful. There also is the problem of evaluating and rating studies of spinal manipulation and other forms of "hands-on" therapy. They do not easily lend themselves to the standard randomized, double-blind, placebo-controlled format, where one group of patients receives the "real thing" and another receives an identical-looking placebo. Given this, it is fair to say that spinal manipulation is a three-star treatment for migraines backed by intriguing evidence.

Finding a Chiropractor

To learn more about chiropractic, or to find a qualified chiropractor in your area, visit the Web site for the American Chiropractic Association (ACA) at www.amerchiro.org.

Butterbur

Rating: ☆☆ = Modest Evidence

An herbaceous plant found in North America, Europe, and Asia, butterbur is so named because the large leaves once were used to wrap butter, so it wouldn't melt in warm weather. Butterbur has a long history of use in folk medicine. It was popular as a treatment for fever and the plague during the Middle Ages and, in later centuries, as a remedy for ulcers, asthma, anxiety, cough, and wounds.

Butterbur extract—which is made from the leaves, roots, and rhizome of the shrub—contains petasin and isopetasin. These substances help quell inflammation and relax smooth muscle spasms.

A small number of studies suggest that butterbur can help prevent migraines:

♦ A paper appearing in the journal *Headache* in 2005 described what happened when 108 children and adolescents, ranging in age from 6 to

17, were given a butterbur root extract (brand name Petadolex) for their migraines.[15] For a period of 4 months, the study participants took a daily dose of between 50 and 150 milligrams of butterbur root extract, depending on their age. The results were positive, with 77 percent of the youngsters showing a 50 percent or greater decrease in the frequency of migraines. The researchers concluded that "butterbur root extract shows potential as an effective and well-tolerated migraine prophylaxis."

The results of this study are similar to those of two other studies that were double-blinded. In other words, neither the patients nor the researchers knew who was receiving the herb and who was receiving a placebo.

♦ In the first of these studies, 60 patients were randomly split into two groups, with one receiving 100 milligrams of butterbur root extract (Petadolex) and the other a placebo every day for 12 weeks.[16] By the end of the 12-week study period, 45 percent of those taking the butterbur root extract reported a 50 percent or greater reduction in the frequency of migraines compared to only 15 percent of those taking the placebo. In addition, those in the butterbur group showed a drop in the average number of attacks per month, from 3.4 to 1.8. The researchers concluded that butterbur root extract may be effective in the prevention of migraines. Figure 17-2 below shows the drop in the number of migraine attacks per month from beginning to end of treatment in the butterbur and placebo groups.

Figure 17-2: Migraine Attacks Drop with Butterbur versus Placebo

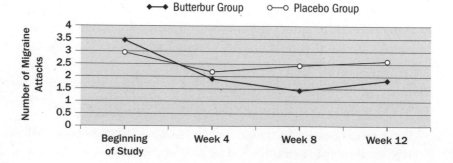

♦ The second study—a larger one involving 245 migraine patients, average age 42—appeared in the journal *Neurology* in 2004.[17] The study participants were randomly divided into three groups and given daily doses of either 150 milligrams or 100 milligrams of butterbur root extract or a placebo. The researchers were primarily interested in whether the herbal extract (supplied by Weber and Weber) would reduce the average number of migraine attacks per month. By the end of the study, the average number of migraine attacks per month had dropped by 48 percent in the group taking 150 milligrams of butterbur root extract, compared to 36 percent in those taking 100 milligrams, and 26 percent in those taking the placebo. The researchers concluded that 150 milligrams of butterbur root extract per day "is more effective than placebo and is well tolerated as a preventive therapy for migraine."

♦ A 2000 study of the effects of butterbur root extract on migraines, which was published in the *International Journal of Clinical Pharmacology and Therapeutics*, also produced positive results.[18] For this randomized, double-blind, placebo-controlled study, 58 migraineurs were given either 100 milligrams of butterbur root extract (Petadolex) or a placebo every day for 12 weeks. At the end of the study period, the average number of headaches per month fell from 3.3 to 1.7 among those taking butterbur root extract, compared to a drop from 2.9 to 2.6 among those on the placebo. The researchers concluded that the butterbur root extract can help prevent migraines.

Summing Up the Evidence for Butterbur

The butterbur/migraine research is intriguing, even though the body of evidence is relatively new and small. At this point, it is fair to say that butterbur is a two-star treatment for migraines backed by modest evidence.

Other Names

Butterbur is known to scientists as *Petasites hybridus* and is referred to in various parts of the world as blatterdock, butterfly dock, exwort, langwort, petasites flower, and umbrella leaves.

Available Forms

Butterbur is available as fresh leaves that can be made into a tea and in capsule or extract form.

How Much Butterbur Is Typically Used

A standard dose of butterbur has not been set. The dosages in successful studies have ranged from 50 to 150 milligrams per day.

Possible Side Effects and Interactions

To date, no side effects have been reported with the use of butterbur. However, the herb does contain compounds called pyrrolizidine alkaloids (PAs), which can be toxic to the liver and possibly carcinogenic. Fortunately, the herb can be processed to remove these compounds. When shopping for a butterbur product, read labels carefully and choose one that is "free of pyrrolizidine alkaloids."

Feverfew

Rating: ☆☆ = Modest Evidence

Feverfew is a perennial plant that grows throughout the world. Ancient Greeks used feverfew as a treatment for headaches as well as "female complaints," nausea, allergies, asthma, headaches, and a number of other ailments. Herbalists have long praised feverfew's effects on headache pain. Nevertheless, it was relegated to the sidelines as a headache remedy with the advent of modern pharmaceutical-based medicine. Interest in the herb picked up again in the 1970s, when more-natural approaches to pain relief came into vogue and reports of feverfew's ability to combat headaches resurfaced.

While feverfew does appear to relieve headache pain, it isn't clear how it does so or which of the active ingredients in the feverfew leaf are the most important. Among the studies of feverfew's effects on migraine pain are the following:

♦ An article published in the *British Medical Journal* in 1985 described a "reverse" study in which feverfew was withdrawn from a group of 17 people who had been taking fresh feverfew leaves daily to help prevent their migraines.[19] For this double-blind, controlled trial, eight of the volunteers were randomly assigned to receive 50 milligrams of feverfew in capsule form every day for 4 weeks. The remaining nine volunteers received a placebo. Those who took the placebo (and thus were no longer using feverfew) experienced a significant increase in the number and severity of migraines, as well migraine-associated vomiting and nausea. Those who continued to take feverfew did not show an increase in the number or severity of their headaches or migraine-associated symptoms.

♦ For a 1988 double-blind, crossover study appearing in the British medical journal *Lancet*, 72 people were randomly assigned to receive either a capsule containing 82 milligrams of feverfew powder or a placebo every day.[20] The study participants ranged in age from 24 to 72, had been suffering from migraines for at least 2 years, and had at least one attack per month. After 4 months, the groups switched treatments; those who had been taking feverfew were given a placebo, and vice versa. On average, the study participants experienced a drop in the number and severity of migraine attacks, as well as in vomiting, while taking feverfew.

♦ Researchers from Poland looked at the effects of feverfew in 24 female migraineurs, ranging in age from 19 to 61.[21] All received 5 milligrams of feverfew sap a day for periods ranging from 30 to 60 days. By the end of the study, one-third of the women scored significantly lower on a scale known as the Migraine Index. Another five also showed improvement, though to a lesser degree.

♦ In 1997 Israeli researchers presented the results of their randomized, double-blind crossover study on migraineurs.[22] Fifty-seven people, ranging in age from 9 to 65, were divided into two groups. Both groups received 100 milligrams of feverfew a day during the 60 days of Phase 1. During Phase 2, one group continued to receive 100 milligrams of feverfew daily, while the other group was given a placebo. In Phase 3, the feverfew group switched to the placebo, and vice versa. By the end of the study, the researchers noted that taking feverfew led to a significant drop in migraine pain, and to a "profound reduction" in nausea, light sensitivity, and other migraine symptoms.

♦ Researchers from the University of Exeter in the United Kingdom scoured the medical literature to find all relevant studies of feverfew and migraines to develop an overview of the herb's effects.[23] For their review article, published in 2000, they looked at six randomized, double-blind, placebo-controlled studies. They were able to conclude that feverfew "is likely to be effective in the prevention of migraine."

Summing Up the Evidence for Feverfew

There are a number of randomized, double-blind, placebo-controlled studies suggesting that feverfew is effective in relieving migraines, although some of them have been criticized for methodological flaws. Despite the possible shortcomings in some of the studies, it is reasonable to say that feverfew is a two-star treatment for migraines based on modest evidence.

Other Names

Feverfew is known to scientists as *Tanacetum parthenium* and by several other names, including altamisa, bachelor's buttons, featherfoil, and Santa Maria.

Available Forms

Feverfew is available in extract, capsule, tablet, tincture, or dried leaf form.

How Much Feverfew Is Typically Used

There is no standard dose for feverfew. A typical supplemental dose is 50 to 100 milligrams of feverfew extract per day.

Possible Side Effects and Interactions

Feverfew can suppress appetite and cause nausea, muscle stiffness, joint pain, and—if you chew the leaves—mouth ulcers. It also may interact with blood-thinning medications such as warfarin (Coumadin). If you're taking any medication, be sure to consult your doctor before adding feverfew to your self-care regimen.

Riboflavin

Rating: ☆☆ = Modest Evidence

The body uses riboflavin—also known as vitamin B_2—to help convert food into energy, support immune function, manufacture blood cells and hormones, and ward off oxidative damage. A shortage of this vitamin can cause soreness and inflammation of the lips and tongue, cracking at the corners of the mouth, itching and burning eyes, depression, and other symptoms.

The notion that riboflavin might be helpful in treating and preventing migraines came about because a lack of mitochondrial energy appears to play a role in triggering migraines, and riboflavin can "rev up" mitochondrial energy. Several studies suggest that riboflavin is indeed effective against migraines:

♦ Forty-nine people suffering from migraines participated in a study published in the journal *Cephalalgia* in 1994. For at least 3 months, all of the participants were given 400 milligrams of riboflavin a day. In addition, 23 were given 75 milligrams of aspirin per day.[24] After 3 to 5 months of treatment, migraine severity had declined by an average of 68 percent for the entire group of volunteers. There was no significant difference between the group that took riboflavin and the group that took riboflavin plus aspirin. In other words, those who took riboflavin alone experienced the same good results as those who took aspirin and riboflavin in combination. The researchers concluded that taking large amounts of riboflavin might "be an effective, low-cost prophylactic treatment of migraine."

♦ In a similar study, published in 2004, German researchers focused on volunteers who had experienced 2 to 8 migraine attacks per month during the 6 months prior to the beginning of the study. All were given 400 milligrams of riboflavin every day for 3 to 6 months. At the 3- and 6-month marks, measurements were taken of headache frequency, duration, and intensity, as well as of the use of abortive drugs (drugs that stop migraines in progress).[25] Headache duration and intensity did not change. However, headache frequency dropped from an average of four attacks per month to two. Also, the use of abortive drugs declined by 35 percent.

Both of these studies were open-label, which means that both the participants and the doctors knew that everyone was receiving riboflavin. Therefore, the findings could have been biased by the placebo effect. They needed to be validated by double-blind, placebo-controlled studies.

♦ Such a double-blind, placebo-controlled study was published in 1998 in the journal *Neurology*.[26] For this study, 55 volunteers were randomly given either 400 milligrams of riboflavin or a placebo every day for 3 months. Those taking riboflavin suffered from fewer migraines and fewer "migraine days." The researchers concluded that "because of its high efficacy, excellent tolerability, and low cost, riboflavin is an interesting option for migraine prophylaxis."

♦ Riboflavin was compared to standard migraine medications in a 2000 study published in the journal *Headache*.[27] This trial was based on the fact that when migraineurs are between attacks, certain changes are detectable in their brains. The researchers were interested in seeing whether riboflavin or standard migraine medicines—metoprolol (Lopressor) and bisoprolol (Zebeta)—would correct these changes. The 26 patients enrolled in the study were given metoprolol, bisoprolol, or 400 milligrams of riboflavin for 4 months. By the end of the study, 55 percent of those taking the medicines and 53 percent of those taking riboflavin experienced a 50 percent or greater drop in headache frequency. However, while the standard medicines seemed to "correct" the brain changes, riboflavin did not. This finding suggests that riboflavin doesn't work the same way the medicines do but does combat migraines by some other mechanism.

Summing Up the Evidence for Riboflavin

The use of riboflavin as a preventive treatment for migraine is exciting for three reasons: It appears to be as effective at preventing migraines as certain standard medications; it has none of the adverse effects seen with standard medications (such as gastrointestinal distress); and it costs far less. Still, relatively few studies of riboflavin and migraines have been published, leading to the conclusion that riboflavin is a two-star treatment for migraines based on modest evidence.

Available Forms

Riboflavin is found in liver, almonds, yogurt, milk, pork, and cooked spinach, among other foods. It also is available in supplement form.

How Much Riboflavin Is Typically Used

There is no set dose of riboflavin for treating migraines. Certain studies have used dosages of 400 milligrams of riboflavin per day.

Possible Side Effects and Interactions

The Institute of Medicine of the National Academy of Sciences has not set a tolerable upper intake for riboflavin. There are no known toxic effects associated with high doses of riboflavin, although taking large amounts for a long period of time may interfere with the metabolism of other B vitamins. As with all supplements and drugs, be sure to read the product label carefully before adding therapeutic amounts of riboflavin to your self-care regimen.

Coenzyme Q_{10}
Rating: ☆☆ = Modest Evidence

An enzyme found throughout the body and in many foods, coenzyme Q_{10} is known to be vitally important to heart health. It increases the oxygen supply to the heart, lowers total cholesterol and "bad" LDL cholesterol, and helps ward off atherosclerosis. It also improves the action of the tiny energy factories called mitochondria that reside inside each cell. But can it do anything for a migraine?

The idea that it can came about because coenzyme Q_{10} shares some energy-metabolizing and energy-improving properties with riboflavin, the vitamin that has shown much promise in combating migraines.

♦ For an open-label trial, researchers from the Jefferson Headache Center of Thomas Jefferson University enlisted 31 migraineurs to take 150 milligrams of CoQ_{10} every day for 3 months.[28] The results were positive, with 61 percent of the volunteers reporting a 50 percent or greater drop in the number of "migraine days." The researchers concluded that "coenzyme Q_{10} appears to be a good migraine preventive." Figure 17-3 on the next page shows the change in headache frequency in individual patients from the time they began receiving CoQ_{10} to the end of the treatment period.

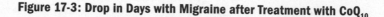

Figure 17-3: Drop in Days with Migraine after Treatment with CoQ$_{10}$

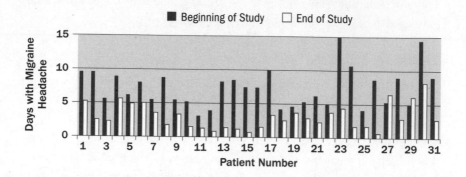

♦ In 2005 the results of a randomized, double-blind, placebo-controlled study were published in the journal *Neurology*.[29] Researchers from the Headache and Pain Unit at University Hospital Zurich, Switzerland, gave daily doses of either 300 milligrams of CoQ$_{10}$ or a placebo to 42 migraine patients. They found that the CoQ$_{10}$ (which had been supplied by MSE Pharmazeutika GmbH) was superior to placebo in reducing the frequency of migraine attacks. Specifically, 47.6 percent of those taking CoQ$_{10}$ showed a 50 percent drop in frequency compared to 14.4 percent of those taking the placebo. In addition, the CoQ$_{10}$ group experienced fewer "migraine days" and fewer days with nausea. The researchers concluded that "CoQ$_{10}$ is efficacious and well tolerated."

Summing Up the Evidence for Coenzyme Q$_{10}$

With only a small amount of research into the effects of CoQ$_{10}$ on migraines to rely on, CoQ$_{10}$ is a two-star treatment for migraines based on modest evidence.

Available Forms

CoQ$_{10}$ is manufactured in the body. You can get additional amounts of the enzyme from supplements and from a variety of foods, including beef, chicken, trout, salmon, oranges, and broccoli. Unfortunately, levels of CoQ$_{10}$ will decrease if you take Lipitor or other statin drugs to combat elevated blood fats and cholesterol, since these drugs interfere with production of the enzyme.

How Much Coenzyme Q_{10} Is Typically Used

There is no standard dose of CoQ_{10}. Some studies used dosages in the range of 150 to 300 milligrams per day.

Possible Side Effects and Interactions

CoQ_{10} can cause stomach upset and reduce blood pressure. It could trigger dangerously low blood pressure if combined with antihypertensive medications such as metoprolol (Lopressor). If you're taking any medication, be sure to consult your doctor before adding CoQ_{10} to your self-care regimen.

18

ALTERNATIVE APPROACHES TO

OSTEOARTHRITIS

Acupuncture	☆☆☆☆
Chondroitin sulfate	☆☆☆☆
Glucosamine	☆☆☆☆
Cetylated fatty acids	☆☆☆
Devil's claw	☆☆☆
SAMe	☆☆☆
Magnets	☆☆
Tai chi	☆☆

Osteoarthritis (OA) is a disease of the cartilage—the tough, rubbery, water-filled substance that caps the ends of the bones within a joint, allowing them to slide easily across each other during movement. Healthy cartilage also functions as a shock absorber, cushioning the bones against the impact created by weight-bearing activity. In OA the cartilage breaks down and becomes dry, cracked, and rough. It may even wear through completely, allowing bones to grind together. Osteoarthritis typically results in joint pain and stiffness that ranges from mild to excruciating, accompanied by limited mobility. Over time, OA damages and may even destroy the affected joint.

SYMPTOMS

The hallmark of OA is joint pain, usually a deep ache that originates in the joint's core. Other symptoms include joint stiffness; limited range of motion; warmth, swelling, and tenderness around the joint; and "crackling" or popping in the joint with movement. Some people develop bony growths at the ends of the fingers (called Heberden's nodes) or on the middle joints of the fingers (called Bouchard's nodes). As cartilage wears away, there is a narrowing of the amount of space between bone ends that can be detected via x-rays.

CAUSES

There are two kinds of osteoarthritis: *primary*, which has no known cause, and *secondary*, which is triggered by another problem.

While the cause of primary OA is uncertain, the end result is very clear: The meshlike substance called collagen that gives cartilage its structure becomes weak and loose, losing its resiliency. When this happens, special water-retaining molecules that are intertwined among the collagen fibers begin to float out of the cartilage and into the joint fluid. The cartilage is no longer able to attract and retain fluid, and so it becomes dry, thin, and vulnerable to damage—a much less effective shock absorber.

Unlike primary OA, secondary OA does have a definitive cause: trauma to the joint. The trauma can result from injury, repetitive motion, damage to the bone ends, excess body weight, or bone disease. Though osteoarthritis may develop soon after the trauma occurs, sometimes it doesn't appear for years or even decades.

With either kind of OA, once the cartilage has been damaged, the body's natural repair processes can make the problem worse. Overproduction of new cartilage to "fix" cracks or tears can create a rough, bumpy area in the cartilage that causes even more irritation within the joint. The body may also overproduce bone when the cartilage has worn through and bone ends begin to grind together. In an attempt to protect the bone, the body makes extra bone in the form of bony spurs or overgrowths—which, unfortunately, grind against the opposing bone even more.

STANDARD TREATMENTS

The standard treatments for OA—whether primary or secondary—include pain-relieving medication, hot and cold packs, proper body alignment, exercise, and weight loss. The pain relievers of choice typically are acetaminophen, when no swelling is present, and nonsteroidal anti-inflammatory drugs (NSAIDs), when swelling is present. Hot and cold packs either relax or numb painful areas; proper body alignment can ease joint wear and tear and protect against further injury; exercise helps lubricate and nourish the joints; and weight loss can alleviate a great deal of the stress and strain on weight-bearing joints.

RATING POPULAR ALTERNATIVE TREATMENTS FOR OSTEOARTHRITIS

Acupuncture

Rating: ☆☆☆☆ = Strong Evidence

The ancient Chinese healing discipline known as acupuncture seeks to treat disease by balancing the flow of energy in the body. The basic theory behind acupuncture is that energy moves through the body along tiny, invisible channels called meridians. If a meridian should become blocked, the flow of energy will slow or stop, causing illness. By inserting very fine needles at specific points where the meridians rise close to the surface of the skin, the energy becomes unblocked and moves freely again. In turn, the body can begin to heal itself.

Acupuncture has a long history as a treatment for pain and other symptoms of osteoarthritis. Its benefits are supported by studies such as these:

♦ The effects of acupuncture were tested on 570 people with OA of the knee for a study published in the *Annals of Internal Medicine* in 2004.[1] For this controlled trial, the volunteers were randomly assigned to receive one of three treatments over the course of 26 weeks: 23 acupuncture treatments, 23 sham acupuncture treatments, or education on self-managing the problems associated with arthritis. (For the sham treatments, either the needles were inserted into the wrong acupuncture points or the points were lightly touched with a plastic needle that was not inserted into the body.) The researchers used the Western Ontario and McMaster Universities Osteoarthritis Index (WOMAC) pain and function scores as the primary tool to monitor the patients' progress. At the end of the treatment period, those receiving true acupuncture had experienced significantly greater improvement in pain and function than those receiving sham acupuncture or education about self-care. In the true acupuncture group, pain scores dropped an average of 40 percent and function scores improved nearly 40 percent compared to the beginning of the study. The researchers concluded that "true traditional Chinese acupuncture is safe and effective for reducing pain and improving physical function in patients with symptomatic knee osteoarthritis who have moderate or greater pain" despite the use of standard medicines. Table 18-1 below summarizes some of the study results.

Table 18-1: After 26 Weeks of Treatment, Acupuncture Is Superior to Sham Acupuncture or Education Alone in Reducing Osteoarthritis Symptoms[2]

AVERAGE CHANGE IN SCORE FROM BEGINNING TO END OF STUDY (LOWER IS BETTER)	CHANGE IN SYMPTOM SCORES FROM BASELINE AFTER 26 WEEKS OF TREATMENT		
	True Acupuncture Group	Sham Acupuncture Group	Education Group
WOMAC pain score	-3.79	-2.92	-1.69
WOMAC function score	-12.42	-9.88	-7.17

♦ Spanish researchers analyzed the effects of acupuncture as a complementary therapy for osteoarthritis of the knee for a 2004 study published in the *British Medical Journal*.[3] Eighty-eight people completed the trial, in which they were randomly assigned to receive 12 sessions of electroacupuncture (acupuncture with transmission of a mild electrical current) plus the standard medicine diclofenac (Cataflam), or 12 sessions of sham acupuncture plus diclofenac. The true acupuncture plus medication produced a greater and statistically significant improvement in symptoms—specifically, relieving pain, reducing stiffness, and improving physical function—compared to sham acupuncture plus medication. The researchers concluded that "acupuncture as a complementary therapy to pharmacological treatment of osteoarthritis of the knee is more effective than pharmacological treatment alone, in terms of reducing pain and rigidity, and improving physical functioning and health-related quality of life." Table 18-2 on the next page summarizes some of the study results.

Table 18-2: Acupuncture plus Drug Reduces Osteoarthritis Symptoms Better Than Sham Acupuncture plus Drug [4]

Rating Scale (Lower Is Better)	True Acupuncture Group	Sham Acupuncture Group
WOMAC total score	9.5	33.4
WOMAC pain score	1.7	6.4
WOMAC stiffness score	0.4	2.1
Pain visual analogue score	10.6	37.2

♦ German researchers published the results of their acupuncture/osteoarthritis study in the prestigious journal *Lancet* in 2005.[5] For this study, which lasted for 8 weeks, 294 people with chronic knee osteoarthritis were randomly assigned to receive either 12 sessions of acupuncture or 12 sessions of sham acupuncture (with needles inserted to a superficial depth at nonacupuncture points) or to have their names put on a waiting list to serve as controls. The researchers were interested in seeing whether acupuncture would relieve osteoarthritis symptoms (as measured by the WOMAC scale) by the end of the treatment period. After 8 weeks, true acupuncture had shown itself to be superior to the other two actions in alleviating OA symptoms. Specifically, the average WOMAC score in the true acupuncture group was 26.9, compared to 35.8 in the sham acupuncture group and 49.6 in the control group.

Summing Up the Evidence for Acupuncture

Although these and many other acupuncture/osteoarthritis studies have produced positive results, a large number of studies have produced equivocal or negative results. In addition, many of the studies have been criticized for involving small numbers of participants and for weaknesses in the study protocols.

Still, the treatment has garnered guarded recommendations from some important health organizations. For example, the World Health Organization has stated that acupuncture has a "therapeutic effect" on osteoarthritis, although further proof of its efficacy and identification of the best treatment approaches are necessary. In its 1997 consensus statement on acupuncture, the National Institutes of Health took note of these limitations but concluded that "acupuncture may be useful as an adjunct treatment or an acceptable alternative to be included in a comprehensive management program" for osteoarthritis.[6]

The debate over the therapeutic value of acupuncture undoubtedly will continue for many years. Based on the World Heath Organization finding, it is fair to say that acupuncture is a four-star treatment for osteoarthritis backed by strong evidence.

Possible Side Effects

When properly administered, acupuncture usually produces no side effects. Occasionally treatment may result in mild bruising or a small amount of bleeding where the needles are inserted. Some people have reported dizziness after treatment as well.

Finding an Acupuncturist

To learn more about acupuncture or to find a certified acupuncturist, visit the Web site for the National Certification Commission for Acupuncture and Oriental Medicine at www.nccaom.org. The commission is the acupuncture profession's equivalent of the American Medical Association.

Chondroitin Sulfate

Rating: ☆☆☆☆ = Strong Evidence

Chondroitin sulfate (CS) is a substance found in human cartilage, as well as in the skin, bone, arterial walls, and corneas. Among several other duties, chondroitin helps the body manufacture molecules called proteoglycans, which in turn help attract water to cartilage and hold it there. The water is important for keeping cartilage moist, slick, and flexible. Chondroitin sulfate also helps to slow the breakdown of collagen, which helps cartilage maintain its strength and structure.

Back in 1966, researchers noted that cartilage affected by osteoarthritis often contained lower amounts of chondroitin sulfate and that any CS in the affected joints may be altered. This finding led researchers to surmise that taking supplemental chondroitin sulfate could help strengthen the cartilage and ease symptoms of OA. The hypothesis has been borne out by a number of studies, including these:

◆ Three hundred people with OA of the knee participated in a double-blind study published in *Arthritis and Rheumatism* in 2005.[7] The volunteers were randomly assigned to receive either 800 milligrams of chondroitin sulfate (brand name Condrosulf) or a placebo every day for 2 years. The researchers were primarily interested in seeing if the supplement could halt the narrowing of joint space—that is, if it could prevent the bones in osteoarthritic joints from moving closer together. After 2 years of treatment, the joint space remained the same, on average, among those in the chondroitin group, while it narrowed among those in the placebo group. The researchers concluded that "long-term treatment with CS may retard radiographic progression [joint space narrowing] in patients with OA of the knee."

◆ A team of European and American researchers looked at the effects of chondroitin sulfate in 84 people with symptomatic OA of the knee for a 2004 double-blind study published in the journal *Osteoarthritis and Cartilage*.[8] The volunteers were randomly assigned to receive either 800 milligrams of chondroitin sulfate (Condrosulf) or a placebo every day for 2 nonconsecutive 3-month periods during the course of a year. At the end of the study, the chondroitin sulfate had significantly reduced symptom scores on the Lequesne's algo-functional index by 36 percent, compared to 23 percent for the placebo. Those taking chondroitin sulfate also experienced a significant drop in the time necessary to walk a measured distance, compared to those taking the placebo. And while joint space declined significantly in the placebo group, there was no change in the chondroitin sulfate group, suggesting that the supplement helped halt the disease process. As the researchers concluded, their study offered evidence that oral chondroitin sulfate "decreased pain and improved knee function."

◆ Italian researchers tested the effects of chondroitin sulfate on osteoarthritis of the hand for their 2004 study.[9] This study looked specifically at the joint erosion that can occur in OA of the hand in its more advanced states. The researchers were particularly interested in the number of eroded joints, as well as in the incidence of the abnormal joint enlargement known as Heberden's nodes and Bouchard's nodes. The 24 volunteers were randomly assigned to receive 800 milligrams of chondroitin sulfate (brand name Control) plus 500 milligrams of the standard drug naproxen (Naprosyn), or just 500 milligrams of naproxen, for 2 years. The chondroitin was taken daily, while the naproxen was taken only as needed. Though joint damage continued to worsen in both groups, the rate of decline was slower among those taking chondroitin. The researchers noted that chondroitin sulfate "was associated with a better clinical course of the disease, which was demonstrated by the improvement in the patients' assessment of their condition."

The chondroitin sulfate/osteoarthritis studies have been pooled for review and meta-analysis several times.

♦ Researchers from Boston University School of Medicine searched for published or unpublished double-blind, randomized, placebo-controlled studies testing chondroitin sulfate's effects on OA for their meta-analysis published in the *Journal of the American Medical Association* in 2000.[10] They statistically merged the results of 15 studies to find that chondroitin sulfate had "moderate to large effects" on OA. The researchers did question the quality of some of the studies and suggested that the results might be exaggerated.

♦ Another review published in the *Journal of Rheumatology* in 2000 pooled the results of seven trials involving 372 people who were taking chondroitin sulfate.[11] The authors of this review found that in studies lasting 4 months or longer, chondroitin sulfate "was shown to be significantly superior to placebo" as measured by the Lequesne Index and pain visual analog scale.

♦ All of the randomized, double-blind, placebo-controlled studies on chondroitin sulfate for knee or hip osteoarthritis published or performed between January 1980 and March 2002 were scrutinized for a review and meta-analysis that appeared in the *Archives of Internal Medicine* in 2003.[12] After using statistical methods to pool the results of the eligible studies, the authors reported that chondroitin sulfate was shown to be effective, triggering improvement in symptom scores on the Lequesne Index, the visual analogue scale for pain, and other assessment tools.

Summing Up the Evidence for Chondroitin Sulfate

Results from a substantial number of studies indicate that chondroitin sulfate not only effectively relieves the symptoms of OA but also may slow or halt progression of the disease—something that standard medicines cannot do. However, the results of other studies have found that chondroitin sulfate is not effective.

The recent large-scale study called GAIT (Glucosamine/Chondroitin Arthritis Intervention Trial), sponsored by the National Institutes of Health, was expected to provide definitive answers by comparing the effects of chondroitin, glucosamine, chondroitin plus glucosamine, the standard drug celecoxib (Celebrex), and placebo in people with OA of the knee. Unfortunately, the results were unclear. Although the combination of chondroitin and glucosamine was the most effective treatment for people with moderate to high levels of OA pain, chondroitin did not relieve symptoms as well as celecoxib. This led researchers to conclude that the combination of glucosamine and chondroitin sulfate "is effective in treating moderate to severe knee pain due to OA."

When weighing the positive and negative findings from the various studies, it's important to remember that chondroitin actually may halt the joint damage caused by OA, which no standard medicine can do. With this in mind, it is fair to say that chondroitin sulfate is a four-star treatment for osteoarthritis backed by strong evidence.

Available Forms

Chondroitin sulfate is available is supplement form.

How Much Chondroitin Sulfate Is Typically Used

There is no standard dose of chondroitin sulfate as a treatment for osteoarthritis. A common dosage in studies is 1,200 milligrams per day.

Possible Side Effects and Interactions

Chondroitin sulfate can cause stomach pain and nausea. It is not known to interact with medications in a significant manner. As with all supplements and drugs, be sure to read and follow label directions when adding chondroitin sulfate to your self-care regimen.

Glucosamine

Rating: ☆☆☆☆ = Strong Evidence

Glucosamine is a natural substance found in the cartilage in joints. The body uses it to make the proteoglycans that help to keep cartilage slick, resilient, and healthy. Glucosamine also slows the breakdown of cartilage and stimulates cells called chondrocytes to produce collagen, which gives cartilage structural strength and integrity.

A number of studies have shown that glucosamine can help relieve symptoms of osteoarthritis. They include the following:

♦ For a 2002 study published in the *Archives of Internal Medicine*, Czech researchers enlisted 202 men and women, ages 45 to 70, with mild to moderate OA of the knee.[13] The participants in this double-blind study were randomly assigned to receive either 1,500 milligrams of glucosamine sulfate (available under the brand names Dona, Viartril-S, and Xicil) or a placebo every day for 3 years. Members of both groups were allowed to take acetaminophen as a "rescue medicine" to control pain, as they deemed necessary. The researchers used x-rays, the WOMAC Index, and other assessment tools to track the progression of OA. At the end of the study, the average amount of space between the bones in the afflicted joints had stayed about the same in the glucosamine group but had narrowed in the placebo group, indicating that glucosamine—but not the placebo—had slowed the progression of OA. In addition, pain and other symptoms improved by up to 20 percent in the glucosamine group but only modestly in the placebo group. The researchers concluded, "This study demonstrates that glucosamine sulfate is the first pharmacologic intervention that retards the progression of osteoarthritis during long-term treatment."

♦ Researchers from the World Health Organization Collaborating Center for Public Health Aspects of Osteoarticular Disorders drew upon the results of two separate randomized, double-blind, placebo-controlled studies to assess the effects of glucosamine sulfate.[14] For the two trials, researchers recruited a total of 319 postmenopausal women and analyzed their osteoarthritic joints after they had taken either 1,500 milligrams of glucosamine (available under the brand names Dona, Viartril-S, and Xicil) or a placebo every day for 3 years. Those in the glucosamine group "showed no joint space narrowing," while those in the placebo group showed modest narrowing. Furthermore, OA symptoms as measured using the WOMAC Index improved in the glucosamine group but showed a trend toward worsening in the placebo group. The researchers concluded that glucosamine sulfate "has [a] disease-modifying effect" and may do more than simply relieve symptoms.

♦ Glucosamine was pitted head-to-head against ibuprofen, a standard drug for treating OA pain and inflammation, in a 1994 study published in *Osteoarthritis and Cartilage*.[15] For this double-blind study, 200 men and women with active OA of the knee were randomly assigned to receive either 1,500 milligrams of glucosamine sulfate or 1,200 milligrams of ibuprofen every day for 4 weeks. The study participants were assessed weekly, with their symptoms monitored using the Lequesne severity index and other scales. The ibuprofen worked faster than the glucosamine; at the end of the first week, 48 percent of the ibuprofen group had responded to treatment, compared to only 28 percent of the glucosamine group. However, from the second week onward, the effects of the two treatments were comparable, with 52 percent of the ibuprofen group and 48 percent of the glucosamine group responding to treatment. Glucosamine was better tolerated, with only 6 percent of those taking glucosamine reporting adverse effects compared to 35 percent of those taking ibuprofen. The researchers concluded that "oral glucosamine sulfate was as effective as ibuprofen in short-term symptom control of patients with active knee OA."

Figure 18-1 below shows the average Lequesne Index scores for the glucosamine and ibuprofen groups. Note that while the score for the ibuprofen group begins to fall immediately, the glucosamine group catches up by the third week, and the scores are the same at the end of the fourth week.

Figure 18-1: Glucosamine Equal to Ibuprofen in Reducing Symptoms of OA

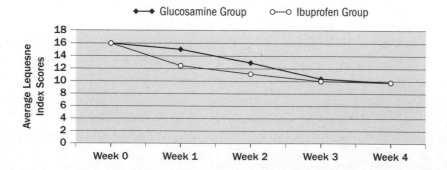

♦ The results of a clinical trial examining the effects of glucosamine on osteoarthritis were presented at the American College of Rheumatology Annual Scientific Meeting in 2005. The name of the trial was GUIDE, which stands for Glucosamine Unum-in-Die (or "glucosamine once a day").[16] Three hundred eighteen people with knee osteoarthritis participated in this double-blind, placebo-controlled study, which was conducted in several cities in Europe. The volunteers were randomly assigned to receive 1,500 milligrams of glucosamine sulfate, 3,000 milligrams of acetaminophen, or a placebo every day for 6 months. All of the groups were allowed to take ibuprofen as needed. The researchers monitored the volunteers' OA symptoms by tracking their scores on the Lequesne Index and other assessment tools. Glucosamine significantly reduced pain, outperforming both acetaminophen and the placebo. The researchers concluded that "glucosamine sulfate at the oral once-daily dose of 1,500 [milligrams] might be the preferred symptomatic medication in knee OA."

Several experts have reviewed the medical literature in an attempt to summarize the evidence for glucosamine.

♦ A 2003 review published in *Drugs and Aging* found that "in short-term clinical trials, glucosamine provided effective symptomatic relief for patients with osteoarthritis of the knee. In addition, glucosamine has shown promising results in modifying the progression of arthritis over a 3-year period."[17]

♦ A review and meta-analysis published in the *Journal of the American Medical Association* in 2000 statistically merged the results of double-blind, randomized, placebo-controlled studies to conclude that glucosamine had "moderate effects" on osteoarthritis.[18] However, the authors of the review questioned the quality of some of the studies and suggested that the results may be exaggerated.

♦ For a 2003 review published in the *Archives of Internal Medicine*, a team of researchers from Belgium and France reviewed all of the randomized, placebo-controlled glucosamine/osteoarthritis studies performed or published between 1980 and early 2002.[19] After using statistical methods to pool the results of the eligible studies, they found a "highly significant efficacy of glucosamine on all outcomes, including joint space narrowing and WOMAC." In other words, glucosamine effectively reduced both the problems that the doctors could measure (such as joint space narrowing seen on x-rays) and the symptoms that the patients could feel (such as pain as evaluated using the WOMAC Index).

Summing Up the Evidence for Glucosamine

Numerous clinical studies and meta-analyses have found glucosamine to be as effective as some standard medications and more effective than placebo at reducing OA symptoms. Some have also suggested that glucosamine may halt the progression of the disease, making it one of only two treatments to do so (the other being chondroitin sulfate). However, there are other studies that have found glucosamine to be no better than placebo. As mentioned earlier, even the large-scale Glucosamine/Chondroitin Arthritis Intervention Trial—which compared the effects of several OA treatments, including glucosamine—was inconclusive. The study, which ended in 2005, found glucosamine in combination with chondroitin sulfate to be the most effective treatment for moderate to intense OA pain. On its own, it didn't relieve symptoms as well as celecoxib (Celebrex).

As with chondroitin sulfate, the fact that glucosamine may halt the joint damage associated with OA should carry some weight when assessing the research evidence. Based on the findings to date, it is fair to say that glucosamine is a four-star treatment for osteoarthritis backed by strong evidence.

Available Forms

Glucosamine is available in supplement form.

How Much Glucosamine Is Typically Used

There is no standard dose of glucosamine for osteoarthritis. A common dosage in studies is 1,500 milligrams per day.

Possible Side Effects and Interactions

Among glucosamine's side effects are nausea, heartburn, constipation, and drowsiness. It also may interfere with the effects of chemotherapy drugs such as doxorubicin (Adriamycin). If you're taking any medication, be sure to consult your doctor before adding glucosamine to your self-care regimen.

Cetylated Fatty Acids

Rating: ☆☆☆ = Intriguing Evidence

A fatty acid is a building block of fat, just as an amino acid is one of the "ingredients" in protein. When what chemists call a natural cetyl alcohol is added to a fatty acid to stabilize the fatty acid, it becomes a cetylated fatty acid. Various CFAs—which go by names such as *cetyl myristoleate* and *cetyl laureate*—have been used alone or in combination as treatments for rheumatoid arthritis, multiple sclerosis, and fibromyalgia, among various other ailments.

Population and clinical studies have shown that people with rheumatoid arthritis respond to treatment with omega-3 fatty acids. In laboratory animals, a form of cetylated monounsaturated fatty acid protected against arthritis. Though the CFAs' exact mechanisms of action have yet to be determined, the theory is that they may help lubricate joints, soften tissues, or reduce inflammation—all of which would be beneficial in cases of OA.

A small number of studies suggest that CFA can help relieve symptoms of osteoarthritis. Among them:

♦ For a 2002 double-blind study that appeared in the *Journal of Rheumatology*,[20] 64 people with osteoarthritis of the knee were randomly assigned to take either a proprietary product containing 2,100 milligrams of CFA (brand name Celadrin) or a placebo every day for 68 days. The volunteers' symptoms and ability to use their knees were evaulated at the beginning of the study and again on days 30 and 68. The results were positive, with the CFA group showing significant improvements in knee range of motion and function, compared to modest improvements in the placebo group.

♦ Forty people with osteoarthritis of the knee participated in a study testing the effects of a topical preparation of CFA (Celadrin) on symptoms of osteoarthritis.[21] For this 2004 study, the volunteers were randomly assigned to receive treatment with a cream containing a CFA blend or a placebo cream. They were instructed to apply a specific amount of cream to both knees twice a day for 30 days. Their osteoarthritis symptoms were measured at the beginning of the study, 30 minutes after applying their first dose of cream, and at the end of the 30-day treatment period. The CFA group experienced improvements in their range of motion, ability to climb stairs, and other tests of knee function. According to the researchers,

"The results of this study provide support for the use of cetylated fatty acids as part of a pain relief treatment in patients with knee OA."

Summing Up the Evidence for Cetylated Fatty Acid

Based on the evidence to date, it is fair to say that cetylated fatty acids are a three-star treatment for osteoarthritis backed by intriguing evidence.

Available Forms

Cetylated fatty acids can be taken orally or applied to affected joints as a topical cream.

How Much Cetylated Fatty Acid Is Typically Used

There is no standard dose of cetylated fatty acids for osteoarthritis. One successful study used an oral dose of 2,100 milligrams per day.

Possible Side Effects and Interactions

No significant side effects or interactions were reported in the small number of CFA studies. As with all supplements and drugs, be sure to read and follow the label directions carefully when using CFA preparations, whether in oral or topical form.

Devil's Claw
Rating: ☆☆☆ = Intriguing Evidence

Known as devil's claw because of the flat, thornlike shape of its fruit, this native of southern Africa has a long history as a treatment for arthritis, indigestion, and other ailments. Devil's claw contains the glycoside harpagoside and other compounds that may help reduce inflammation, ease pain, and increase joint mobility. Germany's Commission E has approved the use of devil's claw to treat rheumatism, loss of appetite, and stomach complaints.

Several studies have suggested that devil's claw may relieve symptoms of osteoarthritis, including these:

♦ Two hundred twenty-seven people enrolled in a study of the effects of devil's claw that was reported in *Phytomedicine* in 2002.[22] Some of the volunteers had osteoarthritis of the knee or hip, while the rest suffered from nonspecific lower back pain. All were treated daily for 8 weeks with a devil's claw extract that provided 60 milligrams of harpagoside (brand name Doloteffin). Their symptoms were tracked using the WOMAC Index and other assessment tools, and they kept diaries to record their pain and any pain medicines they took. After comparing changes in the intensity of symptoms and analyzing the diaries, the researchers concluded that between 50 and 70 percent of the volunteers benefited (through a reduction in pain and/or disability) from this brand of devil's claw extract. In addition, they experienced few side effects.

♦ For a double-blind study published in *Phytomedicine* in 2000, French researchers compared devil's claw to diacerhein (an arthritis drug used in France and Italy) in 122 people suffering from osteoarthritis of the hip or knee.[23] The volunteers were randomly assigned to receive 2,610 milligrams of a standardized devil's claw powder (brand name Harpadol) or 100 milligrams of diacerhein every day for 4 months. Pain and functional disability were measured using a visual analogue scale, while the severity of arthritis was tracked using the Lequesne Index. The results were positive, with both devil's claw and the drug producing "significant improvement" in spontaneous pain, and "a progressive and significant reduction in the Lequesne functional index." There was no statistical difference between the herb and the drug in terms of performance. The primary difference was that those taking devil's claw needed significantly fewer standard medications to control their pain. The researchers concluded that devil's claw and the standard drug "are equally effective in the treatment of osteoarthritis of the knee or the hip."

♦ A 2004 review article published in *BMC Complementary and Alternative Medicine* gathered studies testing the efficacy of devil's claw in reducing the symptoms of osteoarthritis.[24] According to the authors of this paper, there is "moderate evidence" that a devil's claw preparation containing 60 milligrams of harpagoside can help relieve symptoms of spinal, hip, and knee osteoarthritis. Table 18-3 on the next page summarizes the results of the devil's claw/osteoarthritis studies used in the review article.

Table 18-3: Overview of Studies on Devil's Claw and Osteoarthritis[25]

Number of Patients	Treated with	Results	Reviewers' Conclusion	Study Citation
50	4 weeks of daily doses of either 2,500 mg devil's claw preparation or standard drug phenylbutazone	Average pain improvement: 80% with devil's claw, 72% with phenylbutazone	This devil's claw preparation is superior to phenylbutazone.	Schruffler, 1980[26]
89	60 days of daily doses of either 2,000 mg devil's claw preparation or placebo	Average pain improvement: 38% with devil's claw, 25% with placebo	This devil's claw preparation is superior to placebo.	Lecomte and Costa, 1992[27]
78	20 weeks of daily doses of either 4,500 mg devil's claw preparation or placebo	Those who responded to treatment by showing sufficient improvement: 90% with devil's claw, 80% with placebo. Also, those taking placebo took considerably more ibuprofen to reduce pain compared to those taking devil's claw.	This devil's claw preparation is superior to placebo.	Biller, 2002[28]
122	16 weeks of daily doses of either 4,500 mg devil's claw preparation or standard drug diacerhein	No statistically significant difference between treatment groups on Lequesne functional index	This devil's claw preparation is as effective as diacerhein.	Chantre et al., 2000[29]
46	20 weeks of daily doses of either 4,500 mg devil's claw preparation or placebo	Those who responded to treatment by showing sufficient improvement: 71% with devil's claw, 41% with placebo	This devil's claw preparation is superior to placebo.	Frerick et al., 2001[30]

Summing Up the Evidence for Devil's Claw

Given what we know about the herb, it is reasonable to say that devil's claw is a three-star treatment for osteoarthritis backed by intriguing evidence.

Other Names

Devil's claw is known to scientists as *Harpagophytum procumbens* and in various parts of the world as grapple plant, griffe du diable, and wood spider.

Available Forms

Devil's claw is available in herb, liquid, powder, tincture, capsule, and tea forms.

How Much Devil's Claw Is Typically Used

There is no standard dose of devil's claw for osteoarthritis. In the successful studies, a typical dosage is 4,500 milligrams per day.

Possible Side Effects and Interactions

Devil's claw can cause diarrhea, nausea, headache, and ringing in the ears. In addition, the herb may increase the effects of blood pressure medicines such as bisoprolol (Zebeta) and diabetes drugs such as glyburide (Micronase), causing blood pressure and/or blood sugar to drop too low. If you're taking any medication, be sure to consult your doctor before adding devil's claw to your self-care regimen.

SAMe

Rating: ☆☆☆ = Intriguing Evidence

Produced in the body from the amino acid methionine, SAMe (short for S-adenosyl-L-methionine) protects DNA and helps the body manufacture the hormone melatonin, which plays an important role in sleep. Therapeutically, SAMe has been used as an anti-inflammatory and a pain reliever. In fact, in Europe it's sold as a drug for these purposes.

Beyond its anti-inflammatory properties, SAMe is believed to boost production of proteoglycans, the molecules that draw water into cartilage. Although how it works is not fully understood, some studies suggest that SAMe is indeed helpful in treating symptoms of osteoarthritis:

♦ In a 1987 study published in the *American Journal of Medicine*, Argentinean researchers enlisted 45 people suffering from osteoarthritis of the knee for a double-blind comparison of SAMe to the standard arthritis drug piroxicam (Feldene).[31] The participants were randomly assigned to receive either 1,200 milligrams of SAMe or 20 milligrams of piroxicam every day for 84 days. By day 28, "both SAMe and piroxicam proved effective in inducing significant improvement in the total pain score." By day 56, both groups were showing reductions in morning stiffness, pain while walking, and other symptoms. The researchers found the effects of the supplement to be comparable to those of the drug, noting that "no significant difference was found between the two treatments in terms of efficacy and tolerability."

♦ Another 1987 double-blind study published in the *American Journal of Medicine* compared SAMe to the standard drug indomethacin (Indocin).[32] The 36 volunteers—all of whom were suffering from osteoarthritis of the knee, hip, and/or spine—were randomly assigned to receive either 1,200 milligrams of SAMe or 150 milligrams of indomethacin every day for 4 weeks. Both SAMe and the drug significantly improved the patients' symptom scores, but SAMe triggered fewer side effects.

♦ SAMe was pitted head-to-head against the standard drug celecoxib (Celebrex) in a 2004 study conducted at the University of California, Irvine.[33] Sixty-one people age 40 or older—all of whom had osteoarthritis of the knee—participated in this randomized, double-blind, crossover trial. The volunteers were assigned to take 1,200 milligrams of SAMe every day for 8 weeks, followed by 200 milligams of celecoxib every day for 8 weeks, or to use the treatments in reverse order over the same period of time. The effects of SAMe and celecoxib on osteoarthritis symptoms were tracked using the Dartmouth COOP Clinical Improvement System and other rating systems, plus a physician's assessment of each volunteer's progress. As shown in Table 18-4 on the opposite page, SAMe proved to be superior to placebo in all measures and equal to the drug in all categories on the COOP scale. The researchers concluded that in people with OA of the knee, "SAMe is equivalent in almost all measures to COX-2 inhibitors (celecoxib) in relieving pain and improving function." They did note that it might take up to a month before SAMe would begin providing relief.

Table 18-4: COOP Scores Show SAMe Superior to Placebo and Comparable to Standard Drug for Osteoarthritis[34]

	Beginning Level	With SAMe	With Celecoxib
Total Score (Lower Scores Are Better)	48.7	39.9*	39.8*
Physical condition	56.2	51.7	51.3
Emotional condition	37.6	33.5	34.8
Daily work	47.1	34.3*	33.9*
Social activities	31.4	29.1	29.6
Pain	70.5	53.0*	50.9*
Change in condition	65.2	49.1*	47.8*
Overall condition	50.0	44.3*	41.3*
Social support	39.0	29.6*	32.6
Quality of life	41.0	34.3*	36.1

*The difference between the beginning level and the after-treatment level is statistically significant.

♦ In 2002, researchers from the University of Maryland School of Nursing conducted a meta-analysis of SAMe's effects on osteoarthritis.[35] While noting that there were only a few qualified randomized, controlled trials to include in their analysis, they found that "SAMe appears to be as effective as NSAIDs in reducing pain and improving functional limitation in patients with OA without the adverse effects often associated with NSAID therapies."

♦ In their 2002 review of the medical literature, the US Department of Health and Human Services Agency for Healthcare Research and Quality noted that "compared to treatment with nonsteroidal anti-inflammatory medications, treatment with SAMe was not associated with a statistically significant difference in outcomes."[36] In other words, SAMe was as effective as these routinely prescribed medicines.

Summing Up the Evidence for SAMe

SAMe generally has performed well in studies comparing it to standard medicines. However, it should be noted that much of the research was conducted in the 1980s, so there is a paucity of studies comparing SAMe to the newer osteoarthritis medicines. With these limitations in mind, it is fair to say that SAMe is a three-star treatment for osteoarthritis backed by intriguing evidence.

Available Forms

SAMe is available in capsule or tablet form.

How Much SAMe Is Typically Used

There is no standard dose of SAMe for osteoarthritis. Dosages used in studies are often in the range of 600 to 1,200 milligrams per day.

Possible Side Effects and Interactions

SAMe's side effects include anxiety, insomnia, and gastrointestinal upset. It should not be taken by anyone who's suffering from bipolar disorder or taking antidepressants, as it can raise the risk of serotonin syndrome with symptoms such as agitation, anxiety, tremors, and rapid heartbeat. These symptoms also may occur when SAMe is combined with dextromethorphan (Robitussin DM), meperidine (Demerol), or pentazocine (Talwin). If you're taking any medication, be sure to consult your doctor before adding SAMe to your self-care regimen.

Magnets

Rating: ☆☆ = Modest Evidence

The ancient Greeks used magnets as a treatment for arthritis. Later, in the Middle Ages, physicians and healers prescribed them for gout, baldness, and poisoning. They also were helpful for drawing arrowheads and spear tips out of the body. Modern medicine relies on magnets to map the brain and to speed the healing of fractured bones that are not mending well. In complementary and alternative medicine, magnets are popular treatments for pain conditions, breathing and circulatory problems, and other ailments.

No one knows exactly why magnets might relieve pain and other symptoms. Perhaps they change the way in which cells function, alter nerve cells' response to pain, change pain perception in the brain, spur white blood cells to reduce inflammation, or raise temperature in the affected area.

Several studies, including the following, offer compelling evidence that magnets might indeed relieve symptoms of osteoarthritis. (For this discussion, you should be familiar with these terms: *Static* or *permanent* magnets have magnetic fields that do not change; *electromagnets* generate a magnetic field only when an electric current is flowing through them; and *pulsing* means to rapidly turn an electromagnetic field on and off.)

♦ One hundred ninety-four men and women participated in a randomized, controlled trial of magnetic bracelets for relieving osteoarthritis pain, presented in the *British Medical Journal* in 2004.[37] The volunteers—all ranging in age from 45 to 80 and having osteoarthritis of the knee or hip—were assigned to receive 12 weeks of treatment by wearing a bracelet containing a standard-strength magnet, a bracelet containing a weak magnet, or a bracelet with nonmagnetic steel washers (which served as the placebo). The WOMAC "A" and visual analogue scales for pain were used to track symptoms and to compare results from one group to the next. As Table 18-5, on page 270, indicates, average pain scores fell more in the standard magnet group than in the weak magnet or placebo magnet groups. The researchers reported finding "evidence of a beneficial effect of magnetic wrist bracelets on the pain of osteoarthritis of the hip and knee," noting that their results "are consistent with previous studies on magnetic therapies and pain." Table 18-5 also shows the effects of both the weak and the strong magnets (as well as the placebo) OA pain, based on the pain scales used in the study.

Table 18-5: Effects of Strong, Weak and Placebo Magnets on Osteoarthritis[38]

PERCENTAGE RESPONDING TO TREATMENT,
ACCORDING TO TREATMENT

	Placebo Magnet Group	Weak Magnet Group	Strong Magnet Group
WOMAC "A" scale for pain			
Walking on flat surface	28%	25%	34%
Walking up or down stairs	17%	19%	29%
At night while in bed	27%	28%	37%
Sitting or lying	25%	34%	37%
Standing up	14%	25%	26%
Visual analogue scale for pain			
High level of improvement	9%	14%	20%
Moderate improvement	22%	42%	37%

♦ For a 2001 study published in *Current Medical Research and Opinion*, researchers from King's College Hospital in London tested the effects of 6 weeks of treatment with magnets on patients with osteoarthritis.[39] Sixty-nine people who had not been sufficiently helped by conventional approaches participated in this double-blind study, in which they were randomly assigned to receive treatment with either magnetic devices providing low-frequency pulsed electromagnetic fields (PEMF) or a placebo. The magnetic devices (brand name Medicur) were used three times a day at varying frequencies. According to statistical analysis of the data, those receiving treatment with magnetic devices showed significant improvements in their WOMAC overall, WOMAC pain, and WOMAC disability scores, as well as on the Euro Quality of Life scale. The researchers concluded that "unipolar magnetic devices are beneficial in reducing pain and disability in patients with knee OA resistant to conventional treatment."

Summing Up the Evidence for Magnets

Drawing conclusions from the magnet/osteoarthritis research is difficult because of the relatively small number of clinical studies as well as differences in the type and strength of magnets, the way in which the magnets were applied to the body, the length of treatment, and so on. With this in mind, it is fair to say that magnets are a two-star treatment for osteoarthritis backed by modest evidence.

Available Forms

The strength of therapeutic magnets is measured in hundreds or thousands of *gauss*. While a refrigerator magnet may have about 60 gauss, a therapeutic magnet could have 6,000 gauss. However, the amount actually transmitted to the skin may be only 1,800 gauss—a figure that declines as the distance from the skin or the amount of wrapping increases.

How to Use Magnets Therapeutically

To find out where to buy therapeutic magnets, what strength you need, and how to use them, your best bet is to consult a physical therapist who's well versed in magnet therapy. Your doctor or local hospital should be able to recommend someone. You also might visit the Web site for the American Physical Therapy Association at www.apta.org.

Possible Side Effects and Interactions

Although the static magnets available to consumers are generally considered safe when applied to the skin, they should not be used by women who are pregnant; by anyone with a pacemaker, defibrillator, insulin pump, or another magnetically controlled or affected device; by those using a patch or another device that delivers medicine through the skin; or by anyone with a sprain, infection, wound, or inflammation.

Tai Chi
Rating: ☆☆ = Modest Evidence

Tai chi is a form of exercise in which controlled, rhythmic movements flow gently and smoothly from one to the next. Its practitioners often describe tai chi as part physical and part spiritual.

As mentioned earlier, standard treatment for osteoarthritis includes exercise to help lubricate and nourish affected joints. Some studies suggest that tai chi may be helpful for this purpose.

♦ The effects of tai chi on osteoarthritis were tested in a 2000 study published in the *Journal of the American Geriatrics Society*.[40] Thirty-three people with osteoarthritis of the spine and/or lower extremities, average age 68, participated in the study. They were randomly assigned to receive tai chi training (two 1-hour sessions per week for 12 weeks) or to attend three "share your experiences" meetings. Those in the latter group, which served as the control, also were contacted by phone every 2 weeks to discuss any problems related to their osteoarthritis. The volunteers' progress was tracked by using assessment tools such as the Arthritis Self-Efficacy Scale and by testing functional abilities such as the amount of time necessary to walk 50 feet or to rise from a chair. The tai chi group showed significant improvements in their symptoms, levels of tension, and satisfaction with their general health. The researchers concluded that "a moderate tai chi intervention can enhance arthritis self-efficacy, quality of life, and functional mobility among older adults with osteoarthritis."

♦ Forty-three women with osteoarthritis, age 55 or older, enrolled in a 2003 study published in the *Journal of Rheumatology*.[41] The volunteers were randomly assigned to participate in a 12-week tai chi exercise program (the tai chi group) or to simply continue receiving their standard treatment (the control group). The researchers measured the volunteers' perception of their symptoms as well as objective measures such as balance and abdominal muscle strength. According to the researchers, the tai chi group experienced "significantly less pain . . . and stiffness . . . in their joints, and reported fewer difficulties with physical functioning." There was no such improvement in subjective symptoms in the control group. As for the objective measurements, "there were significant improvements in balance . . . and abdominal muscle strength . . . for the tai chi exercise group" but not for the control group.

Summing Up the Evidence for Tai Chi

The idea that tai chi might help relieve symptoms of osteoarthritis certainly makes sense, for we know that gentle exercise can help relieve joint pain while improving overall strength and balance, thus leading to an improvement in physical symptoms and a decline in the perception of illness. However, with only a limited number of scientific studies to support its therapeutic effects, it is best to say that tai chi is a two-star treatment for osteoarthritis based on modest evidence.

Possible Side Effects

When performed properly, tai chi is considered a safe form of physical activity. Still, anyone with arthritis should practice tai chi only with a physician's knowledge and consent.

Finding a Tai Chi Instructor

To locate a tai chi class near you, visit the Web site for the Tai Chi Network at www.taichinetwork.org and click on "Teachers." Tai chi videos especially for people with arthritis are available from Tai Chi Productions at www.taichiproductions.com.

19

ALTERNATIVE APPROACHES TO

OSTEOPOROSIS

Ipriflavone ☆☆☆
Soy isoflavones ☆☆☆
Vitamin K$_2$ ☆☆☆
Tai chi ☆☆

Osteoporosis is a disease that causes a decline in the mass and density of bones, leaving them thin, porous, weak, and vulnerable to fracture. Some 10 million Americans currently have osteoporosis, which causes some 1.5 million snapped wrists, broken hips, crushed vertebrae, or other bone fractures every year. Another 34 million Americans have low bone mass, putting them at risk for developing the disease. Women are the most likely victims: Approximately 80 percent of those with osteoporosis are female. What's more, according to the National Osteoporosis Society, nearly half of all American women over age 50 are expected to suffer an osteoporosis-related fracture at some time during their lives.

Osteoporosis is a significant cause of disability and a possible cause of mortality. Nearly half of the 300,000 people a year who break a hip because of osteoporosis will become permanently dependent on canes or walkers to get around. One in five will end up in a nursing home. Approximately 20 percent of patients with hip fractures die within a year, usually due to fracture complications. Also, epidemiological studies show that those with osteoporosis are at higher risk for dying from heart disease or stroke.

SYMPTOMS

Called the "silent disease" because it produces no obvious symptoms until it's quite advanced, osteoporosis can go undetected for years. Often a bone fracture is the first indication that something is wrong. Besides broken bones, the signs of advanced osteoporosis can include a curved spine, stooped posture, a "dowager's hump" (a rounded hump in the upper back), a loss of height, and severe back pain—all of which are the result of vertebrae that have collapsed under the strain of holding up the body.

CAUSES

Although the exact cause of osteoporosis has not been established, certain factors can contribute to development of the disease. They include age; gender (being female); a family history of fractures; a small, thin frame; estrogen deficiency; irregular menstruation; premature menopause; anorexia nervosa; long periods of bed rest; a low lifetime intake of calcium; excessive intake of vitamin A, protein, wheat bran, sodium, phosphorus, or caffeine; certain medications, including corticosteroids, anticonvulsants, and chemotherapy; certain medical conditions; lack of weight-bearing exercise; cigarette smoking; and excessive alcohol consumption.

Strangely enough, both too little and too much vitamin D can contribute to osteoporosis. Without enough vitamin D, the body cannot absorb calcium efficiently. With too much, the process of bone breakdown speeds up.

STANDARD TREATMENTS

Treatment of osteoporosis is most effective if it begins before the onset of the disease—by building the strongest, densest bones possible during peak bone-building years (up to about age 20) and doing everything possible to maintain bone mass and density thereafter. This means consuming a diet rich in calcium and vitamin D, engaging in plenty of weight-bearing and resistance-training exercise, and avoiding smoking and excessive alcohol consumption.

To detect osteoporosis in its earliest stages, a baseline bone density test should be performed at menopause and every 1 to 2 years thereafter. For existing cases of osteoporosis or declining bone mass, doctors typically recommend all of the preventive measures listed above plus medication. Biphosphonate drugs such as alendronate (Fosamax), ibandronate (Boniva), and risedronate (Actonel) can help increase bone mass and reduce bone loss and fracture risk. Calcitonin (Miacalcin), a naturally occurring thyroid hormone, also can help reduce bone loss. Raloxifene (Evista), a nonsteroidal drug that acts on estrogen receptors, increases bone mineral density specifically in the hip and spine.

RATING POPULAR ALTERNATIVE TREATMENTS FOR OSTEOPOROSIS

Ipriflavone

Rating: ☆☆☆ = Intriguing Evidence

Ipriflavone is a laboratory-manufactured derivative of daidzin, a substance found in soy. Though ipriflavone has been used in Japan and Italy for many years to preserve bone strength and density in postmenopausal women, the supplement has become available in the United States only recently. It is thought to encourage the action of cells that build new bone, while discouraging the action of cells that break down and absorb old bone.

A number of studies conducted in Japan and Europe have shown that ipriflavone can help slow the rate of bone loss in osteoporosis. For example:

◆ Researchers from the University of Parma in Italy looked at the effects of ipriflavone in 28 women over age 65 with x-ray evidence of at least one osteoporotic vertebral fracture.[1] For this double-blind study, the volunteers were randomly assigned to receive either 600 milligrams of ipriflavone or a placebo every day for a year. All were also given 1,000 milligrams of calcium daily, in supplement form. At the end of the treatment period, the women taking ipriflavone showed a statistically significant increase of 6 percent in bone mineral density at the distal radius (lower arm) bone. In contrast, those taking the placebo showed a small decrease in bone mineral density.

◆ One hundred thirty-four postmenopausal women completed a study published in *Calcified Tissue International* in 1997 that compared ipriflavone to placebo.[2] For this double-blind study, the women were randomly assigned to take either 600 milligrams of ipriflavone (brand name Osteofix) or a placebo every day for 2 years. Bone density in the vertebrae as well as biochemical markers of bone turnover were measured at the beginning of the study and every 6 months thereafter. The ipriflavone group showed an average 1 percent increase in vertebral bone density at the end of the 2-year study period, compared to a significant drop in vertebral bone density among the placebo group.

♦ In 1999 Japanese researchers published the results of a randomized study involving 60 women with postmenopausal-related osteoporosis or osteopenia (poorly mineralized bone that can set the stage for osteoporosis).[3] The women were randomly assigned to receive either 600 milligrams of ipriflavone or 800 milligrams of calcium lactate every day for 1 year. Lumbar (lower spine) bone mineral density remained stable among those taking ipriflavone, although it declined significantly among those taking calcium. Also, urinary levels of deoxypyridinoline (a marker of bone breakdown) were significantly lower in the ipriflavone group but not in the calcium group. The researchers concluded that ipriflavone treatment "suppresses bone resorption."

Summing Up the Evidence for Ipriflavone

In general, ipriflavone has fared well in extensive tests conducted throughout Europe and Japan over the past several years. Yet the Ipriflavone Multicenter European Fracture Study, the results of which were published in the *Journal of the American Medical Association* in 2001, found that 3 years of treatment with ipriflavone did not improve bone mineral density or reduce fracture risk.[4] It's difficult to make a definitive statement in the face of such "dueling studies." Taking into consideration both the substantial number of positive studies of ipriflavone for osteoporosis and its possible potential for weakening the immune system (see below), it is best to say that ipriflavone is a three-star treatment for osteoporosis backed by intriguing evidence.

Available Forms

Ipriflavone is available in supplement form.

How Much Ipriflavone Is Typically Used

There is no standard dose of ipriflavone for osteoporosis. Some studies have used supplemental dosages of 600 milligrams per day.

Possible Side Effects and Interactions

Ipriflavone's side effects include diarrhea, stomach pain, and dizziness. At least one study has suggested that the supplement may weaken immune function. In addition, it may increase the effects of immunosuppressant drugs such as basiliximab (Simulect). When taken in combination with theophylline (TheoDur), it may increase blood levels of the drug. If you're taking any medication, be sure to consult your doctor before adding ipriflavone to your self-care regimen.

Soy Isoflavones

Rating: ☆☆☆ = Intriguing Evidence

A popular food in Japan and other Asian countries, soy contains phytoestrogens, substances that act like a mild form of estrogen. Phytoestrogens are able to "plug into" estrogen receptors on various cells, delivering a small amount of this vital hormone to the cells. This characteristic can be beneficial for osteoporosis and other conditions related to estrogen deficiency because it increases estrogen levels.

Estrogen has a direct connection to bone tissue, in that estrogen receptor sites are present on both bone-building and bone-breakdown cells. Many experts believe that estrogen extends the life of the bone-building cells and shortens the life of the bone-breakdown cells. It also plays a role in the absorption of calcium and phosphorus and the deposition of these important minerals into bones.

Observational studies have suggested that in general, women who consume large amounts of soy experience fewer bone fractures than women who do not.[5] This finding has led researchers to hypothesize that soy, or the phytoestrogens in soy (called isoflavones), may help slow the bone loss associated with menopause and lowered estrogen levels. Here are some of the interesting studies suggesting that soy or soy isoflavones do help slow osteoporosis:

+ A 2000 study published in the *American Journal of Clinical Nutrition* looked at the effects of soy protein with isoflavones on bone loss in perimenopausal women.[6] (Perimenopause is the 4- to 8-year phase preceding the final menstrual period, during which estrogen and progesterone levels begin to fluctuate and decline.) For 24 weeks, the 69 women in the study were randomly assigned to consume daily portions of soy containing a large amount of isoflavones; soy containing a very small amount of isoflavones; or whey, which contains no isoflavones and served as a control.

(The soy protein was supplied by Protein Technologies International.) At both the beginning and the end of the study, the researchers took measurements of bone mineral density and bone mineral content at the women's lumbar spines. An analysis of the results showed that the soy containing a large amount of isoflavones reduced bone loss from the women's lumbar spines, while both the soy with a very small amount of isoflavones and the whey did not. The researchers concluded that "isoflavones attenuated bone loss from the lumbar spine in estrogen-deficient perimenopausal women who may otherwise be expected to lose 2 [to] 3 [percent] of bone per year."

♦ Chinese researchers recruited women who already had entered menopause for a similar study published in the *Journal of Endocrinology and Metabolism* in 2003.[7] The 203 women participating in this randomized, double-blind, controlled trial ranged in age from 48 to 62, and all had entered menopause within the past 10 years. They were randomly assigned to take high-dose isoflavones (80 milligrams), mid-dose isoflavones (40 milligrams), or a placebo (no isoflavones) for 1 year. (The isoflavones were provided by Acatris Holding BV.) All participants also took calcium and vitamin D supplements. Bone mineral density and bone mineral content at the hip, spine, and whole body were measured at the beginning and the end of the study. An analysis of the results showed that the higher dose of isoflavones significantly slowed the loss of bone mineral content in the hip compared to the mid-dose isoflavones and placebo. The researchers concluded that "soy isoflavones have a mild, but significant, independent effect on the maintenance of" bone mineral content in the hips of women who have gone through menopause within the last 10 years.

♦ Danish researchers conducted a 2-year randomized, double-blind, placebo-controlled study looking at the effects of soy isoflavones on postmenopausal Caucasian women.[8] The women were randomly assigned to receive one of four treatments: soy milk with isoflavones; transdermal progesterone (a progesterone cream that is rubbed on the skin); soy milk with isoflavones plus transdermal progesterone; or a placebo. They also were given vitamin and mineral supplements, including calcium. The bone mineral content and bone mineral density in the lower spine and hip were measured at the beginning of the study and again 2 years later. The results, published in 2004, showed that bone loss in the lower spine was slowed by the progesterone but prevented by the soy milk with isoflavones. Oddly enough, the combination of progesterone and soy milk resulted in a faster rate of bone loss than either treatment alone, although not as fast as seen with the placebo. The researchers concluded that "daily intake of two glasses of soy milk containing 76 [milligrams of] isoflavones prevents lumbar spine bone loss in postmenopausal women."

Summing Up the Evidence for Soy Isoflavones

While a solid body of research indicates that soy isoflavones can prevent bone loss in animals, studies involving humans have yielded conflicting results. This may be because some of the studies were conducted over short periods of time, involved women of different ethnic backgrounds and in different phases of menopause, and tested different soy preparations. With these limitations in mind, it is fair to say that soy isoflavones are a three-star treatment for osteoporosis backed by intriguing evidence.

Available Forms

Soy is available as soybeans, soy flour, soy milk, soy oil, tofu, miso, tempeh, and natto, among other foods. Soy isoflavones also come in extract form.

Amount of Soy Isoflavones Typically Used

There is no standard dose of soy, although supplemental doses may be as high as 80 grams of soy isoflavones per day.

Possible Side Effects and Interactions

Soy's side effects include constipation, nausea, and insomnia. It can trigger an allergic reaction in some people.

Those with breast cancer or a family history of breast cancer should be very cautious about using soy products because of conflicting information about whether soy has a positive or negative effect on the disease. The use of soy isoflavone extract is not recommended, as too many soy chemicals may inhibit mineral absorption, thyroid function, and/or cognitive function.

Soy may compete with estrogen replacement therapy, altering the effects of treatment. It also may interfere with tamoxifen (Nolvadex). If you're taking any medication, be sure to consult your doctor before adding therapeutic amounts of soy to your self-care regimen.

Vitamin K$_2$

Rating: ☆☆☆ = Intriguing Evidence

In 1939 a Danish biochemist and physiologist named Carl Peter Henrik Dam, Ph.D., discovered a factor in the fatty components of food that aids in the clotting of blood. He named this substance the "koagulation vitamin." For his discovery, he was awarded the Nobel Prize for Physiology or Medicine in 1943.

Today we refer to this substance as vitamin K, although it actually is a group of three related substances rather than just a single vitamin. Vitamin K$_1$, also known as phylloquinone, is found in plants; K$_2$ is a group of compounds called menaquinones, which are produced by bacteria in the human digestive tract; and K$_3$ or Menadione is a synthetic variant of the vitamin. In addition to helping blood to clot, vitamin K may help keep artery linings flexible and healthy, encourage the death of certain cancer cells, and activate a protein that helps bones retain calcium. It is the K$_2$ form of the vitamin that's important for building bones.

With research to suggest that vitamin K$_2$ helps calcium keep bones strong, scientists wondered if supplemental K$_2$ might prevent or even reverse osteoporotic bone loss. Some studies, including the three that follow, suggest that is indeed the case. All of the studies used a form of vitamin K$_2$ called menatetrenone.

♦ For a 2000 study, Japanese researchers tested the effects of vitamin K$_2$ in 241 people with osteoporosis.[9] For this open-label study, the volunteers were randomly assigned to receive either 45 milligrams of vitamin K$_2$ (as menatetrenone, brand name Gla-kay) plus 150 milligrams of elemental calcium or just calcium every day for 2 years. Lumbar bone mineral density was measured at the beginning of the study and again at months 6, 12, and 24. The researchers were primarily interested in whether vitamin K$_2$ would prevent new bone fractures and how it would affect lumbar bone density. At the 24-month mark, the vitamin K$_2$ group had experienced fewer fractures and a smaller loss of lumbar bone mineral density than the calcium-only group (1 percent versus 3.3 percent). According to the researchers, "These findings suggest that vitamin K$_2$ treatment effectively prevents the occurrence of new fractures."

♦ Seventy-two women with osteoporosis, all of whom had entered menopause at least 5 years previously, participated in a 2001 study comparing the effects of vitamin K_2 to a standard drug and to calcium.[10] The volunteers were randomly assigned to receive daily doses of 45 milligrams of vitamin K_2 (as menatetrenone), 200 milligrams of the biphosphonate bone-building drug etidronate (Didronel), or 2,000 milligrams of calcium lactate. Bone mineral density in the forearms of the volunteers was measured at the beginning of the study and again at months 6, 12, 18, and 24. As expected, the drug increased bone mineral density. But vitamin K_2 also triggered a "significant increase" compared to calcium. The researchers concluded that vitamin K_2 "may have the potential to reduce osteoporotic vertebral fractures in postmenopausal women with osteoporosis."

◆ The bone-preserving effectiveness of vitamin K_2 when combined with vitamin D was tested in a 2002 study of 172 postmenopausal women suffering from either osteoporosis or osteopenia.[11] The women were randomly assigned to receive vitamin K_2, vitamin D, vitamin K_2 plus vitamin D, or dietary therapy (the placebo). Bone mineral density measurements were taken at the beginning of the study, and again at months 6, 12, 18, and 24. Analysis of the results after 2 years of treatment showed that vitamin K_2 produced a slight increase in bone mineral density, while the combination of vitamin K_2 plus D produced a marked increase.

Summing Up the Evidence for Vitamin K_2

Much of the positive research on the use of vitamin K_2 for osteoporosis comes from Japan, where menatetrenone is standard treatment for osteoporotic osteopenia.[12] Based on the available evidence, it is reasonable to say that this form of vitamin K_2 is a three-star treatment for osteoporosis backed by intriguing evidence.

Available Forms

Humans and animals normally convert some ingested K_1 to K_2. Vitamin K_1 is found in a variety of plant foods, including kale, broccoli, parsley, spinach, soybean oil, and canola oil. Vitamin K_2 (menatetrenone) supplements are available in health food stores and through online vitamin stores.

How Much Vitamin K_2 Is Typically Used

There is no standard dose of vitamin K_2 for osteoporosis. Studies have used supplemental doses in the range of 45 milligrams of vitamin K_2 (menatetrenone) per day.

Possible Side Effects and Interactions

Vitamin K$_2$ can enhance the effects of blood-thinning medications such as warfarin (Coumadin), increasing the risk of excessive bleeding and bruising. If you're taking any medication, be sure to consult your doctor before adding therapeutic amounts of vitamin K$_2$ to your self-care regimen.

Tai Chi

Rating: ☆☆ = Modest Evidence

Tai chi is a *soft* Chinese martial art, which means that it is performed with the muscles as relaxed as possible—in contrast to the *hard* martial art styles, in which the muscles are tense. Tai chi involves slow, controlled, rhythmic movements and emphasizes relaxed breathing, a straight spine, and a natural range of motion.

A few studies have explored the effects of tai chi on bone loss in osteoporosis. For example:

♦ Researchers from the Chinese University of Hong Kong conducted a case-control study to test the effects of tai chi in 34 postmenopausal women.[13] Seventeen of the women already were practicing tai chi on a regular basis, while the remaining 17 were not regular exercisers. These women served as the control group. For 1 year, the tai chi group continued their practice for at least 3½ hours per week, while the control group refrained from exercise. Bone mineral density at the lumbar spine and femur was measured at the beginning of the study and again a year later. In the first measurement, those who practiced tai chi "had significantly higher" bone mineral density than those who did not. A year later, both groups of women had generalized bone loss, but those practicing tai chi had a lower rate of loss. The researchers concluded that "regular tai chi exercise may help retard bone loss of the weight-bearing bones in postmenopausal women."

♦ A randomized trial testing the effects of tai chi on osteoporosis was published in the *Archives of Physical Medicine and Rehabilitation* in 2004.[14] One hundred thirty-two postmenopausal women—average age 54, with no history of participating in physical exercise for more than 30 minutes per week—were randomly assigned to either a tai chi practice group or a sedentary control group. All of the volunteers had entered menopause within the previous 10 years. Those assigned to the tai chi group participated in supervised exercise sessions for 45 minutes a day, 5 days a week, for 1 year, while the other group remained sedentary. Bone mineral density at the lumbar spine and femur was measured at the beginning of the study and again after 12 months. Both groups of women suffered from general bone loss, but among those in the tai chi group, bone loss occurred at a slower rate. The researchers concluded that tai chi exercise "is beneficial for retarding bone loss in weight-bearing bones" among women in the early years of menopause.

Summing Up the Evidence for Tai Chi

Given the few published studies of acceptable quality, it is perhaps best to say that tai chi is a two-star treatment backed by modest evidence.

Finding a Tai Chi Instructor

To find a tai chi class near you, visit the Tai Chi Network Web site at www.taichinetwork.org, and click on "Teachers." If you have osteoporosis, please be sure to consult your doctor and obtain his or her consent before beginning tai chi practice.

20

ALTERNATIVE APPROACHES TO

PIMPLES

Acupuncture	☆☆☆☆
Guggul	☆☆
Tea tree oil	☆☆
Zinc	☆☆
Olive leaf	☆

Many teenagers wrestle with pimples, more technically known as acne. The appearance of blackheads, whiteheads, and other skin lesions on the face, neck, chest, back, shoulders, and upper arms begins in the sebaceous hair follicles, which are visible as the little openings in the skin known as pores. Inside each follicle, sebaceous glands produce oil (sebum) that travels upward through the pore to the skin's surface, where it helps keep the skin moist. Along the way, the sebum mixes with dead skin cells, which are shed through the pore.

If shedding occurs unevenly or too rapidly, dead skin cells can stick together and plug up the pore. The cells and sebum become trapped inside the pore and promote the growth of *Propionibacterium acnes,* bacteria that normally reside inside the follicle. The follicle swells, and the body sends white blood cells to fight the trapped bacteria. The result is the raised skin eruption that we commonly call a pimple.

Almost 90 percent of teenagers are affected by acne to some extent. It also can be seen in adults in their twenties, thirties, or even forties. Although acne does not represent a health threat for most people, it can be disfiguring, upsetting, and tough to live with. In some cases, it can lead to scarring.

SYMPTOMS

Acne appears on the skin as whiteheads, blackheads, papules, pustules, cysts, or nodules. When the sebum-and-bacteria blockage stays beneath the surface of the skin, it forms a *whitehead*, a bump that is not inflamed but has a white center. When the blockage surfaces through a partially open pore, the trapped sebum and bacteria turn dark due to the melanin in the skin. This is what's known as a *blackhead*. A *papule* is a small, solid, red bump on the surface of the skin. A *pustule* is a whitehead that has become inflamed; a *cyst* is a larger version of a pustule—also inflamed (sometimes severely) and involving deeper layers of the skin. A *nodule* is a deep, solid, inflamed collection of tissue. Both cysts and nodules can cause tissue damage that leads to scarring.

CAUSES

Many factors can contribute to the development of pimples, including an increase in the shedding of dead skin cells, which can clog pores; an overproduction of sebum; a rise in hormone levels (particularly androgens such as testosterone), which increase the production of sebum; the growth of *P. acnes* bacteria; genetics; and a strong inflammatory response.

STANDARD TREATMENTS

The standard treatment for pimples is to wash the affected area twice a day with a mild soap and apply a topical antibacterial agent such as clindamycin, erythromycin, or benzoyl peroxide. Prescription topical medications such as tretinoin can help unclog pores. More severe acne may require treatment with oral antibiotics such as tetracycline, doxycycline, or erythromycin. For the most severe cases, doctors may prescribe oral isotretinoin—although it has potentially serious side effects, including damage to blood cells and the liver and the potential to harm a developing fetus.

RATING POPULAR ALTERNATIVE TREATMENTS FOR PIMPLES

Acupuncture

Rating: ☆☆☆☆ = Strong Evidence

Acupuncture, the ancient Chinese healing discipline, has been in use for thousands of years as a treatment for pain and disease. But can this therapy—which involves the insertion of very fine needles into specific points on the body to release blocked energy—do anything for acne? A surprising amount of research suggests that the answer is yes. The English-language literature contains many reports of successful treatment of acne with acupuncture. They include the following:

♦ In a 1990 paper published in the *Journal of Traditional Chinese Medicine*, a researcher from the Wuhan Hospital of Traditional Chinese Medicine in China administered acupuncture to 80 people suffering from acne.[1] The acupuncture points were individually selected for each patient. Sixty-two of the 80 experienced a "clinical cure," meaning that the skin cleared and other symptoms were controlled. In another 11, the treatment was "markedly effective," while in the remaining 7 it had no effect.

♦ A 1993 paper published in the Journal of Traditional Chinese Medicine reported on 98 people, ranging in age from 15 to 28, who were suffering from acne.[2] They were given acupuncture treatments every 2 to 3 days for 3 weeks. Fifty-four of the volunteers were considered cured, 42 were improved, and 2 were not helped.

Summing Up the Evidence for Acupuncture

Many of the studies testing the efficacy of acupuncture for acne have taken place in non-English-speaking countries, making a thorough analysis of the scientific literature difficult. The two papers mentioned above describe case series, not studies comparing acupuncture to another treatment or to placebo. However, the World Health Organization reviewed the scientific literature and concluded that acupuncture has a "therapeutic effect" on acne vulgaris. Based on this recommendation, it is fair to conclude that acupuncture is a four-star treatment for pimples backed by strong evidence.

Possible Side Effects

When properly administered, acupuncture usually produces no side effects. There have been reports, though rare, of mild bruising or a small amount of bleeding where the needles are inserted. Some people have experienced dizziness after treatment.

Finding an Acupuncturist

To learn more about acupuncture, or to find a certified acupuncturist in your area, visit the Web site for the National Certification Commission for Acupuncture and Oriental Medicine (NCCAOM) at www.nccaom.org. The commission is the acupuncture profession's equivalent of the American Medical Association.

Guggul

Rating: ☆☆ = Modest Evidence

A resin produced by the mukul mirth tree, guggul is a traditional Indian remedy that has been used to treat skin disorders, joint pain, urinary problems, and other ailments. Its active ingredients include Z-guggulsterone and E-guggulsterone. Guggul may be further refined to a form known as gugulipid, which contains various substances that may lower cholesterol and help combat obesity.

Some studies have suggested that guggul could reduce the secretion of sebum associated with pimples. So the resin has been put to the test as an acne remedy.

♦ Indian researchers enlisted 20 people with nodulocystic acne (a severe form of acne affecting the face, chest, and back that leads to scarring) for their study comparing gugulipid to the standard medicine tetracycline.[3] The participants—ranging in age from 16 to 25—were randomly assigned to receive either gugulipid providing 25 milligrams of guggulsterones or 500 milligrams of tetracycline, twice a day for 3 months. Both gugulipid and the drug performed well, with gugulipid reducing inflammatory lesions by 68 percent and noninflammatory lesions by 11.8 percent, compared to 65.2 percent and 10.5 percent for the drug. Table 20-1 below shows the percentage of people in the gugulipid and standard medicine groups who had an excellent, good, or poor response to treatment.

Table 20-1: Gugulipid and Tetracycline
Both Reduce Inflammatory Acne Lesions[4]

**PERCENTAGE OF PATIENTS IN EACH TREATMENT GROUP
WITH REDUCTION OF INFLAMMATORY LESIONS**

	Excellent Reduction	Good Reduction	Poor Reduction
Gugulipid	30%	70%	0%
Tetracycline	20%	60%	20%

Summing Up the Evidence for Guggul

This single study is intriguing but not enough to allow for a definitive conclusion. Given the limited evidence available thus far, it is fair to say that guggul is a two-star treatment for pimples backed by modest evidence.

Available Forms

Guggul is available in supplement form.

How Much Guggul Is Typically Used

There is no standard dose of guggul. The study above used a supplemental dose of 50 milligrams of guggulsterones per day.

Possible Side Effects and Interactions

Guggul's side effects include headaches, vomiting, diarrhea, and hiccups. It may interfere with the absorption of blood pressure medicines such as diltiazem (Cardizem). Taken in combination with anticoagulants such as fondaparinux (Arixtra), guggul may increase the risk of bruising and bleeding. If you're on any medication, be sure to consult your doctor before adding guggul to your self-care regimen.

Tea Tree Oil

Rating: ☆☆ = Modest Evidence

A product of the leaves of a small tree native to Australia, tea tree oil has been used by Aboriginal tribes for hundreds of years as an all-purpose health remedy. The oil, which is extracted from the leaves through the process of steam distillation, contains a variety of substances with antibacterial, antiyeast, and other therapeutic properties. It has been used as a treatment for wounds, burns, cuts, lice, athlete's foot, insect bites, vaginal infections, toothache, and other ailments. It also shows promise for acne, as the following study suggests:

◆ One randomized, single-blind 1990 study has compared tea tree oil to benzoyl peroxide lotion, a standard treatment for acne.[5] Researchers from Royal Prince Alfred Hospital in Australia randomly assigned 124 people with mild to moderate acne—average age 19.7—to receive treatment with either 5 percent tea tree oil gel (supplied by Lederle Laboratories) or 5 percent benzoyl peroxide lotion. The numbers of inflamed and noninflamed acne lesions were counted at the beginning of the study and then monthly for 3 months. Both treatments were effective, although it took longer for the tea tree oil to work. However, only 44 percent of those using tea tree oil reported skin discomfort, compared to 79 percent of those using benzoyl peroxide. The researchers concluded that this tea tree oil preparation was "an effective topical treatment for acne."

Summing Up the Evidence for Tea Tree Oil

This study is intriguing, but it is only the first step in marshaling evidence to support the use of tea tree oil for pimples. At this point, the best we can say is that tea tree oil is a two-star treatment for pimples backed by modest evidence.

Other Names

Tea tree's scientific name is *Melaleuca alternifolia*. It has several other common names, including Australian tea tree oil and oil of Melaleuca.

Available Forms

Tea tree oil is available as an ointment, cream, lotion, and soap.

How Much Tea Tree Oil Is Typically Used

There is no standard dose of tea tree oil. The study cited on page 290 used tea tree oil with a 5 percent concentration.

Possible Side Effects

Tea tree oil can cause skin irritation and rash in people who are sensitive to it. Therefore, before using tea tree oil, you may want apply it to a small patch of skin (perhaps the inside of the elbow) and wait for 24 hours to see if a reaction occurs. When you begin treatment, be sure to read and follow the label directions of the tea tree product you choose.

Zinc

Rating: ☆☆ = Modest Evidence

Zinc is a trace mineral that plays important roles in normal growth and development, immunity, wound healing, reproduction, and many other bodily functions. Every single cell in the body needs zinc, although it's found in the largest concentrations in the bones, eyes, kidneys, liver, pancreas, prostate gland, and skin.

Zinc deficiency has been linked to several skin disorders. Research dating back to the 1970s has pointed to a possible link between low zinc levels and acne.[6] A number of studies suggest that taking supplemental zinc may help clear the problem. For example:

♦ A 1977 study presented in the *British Journal of Dermatology* compared daily doses of 400 milligrams of oral zinc sulphate to a placebo in the treatment of 91 people ranging in age from 13 to 37, all with acne vulgaris.[7] After 12 weeks, the 48 people taking zinc showed "significantly better results" (according to the doctors' and patients' subjective evaluations) than the 43 taking the placebo. Seventy-five percent of those in the zinc group were satisfied with the results of their treatment.

♦ Another study, presented in the *Archives of Dermatology* in the same year, examined the effects of zinc and vitamin A on acne in 64 volunteers ranging in age from 13 to 25.[8] The volunteers were randomly divided into four groups and given one of the following treatments: 600 milligrams of oral zinc sulfate (brand name Solvezink); 300,000 to

400,000 IU of vitamin A; both zinc and vitamin A, in the same amounts; or a placebo. The researchers counted the number of acne lesions on each of the volunteers at the beginning of the study and again after 4 weeks. Those taking zinc—whether alone or in combination with vitamin A—showed a "significant decrease in the number of papules, pustules," and other indications of acne. Adding vitamin A to zinc did not confer additional benefits in this study.

♦ Zinc was compared to oxytetracycline—a standard drug treatment for acne—in a double-blind study conducted by Swedish researchers.[9] The 37 people who enrolled in the study, all with moderate to severe facial acne, were randomly assigned to receive either 600 milligrams of oral zinc sulfate (Solvezink) or 250 to 750 milligrams of oxytetracycline every day for 12 weeks. Acne scores fell approximately 70 percent in both groups. The mineral and the drug were equally effective, with the researchers reporting that "no difference in effect between the treatments was seen."

Summing Up the Evidence for Zinc

These and other studies have suggested that zinc is helpful in treating pimples. However, several studies have produced equivocal results. Based on the current state of information, it is fair to say that zinc is a two-star treatment for pimples backed by modest evidence.

Available Forms

Food sources of zinc include oysters, chicken leg, pork tenderloin, plain yogurt, pecans, and cashews. The mineral also is available in supplement form.

How Much Zinc Is Typically Used

The Food and Nutrition Board has set the Recommended Dietary Allowance for zinc at 11 milligrams for men ages 19 and older and 8 milligrams for women ages 19 and older. Some studies have produced good results using 600 milligrams of zinc sulfate per day.

Possible Side Effects and Interactions

The Food and Nutrition Board of the Institute of Medicine has set a tolerable upper intake for zinc at 40 milligrams per day for adults. Taking excessive amounts of zinc can lower levels of "good" HDL cholesterol and weaken the immune system. It also can impair copper absorption. If high-dose treatment continues for more than a month, it's best to take 2 milligrams of copper along with zinc.

Zinc may hamper the absorption of antibiotics such as ciprofloxacin (Cipro), reducing the level of the drug in the body. If you're taking any medication, be sure to consult your doctor before adding therapeutic amounts of zinc to your self-care regimen.

Olive Leaf

Rating: ☆ = Preliminary Evidence

Long used for pneumonia, severe diarrhea, and various types of infection, olive leaf extract is now being studied as a treatment for acne. Research involving laboratory animals already has suggested that olive leaf extract may play a role in lowering blood pressure, preventing irregular heartbeat, and reducing inflammation. It also may be helpful in combating bacterial, viral, parasitic, and fungal infections.

The theory that olive leaf extract can help combat pimples is based on studies of its antibacterial action. If it can slow the growth of bacteria in follicles, it may help keep pimples under control.

This early work is promising, and there have been numerous reports of success using olive leaf extract against acne. But more research is necessary. For now, it is fair to say that olive leaf extract is a one-star treatment for pimples backed by preliminary evidence.

Available Forms

Olive leaf extract can be found in liquid, tincture, tablet, and capsule form. Some people make a tea from the loose leaves.

How Much Olive Leaf Is Typically Used

There is no standard dose of olive leaf extract for pimples. A typical dosage is two 500-milligram capsules, three or four times daily. Some people may require up to 10 to 12 capsules per day for optimal results. Look for a product that's standardized to oleuropein content, 20 percent or higher.

Possible Side Effects and Interactions

There have been no reports of significant side effects with olive leaf extract. It may interact with diabetes medications such as glyburide (Dia-Beta), causing blood sugar to drop too low. If you're taking any medication, be sure to consult your doctor before adding olive leaf extract to your self-care regimen.

21

ALTERNATIVE APPROACHES TO

PMS

Acupuncture	☆☆☆☆
Chasteberry	☆☆☆☆
Calcium	☆☆☆
Homeopathy	☆☆
Qi gong	☆☆

PMS is a cornucopia of physical and psychological symptoms that can occur between 1 and 14 days prior to menstruation. These symptoms typically disappear once the menstrual period begins and do not return for the next 2 to 3 weeks, although those who are nearing menopause may have symptoms that continue through and after menstruation. It's estimated that 85 percent of women of childbearing age suffer from PMS at least some of the time, and 40 percent suffer from it regularly. Ten to 15 percent experience severe symptoms that seriously disrupt their lives.

SYMPTOMS

Perhaps as many as 200 symptoms have been attributed to PMS. Among the most common are physical symptoms such as bloating, breast tenderness and swelling, headaches (including migraines), acne, backaches, cravings for sweets, fatigue, joint pain, and weight gain; psychological symptoms such as mood swings, irritability, anxiety, and depression; and behavioral symptoms such as crying, binge eating, aggressiveness, and hostility. Slightly less common are symptoms such as constipation, diarrhea, hypersensitivity to sound, shakiness, and heaviness in the legs. During the "PMS phase" (the 2 weeks prior to menstruation), symptoms of chronic conditions such as seizure disorders, lupus, rheumatoid arthritis, and allergies may become worse.

How can a woman tell if her lower back pain and irritability are signs of PMS or something entirely different? There are three hallmarks of PMS: (1) The symptoms appear within 2 weeks prior to the beginning of the menstrual period; (2) certain symptoms may occur all month, but they are markedly worse during the week or two before the onset of menstruation; and (3) symptoms clear up or are markedly improved once the menstrual period begins.

CAUSES

Most experts believe that PMS is the result of fluctuations or imbalances in the female hormones estrogen and progesterone. During ovulation (which occurs about 2 weeks before menstruation), estrogen levels drop somewhat, triggering premenstrual symptoms in some women. But the majority of women experience PMS about a week after ovulation, when both estrogen and progesterone levels drop precipitously (about day 23 of the menstrual cycle, counting the start of menstruation as day 1). Estrogen and progesterone keep each other in balance; when there is too much or too little of either hormone, it disrupts this balance. PMS is thought to be at least partially due to estrogen levels that are too high and/or progesterone levels that are too low.

STANDARD TREATMENTS

The standard treatments for PMS typically involve lifestyle changes that are intended to alleviate symptoms. For example, reducing salt intake may help ease bloating, breast tenderness or swelling, and weight gain. Avoiding caffeine may help minimize nervousness and agitation. Exercise and stress reduction techniques as well as consuming a healthy diet (three meals plus snacks, spread out over the course of a day) can help counteract anxiety, depression, irritability, binge eating, and a craving for sweets.

Depending on the severity of symptoms, certain medications may be recommended. These include nonsteroidal anti-inflammatory drugs (NSAIDs) for headaches, joint pain, and other pains; combination oral contraceptives (estrogen plus progestin) for breast tenderness and appetite changes; antidepressants such as fluoxetine, paroxetine, and sertraline for irritability and depression; and antianxiety medications such as buspirone and alprazolam for anxiety and nervousness.

RATING POPULAR ALTERNATIVE TREATMENTS FOR PMS

Acupuncture

Rating: ☆☆☆☆ = Strong Evidence

Acupuncture—the ancient Chinese healing art that involves inserting needles into various points on the body to unblock the flow of qi (pronounced "chee"), or life energy—has long been used to alleviate premenstrual symptoms. Its effectiveness has been the subject of several small controlled trials, including these:

♦ For a 2002 study published in the *Archives of Gynecological Obstetrics*, Croatian researchers randomly placed 35 women suffering from PMS into either an acupuncture group or a placebo group.[1] The women began treatment at about day 14 of the menstrual cycle (counting the start of menstruation as day 1). Those in the acupuncture group received seven acupuncture treatments, 30 minutes every other day. Those in the placebo group followed the same schedule but were given a sham procedure that appeared to be real acupuncture but was not. The acupuncture treatments were considered successful if PMS no longer occurred, acupuncture and/or medicine was no longer necessary, or premenstrual symptoms disappeared within a year after the end of treatment. The success rate in the acupuncture group was 77.8 percent, compared to only 5.9 percent in the sham acupuncture group.

♦ An interesting study combined acupuncture with acupoint injections, in which herbs or vitamins are administered directly into acupuncture points.[2] For this 2005 study, Chinese researchers divided 102 women with PMS into two groups. One group received acupuncture plus acupoint injection once every 3 days, beginning 10 days before menstruation. The other group received the standard medicines diazepam (Valium) and oryzanol (Gamma-O), which is made from plant sterols that relieve pain by triggering the release of hormones called endorphins. This second group served as the control. The results were positive and statistically significant, with the acupuncture/acupoint group showing a 92.6 percent effectiveness rate compared to a 75 percent effectiveness rate in the control group.

♦ A 2005 review written by researchers from the China Academy of Traditional Chinese Medicine found eight controlled studies involving slightly more than 800 women and examining the effectiveness of various types of acupuncture treatment for PMS.[3] These researchers noted that in seven of eight studies, acupuncture proved superior to standard Western medicine or Chinese herbs.

Summing Up the Evidence for Acupuncture

Although these and many other acupuncture/PMS studies have produced positive results, a large number of studies have produced equivocal or negative results. And many of the studies have been criticized for small numbers of participants and weaknesses in the study protocols. On the other hand, the World Health Organization has said that acupuncture has a therapeutic effect on PMS, though more proof is necessary.[4] Based on the strength of the World Health Organization finding, it is fair to say that acupuncture is a four-star treatment for PMS backed by strong evidence.

Possible Side Effects

When properly administered, acupuncture usually produces no side effects, although in a few cases there may be slight bruising, a small amount of bleeding, or some dizziness.

Finding an Acupuncturist

To learn more about acupuncture, or to find a certified acupuncturist in your area, visit the Web site for the National Certification Commission for Acupuncture and Oriental Medicine (NCCAOM) at www.nccaom.org. The commission is the acupuncture profession's equivalent of the American Medical Association.

Chasteberry

Rating: ☆☆☆☆ = Strong Evidence

A shrub native to the Mediterranean area, chasteberry has a long history of medicinal use. The Greek physician Hippocrates prescribed it for menstrual difficulties, while medieval monks used it to help reduce their sex drive so that they could more easily adhere to their vows (thus the name *chaste-berry*). The herb also has been said to suppress appetite, control flatus, and treat insomnia.

Although chasteberry's mechanism of action is not well understood, some experts believe that it can help correct female hormonal imbalances by stimulating the pituitary gland at the base of the brain to produce more luteinizing hormone (LH). This, in turn, prompts the ovaries to produce more of the hormone progesterone, helping to balance the ratio of estrogen to progesterone—and possibly easing PMS and other menstrual problems in the process.

Some studies seem to confirm that chasteberry may be helpful in relieving premenstrual symptoms. They include the following:

♦ A 2001 study published in the *British Medical Journal* compared the effects of chasteberry to placebo in 170 women, average age 36, who suffered from PMS.[5] For this double-blind study, the women were randomly assigned to receive either 20 milligrams of chasteberry fruit extract in tablet form or a placebo every day over the course of three consecutive menstrual cycles. Throughout the study, the volunteers assessed their symptoms, including irritability, headaches, and breast fullness. Fifty-two percent of the women taking chasteberry responded with at least a 50 percent improvement in overall symptoms, compared to only 24 percent of those taking the placebo. The researchers concluded that chasteberry extract "is an effective and well-tolerated treatment for the relief of symptoms of the premenstrual syndrome." Table 21-1 on page 300 shows the rate of reduction in specific symptoms of PMS by chasteberry and placebo. Note that chasteberry outperformed the placebo in reducing every symptom.

Table 21-1: Chasteberry Outperforms Placebo in Reducing PMS Symptoms[6]

SYMPTOMS	AVERAGE CHANGE IN SYMPTOM SCORE	
	Chasteberry	Placebo
Irritability	-28.9%	-18.2%
Mood alteration	-28.7%	-17.6%
Anger	-22.1%	-11.7%
Headache	-17.8%	-5.9%
Breast fullness	-18.6%	-9.4%

♦ German researchers conducted a large-scale study to determine the effectiveness of a chasteberry extract (brand name Femicur) in 1,634 women suffering from PMS.[7] The average volunteer was 35.8 years old and had been suffering from premenstrual symptoms for nearly 3 years. For this open, uncontrolled study, the volunteers were given 40 milligrams of *Vitex agnus* (chasteberry) extract every day. By the end of the three-cycle treatment period, PMS symptoms had vanished in 42 percent of the women and improved in another 51 percent. Figure 21-1 below shows the decline in premenstrual symptoms after treatment with chasteberry.

Figure 21-1: Chasteberry Reduces PMS Symptoms

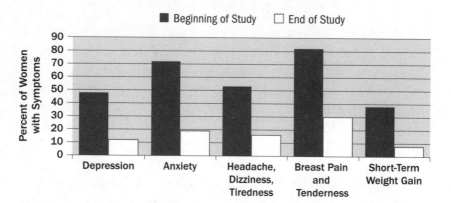

Summing Up the Evidence for Chasteberry

Only a few randomized, controlled studies of chasteberry as a treatment for PMS have been published in English, making it difficult to arrive at an independent appraisal of the herb. But given that Germany's Commission E has approved the use of chasteberry for PMS, it is reasonable to designate it as a four-star treatment backed by strong evidence.

Other Names

Chasteberry's scientific name is *Vitex agnus castus*. It has several other common names, including agnolyt, chaste tree, gattilier, monk's pepper, and vitex.

Available Forms

Chasteberry is available in fluid and solid extract, powder, capsule, tea, and tincture form.

How Much Chasteberry Is Typically Used

There is no standard dose of chasteberry to treat PMS. Successful studies have used dosages in the range of 20 to 40 milligrams per day.

Possible Side Effects and Interactions

Chasteberry can cause acne, rash, headache, and irregular menstrual bleeding. It may interfere with the effectiveness of oral contraceptives such as ethinyl estradiol and desogestrel (Cyclessa) and may increase the risk of side effects when combined with Parkinson's medications such as carbidopa (Lodsoyn). If you're taking any medication, be sure to consult your doctor before adding chasteberry to your self-care regimen.

Calcium

Rating: ☆☆☆ = Intriguing Evidence

Calcium, the mineral with a reputation for building strong bones, also performs a wide variety of other bodily functions. It aids in muscle contraction, nerve signal transmission, and wound healing and supports various enzyme systems. It also helps ease muscle cramps, insomnia, depression, anxiety, and water retention—all of which are common premenstrual symptoms.

As far back as 1930, it was noted that calcium levels in the blood were lower during the premenstrual phase of the cycle than they were during the postmenstrual phase, leading to the theory that increasing calcium levels might reduce PMS symptoms.[8] Several studies of the effects of calcium on PMS have found this to be true, including the following:

♦ For a 2005 case-control study presented in the *Archives of Internal Medicine,* researchers compared calcium intake to the risk of developing PMS.[9] More than 3,000 women ranging in age from 27 to 44, none of whom had PMS, were tracked for 10 years. During this decade, 1,057 developed PMS while 1,968 either did not or had only minimal premenstrual symptoms. When the researchers analyzed their data, they determined that the women consuming the largest amount of calcium were about 30 percent less likely to develop PMS than those consuming the smallest amount.

♦ Thirty-three women with recurrent PMS symptoms enrolled in a study comparing the effects of calcium supplementation to placebo.[10] The volunteers were randomly divided into two groups, with one group receiving 1,000 milligrams of calcium carbonate (Oscal 500) and the other receiving a placebo every day for 3 months. Then the groups switched treatments for 3 months, with those in the calcium group taking the placebo and vice versa. Seventy-three percent of the volunteers reported that they had fewer PMS symptoms, especially water retention and pain, while taking calcium. The researchers concluded that "calcium supplementation is a simple and effective treatment for premenstrual syndrome."

♦ A 1998 study published in the *American Journal of Obstetrics and Gynecology* looked at the effects of calcium on 466 women between ages 18 and 45 with moderate to severe PMS.[11] For this double-blind study, the women were randomly assigned to receive either 1,200 milligrams of elemental calcium (Tums E-X) or a placebo every day over the course of three menstrual cycles. Seventeen PMS symptoms were tracked and compiled into a symptom complex score. By the third cycle, the total symptom complex scores had dropped by 48 percent in the calcium group, compared to 30 percent in the placebo group. The researchers noted that "calcium supplementation is a simple and effective treatment in premenstrual syndrome."

Summing Up the Evidence for Calcium

A fair number of studies have found an inverse relationship between calcium intake and PMS. That is, a low intake of calcium raises the risk of developing PMS, while a high intake lowers the risk. This fact—combined with the results of studies showing that supplemental calcium reduces premenstrual symptoms, plus the value of calcium supplementation for overall health—suggests that the mineral is a three-star treatment for PMS backed by intriguing evidence.

Available Forms

Calcium is found in a variety of foods, including dairy products, canned salmon or sardines with bones, dried figs, smoked oysters, spinach, tofu, broccoli, almonds, and papaya. The mineral also is available in supplements, often as calcium carbonate or calcium citrate. Of the two, calcium carbonate is less expensive and contains more calcium per pill. On the other hand, calcium citrate is less constipating, and according to some studies, it may be better absorbed.

How Much Calcium Is Typically Used

There is no standard dose of calcium as a treatment for PMS. Studies have used dosages ranging from 1,000 to 1,200 milligrams per day.

Possible Side Effects and Interactions

The Food and Nutrition Board of the Institute of Medicine has set a tolerable upper intake for calcium at 2,500 milligrams per day for adults. Taking excessive amounts can lead to kidney damage. Other possible side effects include belching, gastrointestinal irritation, and constipation.

Calcium may reduce the effectiveness of aspirin and other medicines for pain; of ciprofloxacin (Cipro) and other antibiotics; and of blood pressure medications such as nisoldipine (Sular). If you're taking any medication, be sure to consult your doctor before adding therapeutic amounts of calcium to your self-care regimen.

Homeopathy

Rating: ☆☆ = Modest Evidence

In homeopathy, the treatment for a given medical condition is a minuscule amount of a substance that would cause symptoms of that very condition in larger amounts. The theory is that the tiny dose will stimulate the body's internal defenses to fend off the illness and/or restore internal balance.

Although many women have used homeopathy to relieve PMS, there is relatively little scientific evidence examining its effectiveness.

♦ One of the most quoted studies was performed by Israeli researchers in 2001.[12] For this double-blind trial, 20 women ranging in age from 20 to

48 and suffering from PMS were randomly assigned to receive either a single dose of a homeopathic medicine or a placebo. The homeopathic medicine was chosen individually for each volunteer, depending on her specific symptoms and personal characteristics. The women were asked to rate their symptoms using a daily Menstrual Distress Questionnaire both before and after treatment. Ninety percent of the women who received homeopathic medicine reported a greater than 30 percent improvement in their symptoms, compared to only 37.5 percent of the women who received the placebo.

Summing Up the Evidence for Homeopathy

Rating the effectiveness of homeopathy is difficult because the treatment is, by design, very individualized. It's virtually impossible to say that a particular homeopathic medicine works or doesn't work, or that one homeopathic medicine is superior to another for PMS.

With this caveat in mind, it is fair to say that homeopathy is a two-star treatment for PMS backed by modest evidence.

Finding a Homeopathic Physician

To learn more about homeopathy, or to find a qualified practitioner, visit the Web site for the National Center for Homeopathy at www.homeopathic.org.

Qi Gong

Rating: ☆☆ = Modest Evidence

Qi gong might be described as the art of drawing vital energy into the body and into life. By combining breathing techniques, concentration, and simple movements, this Chinese discipline may be helpful in treating stress, pain, and elevated blood pressure, among a number of other ailments.

Some studies have examined qi gong's effects on PMS. Among them:

♦ A 2004 study published in the *International Journal of Neuroscience* compared a form of qi gong called qi therapy to doing nothing in 46 women with PMS.[13] The volunteers were given nine sessions of qi therapy over the course of two menstrual cycles, or were simply placed on a waiting list to serve as controls. Qi therapy had a significant positive effect on pain and water retention and produced significant but short-term reductions in anxiety and depression.

♦ In 2004, Korean researchers published the results of their study of the effects of qi therapy on 36 women with PMS in the *Journal of Alternative and Complementary Medicine*.[14] All of the women suffered from at least two severe PMS symptoms, such as pain, water retention, or behavioral changes. The volunteers were randomly assigned to receive either four sessions of qi therapy per cycle for two menstrual cycles or a placebo therapy. According to the researchers, those receiving qi therapy showed "significant improvements in the symptoms of negative feeling, pain, water retention, and total PMS symptoms."

Summing Up the Evidence for Qi Gong

Only a small number of well-designed studies support qi gong's efficacy, making it difficult to draw a definitive conclusion about this ancient healing art. Given that it is noninvasive, and that its combination of breathing techniques, meditation, and simple movement can reduce or relieve stress, qi gong certainly may have therapeutic benefits for many ailments. It may be best to say that qi gong is a two-star treatment for PMS backed by modest evidence.

Finding a Qi Gong Practitioner

You can find lists of qi gong practitioners and teachers at the National Qigong Association Web site (www.nqa.org) and similar sites.

22

ALTERNATIVE APPROACHES TO
PROSTATE ENLARGEMENT

Beta-sitosterol ☆☆☆☆
Pygeum ☆☆☆☆
Saw palmetto ☆☆☆☆
Rye grass pollen ☆☆

Prostate enlargement—also known as benign prostatic hyperplasia (BPH)—is an abnormal growth of the prostate that is not due to cancer or infection. The prostate is a walnut-shaped gland that contributes fluid as sperm arises from the testicles and helps expel semen during ejaculation. The prostate sits right underneath the bladder and is wrapped around the urethra, the tube that carries urine out of the body. When the prostate gland grows, it can push up against the bladder and tighten its grip on the urethra, causing urinary and/or sexual difficulties. Prostate enlargement is surprisingly common and will affect almost every man if he lives long enough.

SYMPTOMS

The first symptoms of BPH typically appear in midlife, although they may occur in adult men at any age. The risk of developing an enlarged prostate increases with age. About 10 percent of men between ages 25 and 30 have BPH, compared to approximately 50 percent of men at age 60 and 90 percent of men age 85 or older.

Symptoms of BPH include difficulty in starting the urine stream; a weak urine stream; urinary flow that starts, then stops, then starts again; dribbling urine; frequent urination; a sense of urgency to urinate; a bladder that does not empty completely; incontinence; and getting up several times during the night to urinate. There may also be a decline in libido, erectile dysfunction, or ejaculatory problems. If BPH becomes severe, it can impair urination, stop the urine flow entirely, cause urinary tract infections and/or bladder stones, and damage the bladder or kidneys.

CAUSES

No one knows for sure what triggers BPH. It may be that with age, the prostate becomes more sensitive to the growth-promoting effects of the male hormones testosterone and dihydrotestosterone. A family history of BPH also slightly increases the risk of developing the condition.

STANDARD TREATMENTS

The least invasive treatment for BPH is "watchful waiting"—that is, keeping an eye on the progress of the condition while delaying powerful medication or surgery until it is absolutely necessary. Medications for BPH fall into two categories: the alpha-blockers such as terazosin (Hytrin), which relax the muscles around the neck of the bladder so that urination is easier, and enzyme inhibitors such as finasteride (Proscar), which reduce the amount of testosterone that converts to dihydrotestosterone.

Minimally invasive treatments such as transurethral microwave therapy, transurethral needle ablation, interstitial laser therapy, and prostatic stents attempt to enlarge the urethra to increase urinary flow. The most invasive treatments are surgeries, which include transurethral resection of the prostate, transurethral incision of the prostate, laser surgery, and open prostatectomy. All of these procedures involve removing part or all of the prostate gland.

RATING POPULAR ALTERNATIVE TREATMENTS FOR PROSTATE ENLARGEMENT

Beta-Sitosterol

Rating: ☆☆☆☆ = Strong Evidence

Found in a variety of plants, beta-sitosterol is a compound that is structurally similar to cholesterol. Concentrated extracts of beta-sitosterol are used to treat elevated cholesterol levels, gallstones, fibromyalgia, tuberculosis, and even the common cold, among numerous other ailments. Beta-sitosterol is added to some brands of margarine to help reduce cholesterol. Some studies suggest that it might have anticancer properties, too.

The following studies have suggested that beta-sitosterol may improve the urological symptoms associated with prostate enlargement.

♦ A 1995 study, presented in the journal *Lancet*, looked at the effects of beta-sitosterol in 200 men with symptomatic BPH.[1] For this double-blind trial, the volunteers were randomly assigned to receive three daily doses of either 60 milligrams of beta-sitosterol or a placebo. The researchers used various measures—including the International Prostate Symptom Score, a modified Boyarsky score, and changes in urine flow and prostate size—to track the patients' progress. After 6 months of treatment, the results were positive. The Boyarsky score (which rates the severity of symptoms) dropped 6.7 points among those taking beta-sitosterol, compared to 2.1 points in the placebo group. The beta-sitosterol group also showed a greater drop in the International Prostate Symptom Score (7.4 compared to 2.1). For these men, urinary peak flow increased while the amount of urine left in the bladder after urinating decreased—changes not seen in the placebo group. The researchers concluded that although beta-sitosterol did not shrink enlarged prostates, the "significant improvement in symptoms and urinary flow parameters show the effectiveness of beta-sitosterol in the treatment of BPH." Table 22-1 below summarizes selected results from the study.

Table 22-1: Beta-Sitosterol Outperforms Placebo in Men with BPH[2]

	BETA-SITOSTEROL GROUP		PLACEBO GROUP	
	Beginning of Study	End of Study	Beginning of Study	End of Study
Modified Boyarsky score (lower score is desirable)	15.0	7.7	14.9	12.2
International Prostate Symptom Score (lower score is desirable)	14.9	7.5	15.1	12.8
Peak urinary flow (increase is desirable)	9.9	15.2	10.2	11.4
Median urinary flow (increase is desirable)	5.7	8.8	5.8	6.2

♦ For a double-blind study that appeared in the *British Urology Journal* in 1997,[3] German researchers gave 177 men with BPH either 130 milligrams of beta-sitosterol (brand name Azuprostat) or a placebo every day for 6 months. Compared to placebo, beta-sitosterol produced significant improvement in urinary symptoms and in symptoms measured by the International Prostate Symptom Score. Scores on this test fell from 16.0 to 7.8 in the beta-sitosterol group, compared to a reduction of 14.9 to 12.1 in the placebo group. The researchers concluded that "beta-sitosterol is an effective option in the treatment of BPH."

♦ The authors of a 1999 review study, published in the *British Journal of Urology International*, searched the medical literature for randomized studies of the effect of beta-sitosterol on symptomatic BPH. The studies were to have lasted at least 1 month and were to compare beta-sitosterol to either a placebo or a drug.[4] The authors found 4 double-blind trials—involving a total of 519 men and lasting from 4 to 26 weeks—that met their criteria. After reviewing these studies, the researchers concluded that "beta-sitosterol improves urological symptoms" in men with BPH. They cautioned, however, that the results were limited because they came from short-term studies that used a variety of beta-sitosterol preparations.

Summing Up the Evidence for Beta-Sitosterol

Although the beta-sitosterol/BPH studies generally have been short-term and involved different "versions" of beta-sitosterol, they have demonstrated the supplement's potential. Although we are lacking the large-scale, long-term trials that are necessary before a definitive conclusion can be drawn, at this point it is fair to say that beta-sitosterol is a four-star treatment for BPH backed by strong evidence.

Other Names

Beta-sitosterol is known by a variety of other names, including angelican, B-sitosterolin, cinchol, sitosterol, and sterolins.

Available Forms

Beta-sitosterol is found in soybeans, wheat germ, and corn oil, among other foods. It is also available in tablet, capsule, and soft gel form.

How Much Beta-Sitosterol Is Typically Used

There is no standard dosage of beta-sitosterol. For men with prostate enlargement, daily doses may range from 60 to 130 milligrams.

Possible Side Effects and Interactions

Beta-sitosterol's side effects include gas, diarrhea, and nausea. Beta-sitosterol is not known to interact with medications in a significant manner. As with all supplements and drugs, be sure to read the label directions carefully before using beta-sitosterol.

Pygeum

Rating: ☆☆☆☆ = Strong Evidence

Some 300 years ago, South African tribes introduced visiting Europeans to the medicinal properties of the *Pygeum africanum* tree. Of great interest was a tea made from the powdered bark of the tree that could help relieve bladder problems, particularly in older men suffering from prostate problems. It took awhile, but in the 1960s pygeum finally found its way to the Western world when an extract taken from its bark began to be used in Europe to treat the urinary difficulties seen in mild to moderate BPH. Scientists have since discovered that certain compounds in pygeum bark may help ease urinary problems by decreasing inflammation and reducing cholesterol deposits in the prostate.

A large number of randomized, controlled trials have investigated the effects of pygeum on BPH. Here is a sampling.

- A 1990 double-blind study involved 263 men in Germany, France, and Austria.[5] The men were randomly assigned to receive either 100 milligrams of pygeum or a placebo every day for 60 days. At the end of the treatment period, urination had "improved in 66 [percent] of the patients treated with *Pygeum africanum* extract," compared with 31 percent of those given the placebo. The superiority of pygeum over placebo was statistically significant.

- A 1999 study published in *Urology* compared the effects of two varying doses of pygeum extract in 209 men with BPH.[6] For this double-blind study, the men were randomly assigned to take either 50 milligrams of pygeum twice daily or 100 milligrams of pygeum once a day for 2 months.

Both doses were effective, with the International Prostate Symptoms Scores falling by 35 to 38 percent and the urinary symptoms improving as well. The researchers concluded that both 50 milligrams twice a day and 100 milligrams once a day of pygeum "proved equally effective and safe."

♦ In 2000, researchers from the Minneapolis Veterans Affairs Center published a meta-analysis of pygeum in the *American Journal of Medicine*.[7] The meta-analysis combined the results of 18 trials involving 1,562 men. All of the studies were randomized, lasted at least 30 days, and compared pygeum to either a placebo or a drug in men with symptomatic BPH. The researchers found that while the men were taking pygeum, they were "more than twice as likely to report an improvement in overall symptoms," with a 19 percent reduction in night-time urination (nocturia), a 23 percent increase in peak urinary flow, and a 24 percent drop in the amount of urine remaining in the bladder after urination was complete. Adverse effects triggered by pygeum "were mild and similar to placebo." The researchers concluded that although the studies were generally short-term and used different pygeum preparations, the evidence indicated that pygeum had a modest but statistically significant ability to improve urinary symptoms in BPH.

♦ A 1995 review prepared by French researchers noted that pygeum has been used in France since 1969 to treat symptoms of mild to moderate BPH.[8] Their paper concluded that "clinical data from 2,262 patients over 25 years of use show that *Pygeum africanum* extract produces subjective and objective improvements in a majority of patients with mild symptomatic BPH." The researchers added that although much of the early data had come from open studies, it has been confirmed by more recent double-blind, placebo-controlled studies.

Summing Up the Evidence for Pygeum

Although the pygeum studies were of relatively short duration and their results are somewhat muddied because different preparations were used, their findings paint a positive picture. Given what we know so far, it is fair to say that pygeum is a four-star treatment for BPH backed by strong evidence.

Available Forms

Pygeum is available in tablet, tincture, or liquid extract form.

How Much Pygeum Is Typically Used

There is no standard dose of pygeum. Supplemental doses of 50 milligrams taken twice a day or 100 milligrams taken once a day have been used to treat symptoms of BPH.

Possible Side Effects and Interactions

Pygeum can cause abdominal pain, lack of appetite, and nausea. It is not known to interact with medications in a significant manner. As with all supplements and drugs, be sure to read the label directions carefully before using pygeum.

Saw Palmetto

Rating: ☆☆☆☆ = Strong Evidence

Saw palmetto, also known as the American dwarf palm tree, is native to the United States. American Indians once used its berries to treat urinary tract and prostate problems. Today, an extract taken from the oil of the saw palmetto berry (often referred to by its botanical name, *Serenoa repens*) is an accepted medical treatment for BPH in Germany, Austria, Italy, and other European countries. Saw palmetto also has been used to relieve inflammation and improve sexual vigor.

A large number of studies suggest that saw palmetto can help relieve symptoms of BPH. For example:

♦ For a 2002 double-blind study published in *European Urology*, 704 men with BPH were randomly assigned to receive daily doses of either 320 milligrams of saw palmetto berry extract (brand name Permixon) or 0.4 milligram of the standard drug tamsulosin (Flomax).[9] After 12 months of treatment, the results were positive for both groups. The International Prostate Symptom Score fell by 4.4 points, with equal improvement in symptoms across the groups. The researchers concluded that this particular brand of saw palmetto extract and the standard medicine "are equivalent in medical treatment of lower urinary tract symptoms in men with BPH, during and up to 12 months of therapy."

♦ For a 1996 double-blind study published in the journal *Prostate*, 1,098 men with moderate BPH were randomly assigned to receive daily doses of either 320 milligrams of saw palmetto berry extract (Permixon) or 5 milligrams of the standard drug finasteride (Proscar).[10] The results produced by the extract and the drug were nearly equal. Saw palmetto improved the International Prostate Symptom Scores by 37 percent, quality of life scores by 38 percent, and peak urinary flow rate by 25 percent, compared to improvements of 39 percent, 41 percent, and 30 percent, respectively, in the same categories for the drug. The researchers concluded that "both treatments relieve the symptoms of BPH in about two-thirds of the patients." They noted that while the drug could shrink an enlarged prostate, saw palmetto could not.

◆ An earlier study was reported as a letter to the editor in the *British Journal of Clinical Pharmacology* in 1984.[11] Ninety-four men suffering from BPH completed the 30-day treatment period. Fifty of the men had been randomly assigned to receive a daily dose of 320 milligrams of saw palmetto berry extract (Permixon); the rest were given a placebo. The researchers found that the improvement associated with saw palmetto "was significantly superior to that achieved with placebo." Table 22-2 below shows selected results from the study. Note that saw palmetto reduced the number of times the men needed to urinate at night and the amount of urine left in the bladder after they had urinated. The herb also increased the urinary flow rate.

Table 22-2: Saw Palmetto Extract Superior to Placebo in Treating Symptoms of BPH[12]

	Before	After	% Difference
Instances of nighttime urination (fewer is better)			
Saw palmetto	3.1	1.7	-45.8
Placebo	3.2	2.7	-15.0
Urine remaining in the bladder after urination (mL) (less is better)			
Saw palmetto	94.7	55.1	-41.9
Placebo	91.3	100.0	+9.3
Flow rate (mL/s) (more is better)			
Saw palmetto	5.4	8.05	+50.5
Placebo	5.0	5.29	+5.0

♦ A 1998 review study published in the *Journal of the American Medical Association* examined the scientific literature on saw palmetto to see if it was indeed effective in relieving symptoms of BPH.[13] The study's authors, who were from the Department of Veterans Affairs in Minneapolis, found 18 randomized, controlled trials involving more than 2,900 men with BPH. The studies, 16 of which were double-blind, lasted from 4 to 48 weeks. The researchers found that when compared to placebo, saw palmetto berry extract improved urinary tract symptom scores, reduced nighttime urination, and improved peak urine flow and the men's own rating of their symptoms. The use of saw palmetto also was compared to the standard drug finasteride (Proscar), with the herb producing "similar improvements in urinary tract symptoms scores . . . and peak urine flow." Though the saw palmetto studies were generally short in duration, followed different protocols, and used different herbal preparations, the authors found sufficient evidence to conclude that saw palmetto can "improve urinary tract symptoms and flow measures in men with BPH." Compared with the drug finasteride, saw palmetto "produces similar improvement in urinary tract symptoms and flow measures" and is associated fewer side effects.

♦ A researcher from the University of Chicago Pritzker School of Medicine conducted a review of the saw palmetto/BPH literature. In the review, which appeared in the *Journal of Urology* in 2000,[14] the author concluded that "a number of placebo-controlled trials have shown significant improvements in symptoms and flow rates" in men with BPH, although the studies have generally been small and short-term.

♦ A 2004 meta-analysis published in the *British Journal of Urology International* looked only at the published studies involving the saw palmetto berry extract Permixon.[15] The authors of this study used statistical methods to "marry" 14 randomized and 3 open trials involving 4,280 patients with BPH, with the various trials lasting from 21 to 720 days. They found that this particular brand of saw palmetto extract produced "a significant improvement in peak flow rate and reduction in nocturia above placebo, and a 5-point reduction in the [International Prostate Symptom Score]."

♦ A 2002 Cochrane review examined 21 randomized trials involving 3,139 men and lasting from 4 to 48 weeks to determine the effects of saw palmetto on BPH.[16] The authors of this review concluded that saw palmetto provided "mild to moderate improvement in urinary symptoms and flow measures" in men with BPH. Compared to the standard drug finasteride, saw palmetto "produced similar improvements in urinary symptoms and flow measure, is associated with fewer adverse treatment effects, and costs less."

Summing Up the Evidence for Saw Palmetto

There is a fairly robust body of research supporting the use of saw palmetto as a treatment for BPH, as well as positive reviews published in the *Journal of the American Medical Association* and the Cochrane Library. In addition, Germany's Commission E has approved the herb as a treatment for prostate complaints. With this in mind, it is safe to say that saw palmetto is a four-star treatment for BPH backed by strong evidence.

Other Names

Saw palmetto is known to scientists as *Serenoa repens* and *Sabul serrulata*. It also goes by various common names, including American dwarf palm tree, cabbage palm, and scrub palm.

Available Forms

Saw palmetto is available as whole berries, extract from the oil of the berry, tea, capsules, and tablets.

How Much Saw Palmetto Is Typically Used

There is no standard dose of saw palmetto. In studies, daily doses have been as high as 320 milligrams of saw palmetto berry extract containing 80 to 90 percent fatty acids.

Possible Side Effects and Interactions

Among saw palmetto's possible side effects are headache, back pain, and impotence. The herb may interact with medicines for pain and inflammation, such as aspirin and diclofenac (Cataflam), increasing the risk of bruising and bleeding. If you're taking any medication, be sure to consult your doctor before adding saw palmetto to your self-care regimen.

Rye Grass Pollen

Rating ☆☆ = Modest Evidence

Extracts of rye grass pollen contain substances that appear to strengthen the ability of the bladder to contract and expel urine while encouraging the urethra to relax and let the urine pass through. These substances may also inhibit the binding of the male hormone 5-alpha-dihydrotestosterone (DHT) to the prostate cells, protecting the prostate from enlargement. Some evidence suggests that rye grass pollen might discourage inflammation. The herb is used to treat prostate infection as well as the pain and symptoms of BPH.

A small number of studies have investigated the effectiveness of rye grass pollen as a treatment for BPH. For example:

♦ Japanese researchers performed an open study of the effects of rye grass pollen extract on 79 men ranging in age from 62 to 89.[17] The men were given 378 milligrams of rye pollen extract (brand name Cernitin) every day for 12 weeks. At the end of the treatment period, their BPH symptoms scores had fallen significantly. The researchers concluded that this particular rye grass pollen extract had mildly beneficial effects on men with BPH. Table 22-3 below shows how much this rye grass pollen extract improved various BPH symptoms.

Table 22-3: Percent Improvement in BPH Symptoms after Taking Rye Grass Pollen Extract[18]

Symptom	% Improvement
Urgency or discomfort	76.9
Dysuria	71.4
Nighttime urination (nocturia)	56.8
Incomplete emptying of bladder	66.2
Prolonged voiding	64.1
Having to wait a while for the urine stream to start (delayed voiding)	62.2
Starting and stopping of the urinary stream (intermittency)	60.6
Postvoid dribbling	42.7

♦ A 1990 study published in the *British Journal of Urology* looked at the effect of rye grass pollen extract on 53 men with difficulty urinating due to BPH.[19] For this double-blind study, some of the men were given rye grass pollen extract (Cernilton), while others received a placebo. At the end of the 6-month treatment period, 69 percent of the men taking rye grass pollen extract reported subjective improvement in their symptoms, compared to 30 percent of those taking the placebo. The researchers concluded that this rye grass pollen extract "has a beneficial effect in BPH and may have a place in the treatment of patients with mild or moderate symptoms of outflow obstruction."

♦ A 1999 review article published in the *British Journal of Urology International* examined published studies of the rye grass pollen extract Cernilton to see if the herbal preparation is effective in relieving symptoms of BPH.[20] The authors of the paper found four studies—three of them double-blind—lasting between 12 and 24 weeks and involving a total of 444 men. The authors noted that although the studies were small, short-term, and of uncertain quality, "the available evidence suggests that Cernilton is well tolerated and modestly improves overall urological symptoms, including nocturia" in men with BPH.

Summing Up the Evidence for Rye Grass Pollen

With but a small body of scientific research supporting the use of rye grass pollen, it is difficult to make a definitive statement about the herb. The existing studies are encouraging, so it seems fair to say that rye grass pollen is a two-star treatment for BPH backed by modest evidence.

Other Names

Rye grass pollen is known to scientists as *Secale cereale* and is referred to by various common names including grass pollen, rye, and rye pollen extract.

Available Forms

Rye grass pollen extract is available in capsule or tablet form.

How Much Rye Grass Pollen Is Typically Used

There is no standard dose of rye grass pollen extract. Supplemental doses may range between 80 and 120 milligrams per day.[21]

Possible Side Effects and Interactions

Rye grass pollen can cause nausea and heartburn. It is not known to interact with medications in a significant manner. As with all supplements and drugs, be sure to read the label directions carefully before using rye grass pollen.

ALTERNATIVE APPROACHES TO
RHEUMATOID ARTHRITIS

Acupuncture ☆☆☆☆☆
Omega-3 fatty acids ☆☆☆☆
Gamma-linolenic acid ☆☆☆
Thunder god vine ☆☆

Rheumatoid arthritis (RA) is an autoimmune disease, which means that the immune system has gone haywire and is attacking the body's own tissues. In the case of RA, the body attacks the joint lining (synovium), restricting movement and causing joint pain, damage, and even destruction.

RA triggers the release of inflammatory substances that cause the entire joint capsule to become swollen, hot, and painful. The cells that make up the joint lining divide and grow abnormally; eventually, they invade the cartilage and bone, causing a thinning of the cartilage and a narrowing of the joint space. Enzymes released along with the inflammatory substances further weaken the cartilage and bone, leading to joint erosion and scarring. Over time, the damaged, deteriorating joint loses its shape and becomes misaligned, causing even more pain and further limiting movement.

Unfortunately, such damage isn't confined to a single joint. RA is a systemic disease, which means that it travels throughout the body and affects tissues and organs in several places. In severe cases, RA may settle in all of the joints. It also can cause inflammation of the membranes surrounding the eyes, heart, lungs, and other internal organs.

SYMPTOMS

The most common symptoms of RA are joint pain, swelling, warmth, or tightness; joints that are affected symmetrically (i.e., both wrists or both ankles); joint stiffness in the morning that lasts for more than an hour; swelling in three or more joints that lasts for 6 weeks or longer; small bumps under the skin (rheumatoid nodules) at pressure points like the elbows or the soles of the feet; and blood tests showing the presence of rheumatoid factor.

In some cases, RA settles in for just a short period, then completely disappears. In other cases it causes occasional flares (painful periods), but the person feels fine the rest of the time. Those with severe RA may experience pain much of the time, exhibit symptoms for many years, and develop serious joint problems.

STANDARD TREATMENTS

The standard treatments for RA include resting the affected joints during a flare, engaging in regular exercise, receiving physical therapy, using joint protection techniques (proper posture, correct lifting, ergonomically correct equipment), applying hot or cold compresses, and taking medication. The most common medications for RA include nonsteroidal anti-inflammatory drugs (NSAIDs) to ease swelling and relieve pain; disease-modifying antirheumatic drugs (DMARDs) to alter the course of the disease and reduce inflammation and joint damage; corticosteroids to suppress the immune system; and biologic response modifiers (BRMs) to quell inflammation and disable one part of the immune system while shoring up other parts.

RATING POPULAR ALTERNATIVE TREATMENTS FOR RHEUMATOID ARTHRITIS

Acupuncture

Rating: ☆☆☆☆☆ = Convincing Evidence

Acupuncture, an important element of traditional Chinese medicine, has been used for thousands of years to prevent and treat disease by balancing energy flow. It's based on the premise that energy moves through the body along invisible channels called meridians. Sometimes, though, the energy becomes blocked. These blockages are thought to be the root of all disease. Acupuncture is believed to treat or prevent disease by releasing blocked energy through the insertion of very fine needles into specific points (called acupoints) along the meridians. With obstructions removed and healthy energy flow restored, the body can begin to heal itself.

Millions of Americans use acupuncture to relieve conditions ranging from asthma to postoperative nausea. Most often, however, it's recommended as a treatment for pain. Some studies have suggested that acupuncture might be helpful in alleviating certain symptoms of rheumatoid arthritis, a very painful condition indeed. For example:

♦ In 1987 Russian researchers conducted a double-blind study involving 15 volunteers with rheumatoid arthritis.[1] Nine of the volunteers were treated with auriculo-electropuncture—that is, electroacupuncture at points on the ear—while the remaining six were treated with a sham procedure (the electroacupuncture device was switched off). At the beginning of the study, 8 indices of the disease—including pain and inflammation—were rated. After 10 treatments, all of those receiving genuine acupuncture showed subjective improvement in all 8 indices of the disease; for 7 of the indices, the improvement was statistically significant. By comparison, only one of the six volunteers receiving the sham procedure showed improvement, while another three showed no improvement and two showed a worsening of symptoms.

♦ Researchers from the University of Manitoba in Winnipeg enlisted 20 people with rheumatoid arthritis who had painful knees for their 1974 study published in the *Journal of Rheumatology*.[2] The volunteers were randomly assigned to one of two groups. For those in group A, one knee was treated with acupuncture and the other with a steroid injection. In group B, one knee was treated with sham acupuncture and the other with a steroid injection. The steroid injection resulted in some improvement in the injected knee, which allowed for comparison with the acupuncture/sham and acupuncture techniques.

The patients' knees were assessed at the beginning of the study, 24 hours after treatment, and periodically for 3 months. The results were positive, with 90 percent of the acupuncture group experiencing a moderate decline in pain, compared to only 10 percent of the sham acupuncture group. The researchers concluded that "acupuncture can relieve pain in the knee in patients with RA for periods of up to 3 months." Table 23-1 below compares the results of acupuncture to placebo treatment.

Table 23-1: True Acupuncture Superior to Sham Acupuncture in Treating Symptoms of Rheumatoid Arthritis[3]

	Acupuncture	Sham Acupuncture
Amount of pain	Moderate decline in 90% of patients	Decline in 10% of patients
Swelling in the treated area	Slight increase in 10% of patients	No difference
Heat in the treated area	No difference	No difference
Range of motion of knee joint	Slight increase in 30% of patients	No difference
How long pain free	1-3 months	Less than 10 hours

♦ In their 2002 publication titled "Acupuncture: Review and Analysis of Reports on Controlled Clinical Trials," the World Health Organization noted that acupuncture has been proven through clinical trials to be an effective treatment for rheumatoid arthritis.[4] It does not fix existing joint damage, but "successful pain relief has been verified in the majority of controlled trials." The WHO added that acupuncture has a beneficial effect on the inflammation and immune system dysfunction that are characteristic of rheumatoid arthritis.

Summing Up the Evidence for Acupuncture

The debate over the efficacy of acupuncture is lively, with some studies claiming that it does work and others claiming that it doesn't. Attempts to clarify the matter are complicated by the fact that a great many of the acupuncture studies are not available in English and cannot be scrutinized. For this reason, it's best—if not ideal—to rely on the findings of major health bodies such as the World Health Organization, which has endorsed acupuncture as an effective treatment for rheumatoid arthritis. With this in mind, it is safe to say that acupuncture is a five-star treatment for symptoms of rheumatoid arthritis backed by convincing evidence.

Possible Side Effects

Acupuncture usually produces no side effects when properly administered. In rare cases, the needles may cause slight bruising or a small amount of bleeding. Some people have reported dizziness after treatment.

Finding an Acupuncturist

To learn more about acupuncture or to find a certified acupuncturist, visit the Web site for the National Certification Commission for Acupuncture and Oriental Medicine (NCCAOM) at www.nccaom.org. The commission is the acupuncture profession's equivalent of the American Medical Association.

Omega-3 Fatty Acids
Rating: ☆☆☆☆ = Strong Evidence

Found primarily in cold-water fatty fish, omega-3 fatty acids are converted in the body to substances called prostaglandins. These are naturally occurring anti-inflammatories can help ease pain and inflammation and suppress certain immune system functions. Knowing this, researchers wondered if omega-3s might reduce the pain and joint stiffness that occur in rheumatoid arthritis, an autoimmune disease with an inflammatory component. Some studies suggest this is true:

> ♦ Researchers enlisted 66 rheumatoid arthritis patients for a double-blind, placebo-controlled study published in *Arthritis and Rheumatism* in 1995.[5] The volunteers were assigned to take daily doses of either an omega-3 fatty acid preparation developed by the National Institutes of Health (130 milligrams per kilogram of body weight) or corn oil. Both groups also took the standard RA medicine diclofenac (Cataflam). Several months into the study, without the volunteers' knowledge, the diclofenac was replaced with a placebo, and the omega-3s with corn oil.

While no improvements were seen in those taking corn oil, those taking omega-3 fatty acids showed "significant decreases" in the number of tender joints, the duration of morning stiffness, and blood levels of interleukin-1 beta—one of the markers of rheumatoid arthritis. Also in the omega-3 group, there was a significant decline in both the patient's and the physician's impression of the overall activity of the disease (such as the amount and duration of flares). The authors reported that certain RA patients taking omega-3s could reduce or even discontinue their pain medication without experiencing disease flares.

♦ A 2000 study published in the *Journal of Rheumatology* looked at the effects of an omega-3 fatty acid preparation (brand name Pikasol) in 50 people suffering from rheumatoid arthritis.[6] For this double-blind, placebo-controlled study, the volunteers were randomly assigned to receive either fish oil containing 60 percent omega-3 fatty acids (40 milligrams per kilogram of body weight) or a placebo every day for 15 weeks. The researchers looked for changes in nine variables, including the duration of morning stiffness, the number of painful joints, and the amount of pain. The researchers found that the omega-3 group experienced significant improvement in six of the nine variables, compared to no significant improvement in the placebo group. The researchers concluded, "The findings add to a considerable body of evidence that dietary fish oil supplements result in improvements in rheumatoid arthritis, without unwanted effects."

♦ Brazilian researchers published the results of their study of the effects of fish oil and olive oil on people with rheumatoid arthritis in the journal *Nutrition* in 2005.[7] The 43 volunteers were randomly assigned to receive one of three daily treatments: 3 grams of fish oil; 3 grams of fish oil plus 9.6 milliliters of olive oil; or a placebo. (The fish oil was supplied by R. P. Scherer do Brasil Encapsulacões Ltda.) Everyone continued taking their regular medications. The researchers measured disease activity at the beginning of the study and again at 12 and 24 weeks. At the end of the study period, those taking fish oil—whether alone or with olive oil—showed statistically significant improvements in the duration of morning stiffness, onset of fatigue, intensity of joint pain, and other indicators of disease activity compared to the placebo group. In addition, there was earlier and greater improvement when olive oil was added to the fish oil. The researchers concluded that "ingestion of fish oil omega-3 fatty acids relieved several clinical parameters" of rheumatoid arthritis.

Several review studies have examined the scientific literature, attempting to draw some conclusion about the value of omega-3 fatty acids for relieving symptoms of rheumatoid arthritis.

♦ A 2000 review presented in the *American Journal of Clinical Nutrition* observed that the benefit most often seen with omega-3 fatty acid supplements "is an improvement in the number of tender joints on physical examination."[8] The review noted that while the response to fish oil is often positive, it is generally moderate.

♦ Another review, published in the *Journal of the American Board of Family Practitioners* in 2005, noted that "fish oil supplementation consistently shows modest clinical improvement and reduction of nonsteroidal anti-inflammatory drug (NSAID) use in randomized clinical trials."[9]

♦ A 2004 review published by the Agency for Healthcare Research and Quality of the US Department of Health and Human Services noted that in six of seven studies, patients taking omega-3 fatty acids were able to cut back on their use of anti-inflammatory drugs or corticosteroids.[10]

♦ For a meta-analysis published in the *Journal of Clinical Epidemiology* in 1995, researchers statistically merged the results of 10 individual randomized, double-blind, placebo-controlled studies involving 395 people.[11] Analysis of the results led to the conclusion that 3 months of treatment with supplementary fish oil significantly reduced the number of tender joints and the duration of morning stiffness in people with rheumatoid arthritis.

Summing Up the Evidence for Omega-3 Fatty Acids

A large body of scientific evidence suggests that while omega-3 fatty acids do not repair joint damage, they can help relieve painful symptoms. Thus, it is fair to say that the omega-3 fatty acids are a four-star treatment for symptoms of rheumatoid arthritis backed by strong evidence.

Available Forms

The best sources of omega-3 fatty acids are cold-water fatty fish such as mackerel, salmon, herring, anchovies, and tuna. As a general rule, the fattier a fish is, the more omega-3s it contains. The human body can manufacture omega-3s from alpha-linolenic acid, which is found in walnuts and flaxseed. Omega-3 fatty acids are also available in supplement form, labeled as fish oil, omega-3, EPA, DHA, or some combination of these.

Amount of Omega-3 Fatty Acids Typically Used

There is no standard dose of omega-3 fatty acids for relieving symptoms of rheumatoid arthritis, although some studies have used 2 to 4 grams of EPA or DHA per day.

Possible Side Effects and Interactions

The omega-3 fatty acids are found in common foods and have been granted Generally Regarded as Safe (GRAS) status by the US government. They can cause prolonged bleeding time, which may be a problem for those who have bleeding disorders, who are taking medicines to thin the blood, or who will be undergoing surgery soon.

Along the same line, the omega-3s may increase the risk of bruising and bleeding when taken with drugs that thin the blood, such as aspirin and heparin (Hep-Lock). In combination with blood pressure medications such as atenolol (Tenormin), they may cause blood pressure to drop too low. If you're taking any medication, be sure to consult your doctor before adding therapeutic amounts of omega-3s to your self-care regimen.

Gamma-Linolenic Acid

Rating: ☆☆☆ = Intriguing Evidence

Gamma-linolenic acid (GLA) is found in the oil of seeds from borage, evening primrose, and black currant plants. It is an essential fatty acid, necessary for normal brain function; regulation of metabolism and development; stimulation of skin and hair growth; bone health; and maintenance of the reproductive system. Therapeutic amounts have been used to treat elevated blood fats, depression, PMS, chronic fatigue syndrome, and psoriasis, among other ailments.

GLA's anti-inflammatory properties have made it a substance of interest in the treatment of rheumatoid arthritis. Since GLA reduces inflammation in animals, some studies have investigated its ability to alleviate certain RA symptoms. Among these studies are the following:

◆ Researchers from the University of Pennsylvania published the results of their double-blind study of GLA in the *Annals of Internal Medicine* in 1993.[12] Thirty-seven adults with rheumatoid arthritis were randomly assigned to receive either 1.4 grams of GLA in the form of borage seed oil (Boracelle capsules) or a placebo every day for 24 weeks. Joint tenderness, joint swelling, and other indications of disease activity were monitored before, during, and after the treatment period. The results were positive, with GLA reducing the number of tender joints by 36 percent and the number of swollen joints by 28 percent. Those taking the placebo either showed no significant improvement or actually got worse. The researchers concluded that GLA produced a "clinically relevant and statistically significant reduction in signs and symptoms of disease activity in patients with rheumatoid arthritis."

◆ A 1996 study published in *Arthritis and Rheumatism* looked at the effects of GLA in 56 people with active rheumatoid arthritis.[13] For this double-blind trial, volunteers were randomly assigned to receive either 2.8 grams of GLA (supplied by Scotia Pharmaceuticals Ltd.) or a placebo on a daily basis. After 6 months of treatment, those taking the GLA showed "statistically significant and clinically relevant reductions in the signs and symptoms of disease activity." In Table 23-2 below, you can see the percentage of improvement in three RA symptoms with GLA and placebo.

Table 23-2: GLA Improves RA Symptoms Better Than Placebo[14]

Percent Improvement in	GLA Group	Placebo Group
Swollen joints (number of)	20.9	8.3
Tender joints (number of)	35.2	11.9
Morning stiffness (minutes of)	55.4	7.9

◆ The Cochrane Library published a review of herbal therapies for rheumatoid arthritis in 2001, including seven studies that compared GLA to placebo.[15] The authors of this review determined that all of the studies "found some improvement" in symptoms of rheumatoid arthritis (joint pain, joint tenderness, and morning stiffness) when GLA was administered, although they noted that the methodology and the quality of the studies varied.

Summing Up the Evidence for Gamma-Linolenic Acid

Although one could question the methodology of certain GLA studies, there is enough evidence to suggest that gamma-linolenic acid is a three-star treatment for symptoms of rheumatoid arthritis backed by intriguing evidence.

Available Forms

GLA is available in supplement form.

How Much Gamma-Linolenic Acid Is Typically Used

There is no standard dose of gamma-linolenic acid for rheumatoid arthritis. Some studies have used supplemental doses ranging from 1 to 2.8 grams per day.

Possible Side Effects and Interactions

Gamma-linolenic acid's side effects include nausea, diarrhea, and belching. GLA may interfere with clotting mechanisms and may increase the risk of bleeding and bruising when combined with anticoagulant or antiplatelet drugs such as NSAIDs or warfarin (Coumadin). If you're taking any medication, be sure to consult your doctor before adding GLA to your self-care regimen.

Thunder God Vine

Rating: ☆☆ = Modest Evidence

Thunder god vine is a flowering, woody shrub that has been used in Traditional Chinese Medicine for more than 400 years as a treatment for rheumatoid arthritis, eczema, leprosy, and other ailments. Extracts of the root of thunder god vine may suppress inflammation and quiet the immune system, which may explain why Chinese medicine practitioners have found it helpful for autoimmune diseases such as rheumatoid arthritis. A small number of studies seem to confirm its therapeutic benefits for RA:

♦ Researchers from the National Institutes of Health performed a randomized, double-blind, placebo-controlled study of people with long-standing rheumatoid arthritis that had not responded to conventional therapy.[16] The volunteers were randomly assigned to receive either 180 milligrams or 360 milligrams of thunder god vine extract or a placebo every day for 20 weeks. Twenty-one of the volunteers completed the study. After 4 weeks, 80 percent of those taking 360 milligrams of the extract and 40 percent of those taking 180 milligrams of the extract showed improvement in their symptoms, while those taking the placebo did not. The researchers concluded that thunder god vine extract shows therapeutic benefit "in patients with treatment resistant" rheumatoid arthritis.

♦ For a 2003 study published in the *Journal of Rheumatology*, 61 patients with rheumatoid arthritis were randomly assigned to use either a topical thunder god vine preparation or a placebo.[17] The results of this 6-week, double-blind study were encouraging: The positive response was eight times greater in the thunder god vine group than in the placebo group. This figure was based on a score derived from changes in the number of swollen or tender joints, grip strength, morning stiffness, and other indicators of rheumatoid arthritis activity.

Summing Up the Evidence for Thunder God Vine

Thunder god vine has received a lot of "buzz" lately, but only a few double-blind, placebo-controlled studies back up its effectiveness. As the research still is in its early stages, it's best to say that thunder god vine is a two-star treatment for symptoms of rheumatoid arthritis backed by modest evidence.

Other Names

Thunder god vine is known to scientists as *Tripterygium wilfordii* and in various parts of the world as Huang-T'eng Ken, Lei Gong Teng, Taso-Ho-Hau, and yellow vine.

Available Forms

Thunder god vine is available in extract and topical form.

How Much Thunder God Vine Is Typically Used

There is no standard dose of thunder god vine as a treatment for rheumatoid arthritis. Oral dosages may range from 180 to 570 milligrams of thunder god vine extract per day. Certain parts of the thunder god vine—such as the leaves and flowers—are poisonous, so be sure to choose a product that is certified as safe.

Possible Side Effects and Interactions

Thunder god vine can cause diarrhea, hair loss, and infertility. It also can weaken the immune system—which means it can enhance the effects of immune-suppressing drugs such as cyclosporine (Sandimmune). If you're taking any medication, be sure to consult your doctor before adding thunder god vine to your self-care regimen.

ENDNOTES

Chapter 3: Alzheimer's Disease

[1] LeBars PL, Katz MM, Berman N, et al. "A placebo-controlled, double-blind, randomized trial of an extract of ginkgo biloba for dementia." North American EGb Study Group. *JAMA* 1997;278(16):1327-1332.

[2] Kanowski S, Herrmann WM, Stephan K, et al. "Proof of efficacy of the ginkgo biloba special extract EGb 761 in outpatients suffering from mild to moderate primary degenerative dementia of the Alzheimer type of multi-infarct dementia." *Pharmacopsychiatry* 1996;29(2):47-56.

[3] Oken BS, Storzbach DM, Kaye JA. "The efficacy of ginkgo biloba on cognitive function in Alzheimer's disease." *Arch Neurol* 1998;55:1409-1415.

[4] Engel RR, Satzger W, Gunther W, et al. "Double-blind cross-over study of phosphatidylserine vs. placebo in patients with early dementia of the Alzheimer type." *Eur Neuropsychopharmacol* 1992;2:149-155.

[5] Amaducci L, and the SMID Group. "Phosphatidylserine in the treatment of Alzheimer's disease: results of a multicenter study." *Psychopharm Bull* 1988;24(1):130-134.

[6] Sano M, Ernesto C, Thomas RG, et al. "A controlled trial of selegiline, alpha-tocopherol, or both as treatment for Alzheimer's disease." The Alzheimer's Disease Cooperative Study. *N Engl J Med* 1997;336(17): 1216-1222.

[7] Morris MC, Evans DA, Tangney CC, et al. "Relation of the tocopherol forms to incident Alzheimer disease and to cognitive change." *Am J Clin Nutr* 2005;81(2):508-514.

[8] Weyer G, Babej-Dolle RM, Hadler D, et al. "A controlled study of 2 doses of ibedenone in the treatment of Alzheimer's disease." Neuropsychobiology 1997;36(2):73-82.

[9] Gutzmann H, Hadler D. "Sustained efficacy and safety of idebenone in the treatment of Alzheimer's disease: update on a 2-year double-blind multi-center study." *J Neural Transm Suppl* 1998;54:301-310.

[10] Gutzmann H, Kuhl KP, Hadler K, et al. "Safety and efficacy of idebenone versus tacrine in patients with Alzheimer's disease: results of a randomized, double-blind, parallel-group multicenter study." *Pharmacopsychiatry* 2002;35(1):12-18.

[11] Adapted from Gutzmann H, Kuhl KP, Hadler K, et al. "Safety and efficacy of idebenone versus tacrine in patients with Alzheimer's disease: results of a randomized, double-blind, parallel-group multicenter study." *Pharmacopsychiatry* 2002;35(1):12-18.

[12] Morris MC, Evans DA, Bienias JL, et al. "Consumption of fish and n-3 fatty acids and risk of incident Alzheimer's disease." *Arch Neurol* 2003; 60:940-946.

[13] Barberger-Gateau P, Letenneur L, Deschamps V, et al. "Fish, meat, and risk of dementia: cohort study." *BJM* 2002;325:932-933.

[14] MacLean CH, Issa AM, Newberry SJ, et al. "Effects of omega-3 fatty acids on cognitive function with aging, dementia, and neurological diseases." Summary, Evidence Report/Technology Assessment No. 114. AHRQ Publication No. 05-E011-1. Rockville, MD: Agency for Healthcare Research and Quality. February 2005.

Chapter 4: Anxiety

[1] Malsch U, Kieser M. "Efficacy of kava-kava in the treatment of non-psychotic anxiety, following pretreatment with benzodiazepines." *Psychopharmacology* (Berl) 2001;157(3):277-283.

[2] Volz HP, Kieser M. "Kava-kava extract WS 1490 versus placebo in anxiety disorders – a randomized placebo-controlled 25-week outpatient trial." *Pharmacopsychiatry* 1997;30(1):1-5.

[3] Boerner JR, Sommer H, Berger W, et al. "Kava-Kava extract LI 150 is as effective as Opipramol and Buspirone in Generalized Anxiety Disorder – an 8-week randomized, double-blind multi-centre clinical trial in 129 out-patients." *Phytomedicine* 2003;10(Suppl 4):38-49.

[4] Adapted from Boerner JR, Sommer H, Berger W, et al. "Kava-Kava extract LI 150 is as effective as Opipramol and Buspirone in Generalized Anxiety Disorder – an 8-week randomized, double-blind multi-centre clinical trial in 129 out-patients." *Phytomedicine* 2003;10(Suppl 4):38-49.

[5] Pittler MH, Ernst E. "Kava extract for treating anxiety." Cochrane Database Syst Rev 2003;(1):CD003383.

[6] Witte S, Loew D, Gaus W. "Meta-analysis of the efficacy of the acetonic kava-kava extract WE1490 in patients with non-psychotic anxiety disorders." *Phytother Res* 2005;19(3):183-8.

[7] Kohnen R, Oswald WD, "The effects of valerian, propranolol, and their combination on activation, performance, and mood of healthy volunteers under social stress conditions." *Pharmacopsychiat* 1988;21:447-448.

[8] Cropley M, Cave Z, Ellis J, et al. "Effect of kava and valerian on human physiological and psychological responses to mental stress assessed under laboratory conditions." *Phytother Res* 2002;16(1):23-27.

[9] Andreatini R, Sartori VA, Seabra ML, et al. "Effects of valepotriates (valerian extract) in generalized anxiety disorder : a randomized placebo-controlled pilot study." *Phytother Res* 2002;16(7):650-654.

[10] Miller HE, Deakin JF, Anderson IM. "Effect of acute tryptophan depletion on CO2 induced anxiety in patients with panic disorder and normal volunteers." *Br J Psychiatry* 2000;176:182-188.

[11] Schruers K, van Diest R, Overbeek T, et al. "Acute L-5-ydroxytrpytophan administration inhibits carbon dioxide-induced panic in panic disorder patients." *Psychiatry Res* 2002;113(3):237-243.

[12] Argyropoulos SV, Hood SD, Adrover M, et al. "Tryptophan depletion reverses the therapeutic effect of selective serotonin reuptake inhibitors in social anxiety disorder." *Biol Psychiatry* 2004;56(7):503-509.

Chapter 5: Asthma

[1] Saoulli, J. "Asthma Sufferers Fight for Breath." CNN.com. May 5, 2005. Accessible at http://www.cnn.com/2005/WORLD/europe/05/05/asthma/index.html.

[2] http://www.cdc.gov/nchs/products/pubs/pubd/hestats/asthma/asthma.htm

[3] http://www.uspharmacist.com/oldformat.asp?url=newlook/files/Tren/ACF2334.htm&pub_id=8&article_id=744

[4] American Academy of Allergy Asthma & Immunology www.aaaai.org

[5] Forastiere F, Pistelli R, Sestini P, et a. "Consumption of fresh fruit rich in vitamin C and wheezing symptoms in children." *Thorax* 2000;55:283-288.

[6] Adapted from Forastiere F, Pistelli R, Sestini P, et a. "Consumption of fresh fruit rich in vitamin C and wheezing symptoms in children." *Thorax* 2000;55:283-288.

[7] Neuman I, Nahum H, Ben-Amotz A. "Reduction of exercise-induced asthma oxidative stress by lycopene, a natural antioxidant." *Allergy* 2000;55(12):1184-1189.

[8] Becker AB, Simons KJ, Gillespie CA, et al. "The bronchodilator effects and pharmacokinetics of caffeine in asthma." *NEJM* 1984;310(12):743-746.

[9] Bara AI, Barley EA. "Caffeine for asthma." The Cochrane Database of Systematic Reviews 2001, Issue 4, Art. No.: CD001112.

[10] Nagakura T, Matsuda S, Shichijyo K, et al. "Dietary supplementation with fish oil rich in -3 polyunsaturated fatty acids in children with bronchial asthma." *Eur Respir J* 2000;16:861-865.

[11] Adapted from Nagakura T, Matsuda S, Shichijyo K, et al. "Dietary supplementation with fish oil rich in -3 polyunsaturated fatty acids in children with bronchial asthma." *Eur Respir J* 2000;16:861-865.

[12] De Luis DA, Armentia A, Aller R, et al. "Dietary intake in patients with asthma: a case control study." *Nutrition* 2005;21(3):320-324.

[13] Okamoto M, Mitsunobu F, Ashida K, et al. "Effect of dietary supplementation with n-3 fatty acids compared with n-6 fatty acids on bronchial asthma." *Intern Med* 2000;39(2):107-111.

[14] Mickleborough TD, Ionescu AA, Rundell KW. "Omega-3 fatty acids and airway hyperresponsiveness in asthma." J Alt Comp Med 2004;10(6): 1067-1075.

[15] Riveron-Garrote M. "Ensayo clinico aleatoriado controlado del tratamento homepatico del asma bronquial." *Boletin Mexiano* 1998;31:54-61. Described in Ullman, Dana. *Homeopathic Family Medicine*. Berkeley, CA: Homeopathic Educational Services, 2005. p82.

[16] Reilly D, Taylor MA, Beattie NG, et al. "Is evidence for homeopathy reproducible?" *Lancet* 1994;344(8937):1601-1606.

[17] Hosseini S, Pishnamazi S, Sadrzadeh SM, et al. "Pycnogenol® in the management of asthma." *Journal of Medicinal Food* 2001;4(4):201-209.

[18] Quotation from "Arizona College of Public Health Study Conducted in Iran Indicates Pycnogenol® Helpful in Management of Asthma." November 26, 2002. Accessible at http://www.ahsc.arizona.edu/opa/news/nov02/asthma. htm. Viewed December 14, 2005.

[19] Lau BHS, Riesen SK, et al. "Pycnogenol® as an adjunct in the management of childhood asthma." *Journal of Asthma* 2004;41(8):825-832.

[20] Adapted from Lau BHS, Riesen SK, et al. "Pycnogenol® as an adjunct in the management of childhood asthma." *Journal of Asthma* 2004;41(8):825-832.

Chapter 6: Colds

[1] Spasov AA, Ostrovskij OV, Chernikov MV, et al. "Comparative controlled study of Andrographis paniculata fixed combination, Kan Jang and an Echinacea preparation as adjuvant, in the treatment of uncomplicated respiratory disease in children." *Phytother Res* 2004;18(1):47-53.

[2] Adapted from Spasov AA, Ostrovskij OV, Chernikov MV, et al. "Comparative controlled study of Andrographis paniculata fixed combination, Kan Jang and an Echinacea preparation as adjuvant, in the treatment of uncomplicated respiratory disease in children." *Phytother Res* 2004;18(1):47-53.

[3] Caceres DD, Hancke JL, Burgos RA, et al. "Use of visual analogue scale measurements (VAS) to assess the effectiveness of standardized Andrographis paniculata extract SHA-10 in reducing the symptoms of common cold. A randomized double-blind placebo study." *Phytomedicine* 1999; 6(4):217-223.

[4] Adapted from Caceres DD, Hancke JL, Burgos RA, et al. "Use of visual analogue scale measurements (VAS) to assess the effectiveness of standardized Andrographis paniculata extract SHA-10 in reducing the symptoms of common cold. A randomized double-blind placebo study." *Phytomedicine* 1999;6(4):217-223.

[5] Hancke J, Burgos R, Caceres D, et al. "A double-blind study with a new monodrug Kan Jang: Decrease in symptoms and improvement in the recovery from common colds." *Phytother Res* 1995;9:559-562.

[6] Adapted from Hancke J, Burgos R, Caceres D, et al. "A double-blind study with a new monodrug Kan Jang: Decrease in symptoms and improvement in the recovery from common colds." *Phytother Res* 1995;9:559-562.

[7] Poolsup N, Suthisisang C, Prathanturarug S, et al. "Andrographis paniculata in the symptomatic treatment of uncomplicated upper respiratory tract infection: systematic review of randomized controlled trials." *J Clin Pharm Ther* 2004;29(1):37-45.

[8] Goel V, Lovlin R, Barton R, et al. "Efficacy of a standardized Echinacea preparation (Echinilin) for the treatment of the common cold: a randomized, double-blind, placebo-controlled trial." *J Clin Pharm Ther* 2004; 9(1):75-83.

[9] Schulten B, Bulitta M, Ballering-Bruhl B, et al. "Efficacy of *Echinacea purpurea* in patients with a common cold. A placebo-controlled, randomized, double-blind trial." *Arzneimittelforschung* 2001;51(2):563-568.

[10] Adapted from Schulten B, Bulitta M, Ballering-Bruhl B, et al. "Efficacy of *Echinacea purpurea* in patients with a common cold. A placebo-controlled, randomized, double-blind trial." *Arzneimittelforschung* 2001; 51(2):563-568.

[11] Lindenmuth GF, Lindenmugt EB. "The efficacy of echinacea compound herbal tea preparation on the severity and duration of upper respiratory and flu symptoms: a randomized, double-blind placebo-controlled study." *J Altern Complement Med* 2000;6(4):327-334.

[12] Barrett B, Vohmann M, Calabrese C. "Echinacea for upper respiratory infection." *J Fam Pract* 1999;48(8):628-635.

[13] Percival SS. "Use of echinacea in medicine." *Biochem Pharmacol* 2000; 60(2):155-158.

[14] Melchart D, Linde K, Fischer P, et al. "Echinacea for preventing and treating the common cold. Cochrane review abstract and plain language summary." Accessible at http://www.cochrane.org/reviews/en/ab000530.html. Viewed December 19, 2005.

[15] Turner RB, Bauer R, Woelkart K, et al. "An evaluation of *Echinacea augustifolia* in experimental rhinovirus infections." *N Engl J Med* 2005;353:341-348.

[16] Barrett RP, Brown RL, Locken K, et al. "Treatment of the common cold with unrefined echinacea: A randomized, double-blind, placebo-controlled trial." *Ann Intern Med* 2002;137:939-946.

[17] Reported in: Turner RB, Bauer R, Woelkart K, et al. "An evaluation of *Echinacea augustifolia* in experimental rhinovirus infections." *N Engl J Med* 2005;353:341-348.

[18] Korant BD, Kauer JC, Butterworth BE. "Zinc ions inhibit replication of rhinoviruses." *Nature* 1974;248:588-590.

[19] Mossad SB, Macknin ML, Mendendorp SV, et al. "Zinc gluconate lozenges for treating the common cold." *Ann Int Med* 1996;125(2):81-88.

[20] Petrus EJ, Lawson KA, Bucci LR, et al. "Randomized, double-masked, placebo-controlled clinical study of the effectiveness of zinc acetate lozenges on common cold symptoms in allergy-tested subjects." *Curr Ther Res* 1998;59(9):595-607.

[21] Adapted from Petrus EJ, Lawson KA, Bucci LR, et al. "Randomized, double-masked, placebo-controlled clinical study of the effectiveness of zinc acetate lozenges on common cold symptoms in allergy-tested subjects." *Curr Ther Res* 1998;59(9):595-607.

[22] Prasad AS, Fitzgerald JT, Bao B, et al. "Duration of symptoms and plasma cytokine levels in patients with the common cold treated with zinc acetate." *Ann Int Med* 2000;133:245-252.

[23] Adapted from Prasad AS, Fitzgerald JT, Bao B, et al. "Duration of symptoms and plasma cytokine levels in patients with the common cold treated with zinc acetate." *Ann Int Med* 2000;133:245-252.

[24] Maiwald LV, Weinfurtner T, Mau J, et al. "Therapy of common cold with a homeopathic combination preparation in comparison with acetylsalicylic acid. A controlled, randomized double-blind study." *Arzneimittelforschung* 1988;38(4):578-582.

[25] Trichard M, Chaufferin G, Nicoloyannis N. "Pharmacoeconomic comparison between homeopathic and antibiotic treatment strategies in recurrent acute rhinopharyngitis in children." *Homeopathy* 2005;94(1):3-9.

[26] Ammerschlager H, Klein P, Weiser M, et al. "Treatment of inflammatory disease of the upper respiratory tract – comparison of a homeopathic complex remedy with xylometazoline." *Forsch Komplementarmed Klass Naturheilkd* 2005;12(1):24-31.

Chapter 7: Constipation

[1] Rao SS, Welcher KD, Pelsang RE. "Effects of biofeedback therapy on anorectal function in obstructive defecation." *Dig Dis Sci* 1997;42(11):2197-2205.

[2] Chiotakakou-Falialou, Kamm MA, Roy AJ, et al. "Biofeedback provides long term benefit for patients with intractable, slow and normal transit constipation." *Gut* 1998;42:517-521.

[3] Adapted from Chiotakakou-Falialou, Kamm MA, Roy AJ, et al. "Biofeedback provides long term benefit for patients with intractable, slow and normal transit constipation." *Gut* 1998;42:517-521.

[4] Emmanuel AV, Kamm MA. "Response to a behavioral treatment, biofeedback, in constipation patients is associated with improved gut transit and autonomic innervation." *Gut* 2001;29:214-219.

[5] Palsson OS, Heymen S, Whitehead WE. "Biofeedback treatment for functional anorectal disorders: a comprehensive efficacy review." *Appl Psychophysiol Biofeedback* 2004;29(3):153-174.

[6] Bassotti G, Chistolini F, Sietchiping-Nzepa F, et al. "Biofeedback for pelvic floor dysfunction in constipation." *BMJ* 2004;328:393-396.

[7] Ernst E. "Abdominal massage therapy for chronic constipation: A systematic review of controlled clinical trials." *Forsch Komplementarmed* 1999;6(3): 149-151.

[8] Jeon SY, Jung HM. "The effects of abdominal meridian massage on constipation among CVA patients." *Taehan Kanho Hakhoe Chi* 2005;35(1):135-142.

[9] Kleessen B, Sykura B, Zunft HJ, et al. "Effects of inulin and lactose on fecal microflora, microbial activity, and bowel habits in elderly constipated persons." *Am J Clin Nutr* 1997;65(5):1397-1402.

[10] Teuri U, Korpela R. "Galacto-oligosaccharides relieve constipation in elderly people." *Ann Nutr Metab* 1998;42(6):319-327.

[11] Koebnick C, Wagner I, Leitzmann P, et al. "Probiotic beverage containing *Lactobacillus casei Shirota* improves gastrointestinal symptoms in patients with chronic constipation." *Can J Gastroenterol* 2003;17(11):655-659.

[12] Ouwehand AC, Lagstrom H, Soumalainen T, et al. "Effect of probiotics on constipation, fecal azoreductase activity and fecal mucin content in the elderly." *Ann Nutr Metab* 2002;46(3-4):159-162.

[13] PRD for Nutritional Supplements, 1st Edition. SS Hendler, Chief Editor. Montvale, NJ, Thomson PDR, 2001. p381.

Chapter 8: Coronary Heart Disease

[1] Hu FB, Bronner L, Willet WC, et al. "Fish and omega-3 fatty acid intake and risk of coronary heart disease in women." *JAMA* 2002;287(14):1815-1821.

[2] Daviglus ML, Stamler J, Orenica AJ, et al. "Fish consumption and the 30-year risk of fatal myocardial infarction." *N Engl J Med* 1997;336(15):1046-1053.

[3] Mozaffarian D, Ascherio A, Hu FB, et al. "Interplay between different polyunsaturated fatty acids and risk of coronary heart disease in men." *Circulation* 2005;111(2):157-164.

[4] Burr MI, Rehily AM, Gilbert JF, et al. "Effects of change in fat, fish, and fibre intakes on death and myocardial reinfarction: diet and reinfarction trial (DART)." *Lancet* 1989;2(8666):757-761.

[5] Singh RB, Niaz MA, Sharma JP, et al. "Randomized, double-blind, placebo-controlled trial of fish oil and mustard oil in patients with suspected acute myocardial infarction: the Indian experiment of infarct survival-4." *Cardiovasc Drugs Ther* 1997;11(3):485-491.

[6] No authors listed. "Dietary supplementation with n-3 polyunsaturated fatty acids and vitamin E after myocardial infarction: results of the GISSI-Prevenzione trial." Gruppo Italiano per lo Studio della Sopravvivenza nell'Infarto miocardico. *Lancet* 1999;354(9177):477-455.

[7] Bucher HC, Hengstler P, Schindler C, et al. "N-3 polyunsaturated fatty acids in coronary heart disease: a meta-analysis of randomized controlled trials." *Am J Med* 2002;112(4):298-304.

[8] Kris-Etherton PM, Harris WS, Appel LJ. "Fish consumption, fish oil, omega-3 fatty acids, and cardiovascular disease." *Circulation* 2002; 106:2747-2757.

[9] Wang C, Chung M, Lichtenstein A, et al. "Effects of Omega-3 Fatty Acids on Cardiovascular Disease." Summary, Evidence Report/Technology Assessment No. 94. AHRQ Publication No. 04-E009-1. Rockville, MD: Agency for Healthcare Research and Quality. March 2004.

[10] Iqbal MP, Ishaq M, Kazmi KA, et al. "Role of vitamins B_6, B_{12} and folic acid on hyperhomocysteinemia in a Pakistani population of patients with acute myocardial infarction." *Nutr Metab Cardiovasc Dis* 2005;15(2):100-108.

[11] Assanelli D, Bonanome A, Pezzini A, et al. "Folic acid and vitamin E supplementa-tion effects of homocysteinemia, endothelial function and plasma antioxidant capa-city in young myocardial-infarction patients." *Pharmacol Res* 2004;49(1):79-84.

[12] Title LM, Cummings PM, Giddens K, et al. "Effect of folic acid and antioxidant vitamins on endothelial dysfunction in patients with coronary artery disease." *J Am Coll Cardiol* 2000;36(3):758-765.

[13] Lau BH, Lam F. Wang-Cheng R. "Effect of an odor-modified garlic preparation on blood lipids." *Nut Res* 1987;7:139-149.

[14] Adapted from Lau BH, Lam F. Wang-Cheng R. "Effect of an odor-modified garlic preparation on blood lipids." *Nut Res* 1987;7:139-149.

[15] Steiner M, Khan AH, Holbert D, et al. "A double-blind crossover study in moderately hypercholesterolemic men that compared the effect of aged garlic extract and placebo administration on blood lipids." *Am J Clin Nutr* 1996;64(6):866-870.

[16] Kannar D, Wattanapenpaiboon N, Savige GS, et al. "Hypocholesterolemic effect of an enteric-coated garlic supplement." *Am J Clin Nutr* 2001;20(3): 225-231.

[17] Budoff M, Takasu J, Flores FR, et al. "Inhibiting progression of coronary calcification using Aged Garlic Extract in patients receiving statin therapy: a preliminary study." *Preventive Medicine* 2004:39:985-991.

[18] Weiss N, Ide N, Abahji T, et al. "Influence of garlic on endothelial dysfunction in hyperhomocysteinemia." Presented at the 2005 Garlic Symposium, April, 2005, Georgetown University Conference Center, Washington, D.C.

[19] Rahman K, Billington D. "Dietary supplementation with aged garlic extract inhibits ADP-induced platelet aggregation in humans." *J Nutr* 2000;130: 2662-2665.

[20] Amagase H, Budoff M, Nihara Y, et al. "Multiple risk factors of cardiovascular diseases and antiatherosclerotic effect of Aged Garlic Extract (Kyolic) as a complementary medication." *FASEB J*, 2004;18(6):600-606.

[21] *PRD for Nutritional Supplements*, 1st ed. SS Hendler, Ed-in-Chief. Montvale New Jersey: 2001. p290-291.

[22] *PRD for Nutritional Supplements*, 1st ed. SS Hendler, Ed-in-Chief. Montvale New Jersey: 2001. p290-291.

[23] Shechter M, Bairey Merz CN, Stuehlinger HG, et al. "Effects of oral magnesium therapy on exercise tolerance, exercise-induced chest pain, and quality of life in patients with coronary artery disease." *Am J Cardiol* 2003;91(5):517-521.

[24] Shechter M, Sharir M, Labrador MJ, et al. "Oral magnesium therapy improves endothelial function in patients with coronary artery disease." *Circulation* 2000;102(19):2353-2358.

[25] Shechter M, Merz CN, Paul-Labrador M, et al. "Oral magnesium supplementation inhibits platelet-dependent thrombosis in patients with coronary artery disease." *Am J Cardiol* 1999,84(2):152-156.

[26] Mukamal KJ, Conigrave KM, Mittleman MA, et al. "Roles of drinking pattern and type of alcohol consumed in coronary heart disease in men." *N Engl J Med* 2003;348(2):109-118.

[27] Mukami KJ, Maclure M, Muller JE. "Prior alcohol consumption and mortality following acute myocardial infarction." *JAMA* 2001;285(15): 1965-1970.

[28] Thun MJ, Peto R, Lopez AD, et al. "Alcohol consumption and mortality among middle-aged and elderly US adults." *N Engl J Med* 1997;337(24): 1705-1714.

[29] Klatsky AL, Armstrong MA, Friendman GD. "Red wine, white wine, liquor, beer, and risk for coronary artery disease hospitalization." *Am J Cardiol* 1997;80(4):416-420.

[30] Stampfer MJ, Colditz GA, Willet WC, et al. "A prospective study of moderate alcohol consumption and the risk of coronary disease and stroke in women." *N Engl J Med* 1988;319(5):267-273.

[31] Goldberg IJ, Mosca L, Piano MR, et al. "Wine and your heart. A science advisory for healthcare professionals from the Nutrition Committee, Council on Epidemiology and Prevention, and Council on Cardiovascular Nursing of the American Heart Association." *Circulation* 2001;103:472-475,

[32] Fernández-Harne E, Martinez-Losa E, Prado-Santamaría M, et al. "Risk of first non-fatal myocardial infarction negatively associated with olive oil consumption: a case-control study in Spain." *Int J Epidemiol* 2002;31:474-480.

[33] Fito M, Cladellas M, de la Torre R, et al. "Antioxidant effect of virgin olive oil in patients with stable coronary heart disease: a randomized, crossover, controlled, clinical trial." *Atherosclerosis* 2005; 181(1):149-158.

[34] Described in Feldman EB. "The scientific evidence for a beneficial health relationship between walnuts and coronary heart disease." *J Nutr* 2002;132:1062S-1101S.

[35] Described in Feldman EB. "The scientific evidence for a beneficial health relationship between walnuts and coronary heart disease." *J Nutr* 2002;132:1062S-1101S.

[36] Described in Feldman EB. "The scientific evidence for a beneficial health relationship between walnuts and coronary heart disease." *J Nutr* 2002;132:1062S-1101S.

[37] Described in Feldman EB. "The scientific evidence for a beneficial health relation-ship between walnuts and coronary heart disease." *J Nutr* 2002;132:1062S-1101S.

Chapter 9: Depression

[1] *The Merck Manual of Medical Information,* 2nd Home Ed. MH Beers, Ed-in-Chief. 2003; p614.

[2] *The Merck Manual of Medical Information,* 2nd Home Ed. MH Beers, Ed-in-Chief. 2003; p614.

[3] From *Runaway Eating.*

[4] Bell KM, Plon L, Bunney WE, et al. "S-adenosylmethionine treatment of depression: a controlled clinical trial." *Am J Psychiatry* 1988; 145(9):1110-1114.

[5] Delle Chiaie R, Pancheri P, Scapicchio P. "Efficacy and tolerability of oral and intramuscular S-adenosyl-L-methionine 1,4-butanedisulfonate (SAMe) in the treatment of major depression: comparison with imipramine in 2 multi-center studies." *Am J Clin Nutr* 2002;76(5):1172S-1176S.

[6] Adapted from Delle Chiaie R, Pancheri P, Scapicchio P. "Efficacy and tolerability of oral and intramuscular S-adenosyl-L-methionine 1,4-butane-disulfonate (SAMe) in the treatment of major depression: comparison with imipramine in 2 multicenter studies." *Am J Clin Nutr* 2002;76(5): 1172S-1176S.

[7] Alpert JE, Papakostas G, Mischoulon D, et al. "S-adenosyl-L-methionine (SAMe) as an adjunct for resistant major depressive disorder." *J Clin Pharmacol* 2004;24(6):1-4.

[8] Bressa GM. "S-adenosyl-l-methionine (SAMe) as an antidepressant: meta-analysis of clinical studies." *Acta Neurol Scand* Suppl 1994;154:7-14.

[9] S-Adenosyl-L-Methionine for Treatment of Depression, Osteoarthritis, and Liver Disease. Summary, Evidence Report/Technology Assessment: Number 64. AHRQ Publication No. 02-E033 August 2002. Agency for Healthcare Research and Quality, Rockville, MD. http://www.ahrq.gov/clinic/epcsums/ samesum.htm.

[10] Hubner WD, Lande S, Podzuweit H. "Hypericum treatment of mild depressions with somatic symptoms." *J Geriatr Psychiatry Neurol* 1994;7(Suppl 1):S12-14.

[11] Philipp M, Kohnen R, Hiller K. "Hypericum extract versus imipramine or placebo in patients with moderate depression: randomized multicenter study of treatment for eight weeks." *BMJ* 1999;319:1534-1539.

[12] Brenner R. Azbel V., Madhusoodanan S, et al. "Comparison of an extract of hypericum (LI 160) and sertraline in the treatment of depression: a double-blind, randomized pilot study." *Clin Ther* 2000;22(4):411-419.

[13] Harrer G, Schmidt U, Kuhn U, et al. "Comparison of equivalence between St. John's wort extract LoHyp-57 and fluoxetine." *Arzneimittelforschung* 1999;49(I):289-296.

[14] Schrader E. "Equivalence of St. John's wort extract (ZE 117) and fluoxetine: a randomized, controlled study in mild-moderate depression." *Int Clin Psychopharmacol* 2000;15(2):61-68.

[15] Linde K, Knuppel L. "Large-scale observational studies of hypericum extracts in patients with depressive disorders – a systematic review." *Phytomedicine* 2005;12(1-2):148-157.

[16] Linde K, Ramirez G, Mulrow C, et al. "St. John's wort for depression—an overview and meta-analysis of randomized clinical trials." *BMJ* 1996; 313:253-258.

[17] Kasper S, Dienel A. "Cluster analysis of symptoms during antidepressant treatment with Hypericum extract in mildly to moderately depressed outpatients. A meta-analysis of data from three randomized, placebo-controlled trials." *Psychopharmacology* 2002;164(3):301-308.

[18] Shelton RC, Keller MG, Gelenberg A, et al. "Effectiveness of St John's wort in major depression: a randomized controlled trial." *JAMA* 2001;285(15): 1978-1986.

[19] Hypericum Depression Trail Study Group. "Effect of *Hypericum perforatum* (St John's wort) in major depressive disorder: a randomized controlled trial." *JAMA* 2002;287(14):1807-1814.

[20] Szegedi A, Kohnen R, Dienel A, et al. "Acute treatment of moderate to severe depression with hypericum extract WS 5570 (St. John's wort): randomised controlled double non-inferiority trial versus paroxetine." *BMJ* 2005;330:503.

[21] See, for example, Hibbeln JR, Salem N. "Dietary polyunsaturated fatty acids and depression: when cholesterol does not satisfy." *Am J Clin Nutr* 1995;62:1-9.

[22] Stoll AL, Severus WE, Freeman MP, et al. "Omega 3 fatty acids in bipolar disorder: a preliminary double-blind, placebo-controlled trial." *Arch Gen Psychiatry* 1999;56(5):407-412.

[23] Nemets B, Stahl Z, Belmaker RH. "Addition of omega-3 fatty acid to maintenance medication treatment for recurrent unipolar depressive disorder." *Am J Psychiatry* 2002;159(3):477-479.

[24] Adapted from Nemets B, Stahl Z, Belmaker RH. "Addition of omega-3 fatty acid to maintenance medication treatment for recurrent unipolar depressive disorder." *Am J Psychiatry* 2002;159(3):477-479.

[25] Peet M, Horrobin DR. "A dose-ranging study of the effects of ethyl-eicosapentaenoate in patients with ongoing depression despite apparently adequate treatment with standard drugs." *Arch Gen Psychiatry* 2002;59(10):913-919.

[26] van Prang HM. "Central monoamine metabolism in depression." II. *Comp Psychiat* 1980;21:44-54.

[27] Takahashi S, Kondo, H Kato N. "Effect of L-5-hydroxytryptophan on brain monoamine metabolism and evaluation of its clinical effect in depressed patients." *J Psychiatr Res* 1975;12:177-187.

[28] Nakajima T, Kudo Y, Kaneko Z. "Clinical evaluation of 5-hydroxy-L-tryptophan as an antidepressant drug." *Folia Psychiatr Neurol Jpn* 1978;32(2);223-230.

[29] Sano I. "L-5-hydroxytryptophan (L-5-HTP) therapy." *Folia Psychiatr Neurol Jpn* 1972;26:7-17.

[30] Shaw K, Turner J, Del Mar C. "Tryptophan and 5-Hydroxytryptophan for depression." *The Cochrane Database of Systematic Reviews* 2002, Issue 1. Art. No.:CD003198.

[31] Docherty JP, Sack DA, Roffman M, et al. "A double-blind, placebo-controlled, exploratory trial of chromium picolinate in atypical depression: effect on carbohydrate craving." *J Psychiatr Pract* 2005;11(5):302-314.

[32] Davidson JR, Abraham K, Connor KM, et al. "Effectiveness of chromium in atypical depression: a placebo-controlled trial." *Biol Psychiatry* 2003;53(3):261-264.

[33] Adapted from Davidson JR, Abraham K, Connor KM, et al. "Effectiveness of chromium in atypical depression: a placebo-controlled trial." *Biol Psychiatry* 2003;53(3):261-264.

[34] Akhondzadeh S, Tahmacebi-Pour N, Noorbala AA, et al. "*Crocus sativus L.* in the treatment of mild to moderate depression: a double-blind, randomized and placebo-controlled trial." *Phytother Res* 2005;19(2):148-151.

[35] Akhondzadeh S, Fallah-Pour H, Afkham K, et al. "Comparison of *Crocus sativus L.* and imipramine in the treatment of mild to moderate depression: A pilot double-blind randomized trial." *BMC Comp Alt Med* 2004;4:12.

[36] Noorbala AA, Akhondzadeh S, Tahmacebi-Pour N, et al. "Hydro-alcoholic extract of *Crocus sativus L.* versus fluoxetine in the treatment of mild to moderate depression: a double-blind, randomized trial." *J Ethnopharmacology* 2005;97:281-284.

Chapter 10: Diabetes

[1] Liu X, Zhou HJ, Rohdewald P. "French maritime pine bark extract Pycnogenol dose-dependently lowers glucose in type 2 diabetic patients." Letter to the editor. *Diabetes Care* 2004;27(3):839.

[2] Spadea L, Balestrazzi E. "Treatment of vascular retinopathies with *Pycnogenol.*" *Phytotherapy Res* 2001;15:219-223.

[3] Liu X, Wei J, Tan F, et al. "Pycnogenol, French maritime pine bark extract, improves endothelial function of hypertensive patients." *Life Sciences* 2004;74:855-862.

[4] *PDR for Nutritional Supplements*, 1st Edition. Hendler SS, Ed-in-Chief. Montvale, NJ: Thompson, 2001. p.20.

[5] Jacob S. Henriksen EJ, Schiemann AL, et al. "Enhancement of glucose disposal in patients with type 2 diabetes by alpha-lipoic acid." *Arzneimittelforschung* 1995;45(8):872-874.

[6] Jacob S, Henriksen EJ, Tritschler HJ, et al. "Improvement of insulin-stimulated glucose-disposal in type 2 diabetes after repeated parenteral administration of thioctic acid." *Exp Clin Endocrinol Diabetes* 1996;104(3):284-288.

[7] Jacob S, Ruus P, Hermann R, et al. "Oral administration of RAC-alpha-lipoic acid modulates insulin sensitivity in patients with type-2 diabetes mellitus: a placebo-controlled pilot trial." *Free Radic Biol Med* 1999;27 (3-4):309-314.

[8] Zeigler D, Nowak H, Kempler P, et al. "Treatment of symptomatic diabetic polyneuropathy with the antioxidant alpha-lipoic acid: a meta-analysis." *Diabet Med* 2004;21:114-121.

[9] Rodriguez-Moran M, Guerrero-Romero F, Lazcano-Burciaga G. "Lipid- and glucose-lowering efficacy of *Plantago* psyllium in type II diabetes." *J Diabetes Complications* 1998;12(5):273-278.

[10] Anderson JW, Allgood LD, Turner J, et al. "Effects of psyllium on glucose and serum lipid responses in men and with type 2 diabetes and hypercholesterolemia." *Am J Clin Nutr* 1999;70:466-473.

[11] Sierra M, Garcia JJ, Fernandez N, et al. "Therapeutic effects of psyllium in type 2 diabetic patients." *Eur J Clin Nutr* 2002;56(9):830-842.

[12] Anderson RA, Cheng N, Bryden NA, et al. "Elevated intakes of supplemental chromium improve glucose and insulin variables in individuals with type 2 diabetes." *Diabetes* 1997;46(11):1786-1791.

[13] Rabinovitz H, Friedensohn A, Leibovitz A, et al. "Effects of chromium supplementation on blood glucose and lipid levels in type 2 diabetes mellitus elderly patients." *Int J Vitam Nutr Res* 2004;74(3):178-182.

[14] Jovanovic L, Gutierrez M, Peterson CM. "Chromium supplementation for women with gestational diabetes mellitus." *J Trace Elem Exp Med* 1999;12:91-97.

[15] Cefalu WT, Hu FB. "Role of chromium in human health and in diabetes." *Diabetes Care* 2004;27(11):2741-2751.

[16] Khan A, Safdar M, Kahn MM, et al. "Cinnamon improves glucose and lipids of people with type 2 diabetes." *Diabetes Care* 2003;26:3215-3218.

[17] Gupta A, Gupta R, Lal B. "Effect of *Trigonella foenum-graecum* (fenugreek) seeds on glycaemic control and insulin resistance in type 2 diabetes mellitus: a double blind placebo controlled study." *J Assoc Physicians India* 2001;49:1057-1061.

[18] Sharma RD, Raghuram TC, Rao NS. "Effect of fenugreek seeds on blood glucose and serum lipids in type I diabetes." *Eur J Clin Nutr* 1990;44(4):301-306.

[19] Vuksan V, Jenkins DJA, Spadafora P, et al. "Konjac-mannan (glucomannan) improves glycemic and other associated risk factors for coronary heart disease in type 2 diabetes." *Diabetes Care* 1999;22(6):913-919.

[20] Chen HL, Sheu WHH, Tai TS, et al. "Konjac supplement alleviated hypercholesterolemia and hyperglycemia in type 2 diabetic subjects—a randomized, double-blind trial." *J Am College Nutr* 2003;22(1):36-42.

[21] Chen HL, Sheu WHH, Tai TS, et al. "Konjac supplement alleviated hypercholesterolemia and hyperglycemia in type 2 diabetes subjects—a randomized, double-blind trial." *J Am College Nutr* 2003;22(1):36-42.

[22] Lalor BC, Bhatnagar D, Winocour PH, et al. "Placebo-controlled trial of the effects of guar gum and metformin on fasting blood glucose and serum lipids in obese, type 2 diabetic patients." *Diabet Med* 1990;7(3):242-245.

[23] Groop PH, Aro A, Stenman S, et al. "Long-term effects of guar gum in subjects with non-insulin-dependent diabetes mellitus." *Am J Clin Nutr* 1993;58(4):513-518.

[24] Gatenby SJ, Ellis PR, Morgan LM, et al. "Effect of partially depolymerized guar gum on acute metabolic variables in patients with non-insulin-dependent diabetes." *Diabet Med* 1996;13(4):358-364.

[25] Goldfine AB, Simonson DC, Folli F, et al. "Metabolic effects of sodium metavanadate in humans with insulin-dependent and non-insulin-dependent diabetes mellitus in vivo and in vitro studies." *J Clin Endocrinol Metab* 1995;80(11):3311-3320.

[26] Boden G, Chen X, Ruiz J, et al. "Effects of vanadyl sulfate on carbohydrate and lipid metabolism in patients with non-insulin-dependent diabetes mellitus." *Metabolism* 1996;45(9):1130-1135.

[27] Tongia A, Tongia SK, Dave M. "Phytochemical determination and extraction of *Momordica charantia* fruit and its hypoglycemic potentiation of oral hypoglycemic drugs in diabetes mellitus (NIDDM)." *Indian J Physiol Pharmacol* 2004;48(2):241-244.

[28] Ahmad N, Hassan MR, Halder H, et al. "Effect of *Momordica charantia* (Karolla) extracts on fasting and postprandial serum glucose levels in NIDDM patients." *Bangladesh Med Res Counc Bull* 1999;25(1):11-13.

[29] Baskaran K, Ahamath B, Shanmugasundaram KR, et al. "Antidiabetic effect of a leaf extract from *Gymnema sylvestre* in non-insulin-dependent diabetes mellitus patients." *J Ethnopharmacol* 1990;30(3):295-305.

[30] Shanmugasundaram ERB, Rajeswari G, Baskaran K, et al. "Use of *Gymnema sylvestre* leaf extract in the control of blood glucose in insulin-dependent diabetes mellitus." *J Ethnopharmacol* 1990;30(3):281-294.

Chapter 11: Diarrhea

[1] Bliss DZ, Jung HJ, Savik K, et al. "Supplementation with dietary fiber improves fecal incontinence." *Nurs Res* 2001;50(4):203-213.

[2] Murphy J, Stacey D, Crook J, et al. "Testing control of radiation-induced diarrhea with a psyllium bulking agent: a pilot study." *Can Oncol Nurs J* 2000;10(3):96-100.

[3] Heather DJ, Howell L, Montana M, et al. "Effect of a bulk-forming cathartic on diarrhea in tube-fed patients." *Heart Lung* 1991;20(4):409-413.

[4] Saavedra JM, Bauman NA, Oung I, et al. "Feeding of *Bifidobacterium bifidum* and *Streptococcus thermophilus* to infants in hospital for prevention of diarrhoea and shedding of rotavirus." *Lancet* 1994;344(8928):1046-1049.

[5] Chouraqui JP, Van Egroo LD, Fichot CJ. "Acidified milk formula supplemented with *Bifidobacterium lactis*: impact on infant diarrhea in residential care settings." *J Pediatr Gastroenterol Nutr* 2004;38(3):288-292.

[6] D'Souza AL, Rajkumar C, Cooke J, et al. "Probiotics in prevention of antibiotic associated diarrhoea: meta-analysis." *BMJ* 2002;324:1361-1364.

[7] Adapted from D'Souza AL, Rajkumar C, Cooke J, et al. "Probiotics in prevention of antibiotic associated diarrhoea: meta-analysis." *BMJ* 2002;324:1361-1364.

[8] Adam J, Barret A, Barret-Bellet C. "Essais cliniques controles en double insu de l'ultra-levure lyophilsee: etude multicentrique par 25 medicins de 388 cas." *Gazette Medicale de France* 1977;84 :2072-2078.

[9] Gotz V, Romankiewicz JA, Moss J, Murray HW. "Prophylaxis against ampicillin associated diarrhoea with *Lactobacillus* preparation." *Am J Hosp Pharm* 1979;36:754-757.

[10] Surawicz CM, Elmer GW, Speelman P, et al. "Prevention of antibiotic-associated diarrhea by *Saccharomyces boulardii*: a prospective study." *Gastroenterology* 1989;96(4):981-988.

[11] Wunderlich PF, Braun L, Fumagalli I, et al. "Double-blind report on the efficacy of lactic acid-producing *Enterococcus* SF68 in the prevention of antibiotic-associated diarrhoea and in the treatment of acute diarrhoea." *J Int Med Res* 1989;17:333-338.

[12] Tankanow RM, Ross MB, Ertel IJ, et al. "Double blind, placebo-controlled study of the efficacy of Lactinex in the prophylaxis of amoxicillin-induced diarrhoea." *DICP, Ann Pharm* 1990;24:382-384.

[13] Orrhage K, Brismar B, Nord CE. "Effects of supplements of *Bifidobacterium longum* and *Lactobacillus acidophilus* on intestinal microbiota during administration of clindamycin." *Microb Ecol Health Dis* 1994;7:17-25.

[14] McFarland LV, Surawicz CM, Greenberg RN, et al. "Prevention of beta-lactam-associated diarrhea by *Saccharomyces boulardii* compared with placebo." *Am J Gastroenterol* 1995;90(3):439-448.

[15] Lewis SJ, Potts LF, Barry Re. "The lack of therapeutic effect of *S Boulardii* in the prevention of antibiotic related diarrhoea in elderly patients." *J Infect* 1998;36:171-174.

[16] Vanderhoof JA, Whitney DB, Antonson DL, et al. "*Lactobacillus GG* in the prevention of antibiotic-associated diarrhea in children." *J Pediatr* 1999;135(5):564-568.

[17] Cremonini F, DiCaro S, Nista EC, et al. "Meta-analysis: the effect of probiotic administration on antibiotic-associated diarrhoea." *Aliment Pharmacol Ther* 2002;16(8):1461-1467.

[18] Rosenfeldt V, Michaelsen KF, Jakobsen M, et al. "Effect of probiotic *Lactobacillus* strains in young children hospitalized with acute diarrhea." *Pediatr Infect Dis J* 2002;21(5):411-416.

[19] Rosenfeldt V, Michaelsen KF, Jakobsen M, et al. "Effect of probiotic *Lactobacillus* strains on acute diarrhea in a cohort of nonhospitalized children attending day-care centers." *Pediatr Infect Dis J* 2002;21(5):417-419.

[20] Shornikova AV, Casas IA, Isolauri E, et al. "*Lactobacillus reuteri* as a therapeutic agent in acute diarrhea in young children." *J Pediatr Gastroenterol Nutr* 1997;24(4):399-404.

[21] Szajewska H, Mrukowicz JZ. "Probiotics in the treatment and prevention of acute infectious diarrhea in infants and children: a systematic review of published randomized, double-blind, placebo-controlled trials." *J Pediatr Gastroenterol Nutr* 2001;33(Suppl 2):S17-S25.

[22] *Van Niel CW, Feudtner C, Garrison MM, et al. "Lactobacillus* therapy for acute infectious diarrhea in children: a meta-analysis." *Pediatrics* 2002;109:678-684.

[23] Adapted from Van Niel CW, Feudtner C, Garrison MM, et al. "*Lactobacillus* therapy for acute infectious diarrhea in children: a meta-analysis." *Pediatrics* 2002;109:678-684.

[24] Simakachorn N, Piochaipat V, Rithipornpaisarn P, et al. "Clinical evaluation of the addition of lyophilized, heat-killed *Lactobacillus acidophilus* LB to oral rehydration therapy in the treatment of acute diarrhea in children." *J Pediatr Gastroenterol Nutr* 2000;30:68-72.

[25] Guandalini S, Penssabene L, Zikri MA, et al. "*Lactobacillus* GG administration in oral rehydration solution to children with acute diarrhea: a multicenter European trial." *J Pediatr Gastroenterol Nutr* 2000;30:54-60.

[26] Shornikova AV, Casas IA, Isolauri E, et al. "*Lactobacillus reuteri* as a therapeutic agent in acute diarrhea in young children." *J Pediatr Gastrointerol Nutr* 1997;24:399-404.

[27] Shornikova AV, Casas IA, Mykkanen H, et al. "Bacterio-therapy with *Lactobacillus reuteri* in rotavirus gastroenteritis." *Pediatr Infect Dis J* 1997;16:1103-1107.

[28] Shornikova AV, Isolauri E, Burkanova L, et al. "A trial in the Karelian Republic of oral rehydration and *Lactobacillus* GG for treatment of acute diarrhea." *Acta Paediatr* 1997;86:460-465.

[29] Kaila M, Isolauri E, Soppi E, et al. "Enhancement of the circulating antibody secreting cell response in human diarrhea by a human *Lactobacillus* strain." *Pediatr Res* 1992;32:141-144.

[30] Pearce JL, Hamilton JR. "Controlled trial of orally administered lactobacilli in acute infantile diarrhea." *J Pediatr* 1974;84:261-262.

[31] Chicoine L, Joncas JH. "Use of lactic enzymes in non-bacterial gastroenteritis." *Union Med Can* 1973;102:1114-1115.

[32] Pereg D, Kimhi O, Tirosh A, et al. "The effect of fermented yogurt on the prevention of diarrhea in a healthy adult population." *Am J Infect Control* 2005;33(2):122-125.

[33] Guarino A, Canani RB, Spagnuolo MI, et al. "Oral bacterial therapy reduces the duration of symptoms and of viral excretion in children with mild diarrhea." *J Pediatr Gastroenterol Nutr* 1997;25(5):516-519.

[34] Vanderhoof JA, Whitney DB, Anlonson DL, et al. "*Lactobacillus GG* in the prevention of antibiotic-associated diarrhea in children." *J Pediatr* 1999;135(5):564-568.

[35] Siitonen S, Vapaatalo H, Salminen S, et al. "Effect of *Lactobacillus GG* yoghurt in prevention of antibiotic associated diarrhea." *Ann Med* 1990;22:57-59.

[36] Gaon D, Garcia H, Winter L, et al. "Effect of *Lactobacillus* strains and *Saccharomyces boulardii* on persistent diarrhea in children." *Medicina (Buenos Aires)* 2003;63(4):293-298.

[37] Tacket CO, Losonsky G, Link H, et al. "Protection by milk immunoglobulin concentrate against oral challenge with enterotoxigenic *Escherichia coli*." *N Engl J Med* 1988;318(19):1240-1243.

[38] Freedman DJ, Tacket CO, Delehanty A, et al. "Milk immunoglobulin with specific activity against purified colonization factor antigens can protect against oral challenge with enterotoxigenic *Escherichia coli*." *Journal of Infectious Diseases* 1998;177(3):662-667.

[39] Sarker SA, Casswall TH, Mahalanabis D, et al. "Successful treatment of rotavirus diarrhea in children with immunoglobulin from immunized bovine colostrum." *Pediatr Infect Dis J* 1998;17(12):1149-1154.

[40] Nord J, Ma P, DiJohn D, et al. "Treatment with bovine hyperimmune colostrum of cryptosporidial diarrhea in AIDS patients." *AIDS* 1990;4(6):581-584.

[41] Plettenberg A, Stoehr A, Stellbrink HJ, et al. "A preparation from bovine colostrum in the treatment of HIV-positive patients with chronic diarrhea." *Clin Investig* 1993;71(1):42-45.

[42] Greenberg PD, Cello JP. "Treatment of severe diarrhea caused by *Cryptosporidium parvum* with oral bovine immunoglobulin concentrate in patients with AIDS." *J Acquir Immune Defic Syndr Hum Retrovirol* 1996;13(4):348-354.

[43] Mitra AK, Mahalanabis D, Ashraf H, et al. "Hyperimmune cow colostrum reduces diarrhoea due to rotavirus: a double-blind, controlled clinical trial." *Acta Paediatr* 1995;84(9):996-1001.

[44] Huppertz HI, Rutkowski S, Busch DH, et al. "Bovine colostrum ameliorates diarrhea in infection with diarrheagenic *Escherichia coli*, shiga toxin-producing *E. Coli*, and *E. coli* expressing intimin and hemolysin." *J Pediatr Gastroenterol Nutr* 1999;29(4):452-456.

[45] Tackett CO, Binion SB, Bostwick E, et al. "Efficacy of bovine milk immuno-globulin concentrate in preventing illness after Shigella flexneri challenge." *Am J Trop Med Hyg* 1992;47(3):276-283.

[46] Ylitalo S, Uhari M, Rasi S, et al. "Rotaviral antibodies in the treatment of acute rotaviral gastroenteritis." *Acta Peadiatr* 1998;87(3):2640267.

[47] McFarland LV, Surawicz CM, Greenberg RN, et al. "A randomized placebo-controlled trial of *Saccharomyces boulardii* in combination with standard antibiotics for *Clostridium difficile* disease." *JAMA* 1994;271(24):1913-1918.

[48] Kotowska M, Albrecht P, Szajewska H. "*Saccharomyces boulardii* in the prevention of antibiotic-associated diarrhoea in children: a randomized double-blind placebo-controlled trial." *Aliment Pharmacol Ther* 2005;21(5):583-590.

[49] Surawicz CM, Elmer GW, Speelman P, et al. "Prevention of antibiotic-associated diarrhea by *Saccharomyces boulardii*: a prospective study." *Gastroenterology* 1989;96(4):981-988.

[50] Kurugol Z, Koturoglu G. "Effects of *Saccharomyces boulardii* in children with acute diarrhea." *Acta Paediatr* 2005;94:44-47.

[51] Sazawal S, Black RE, Bhan MK, et al. "Zinc supplementation in young children with acute diarrhea in India." *N Engl J Med* 1995;333(13):839-844.

[52] Muller O, Becher H, van Zweeden AB, et al. "Effect of zinc supplementation on malaria and other causes of morbidity in west African children: randomised double blind placebo controlled trial." *BMJ* 2001;322:1-6.

[53] Bhutta ZA, Bird SM, Black RE, et al. "Therapeutic effects of oral zinc in acute and persistent diarrhea in children in developing countries: pooled analysis of randomized controlled trials." *Am J Clin Nutr* 2000;72:1516-1522.

[54] Alam NH, Meier R, Sarker SA, et al. "Partially hydrolysed guar gum supplemented comminuted chicken diet in persistent diarrhoea: a randomised trial." *Arch Dis Child* 2005;90(2):195-199.

[55] Spapen H, Diltoer M, Van Malderen C, et al. "Soluble fiber reduces the incidence of diarrhea in septic patients receiving total enteral nutrition: a prospective, double-blind, randomized, and controlled trial." *Clin Nutr* 2001;20(4):301-305.

[56] Rushdi TA, Pichard C, Khater YH. "Control of diarrhea by fiber-enriched diet in ICU patients on enteral nutrition: a prospective randomized controlled trial." *Clin Nutr* 2004;23(6):1344-1352.

[57] Jacobs J, Jiminez LM, Gloyd SS. "Treatment of acute childhood diarrhea with homeopathic medicine: a randomized clinical trial in Nicaragua." *Pediatrics* 1994;93(5):719-725.

[58] Jacobs J, Jimenez LM, Malthouse S, et al. "Homeopathic treatment of acute childhood diarrhea: results from a clinical trial in Nepal." *J Altern Complement Med* 2000;6(2):131-139.

[59] Jacobs J, Jonas WB, Jiminez-Perez M, et al. "Homeopathy for childhood diarrhea: combined results and metaanalysis from three randomized, controlled trials." *Pediatr Infect Dis J* 2003;22:229-234.

Chapter 12: Fibromyalgia

[1] Deluze C, Bosia L, Zirbs A, et al. "Electroacupuncture in fibromyalgia: results of a controlled trial." *BMJ* 1992;305(6864):1249-1252.

[2] Sprott H, Jeschonneck M, Grohmann G, et al. "Microcirculatory changes over the tender points in fibromyalgia patients after acupuncture therapy (measured with laser-Doppler flowmetry)." *Wein Klin Wochenschr* 2000;112(13):580-586.

[3] Sprott H, Franke S, Kluge H, et al. "Letter to the Editor. Pain treatment of fibromyalgia by acupuncture." *Rheumatol Int* 1998;18(1):35-36.

[4] World Health Organization. "3. Diseases and disorders that can be treated with acupuncture." Accessible at http://www.who.int/Medicinedocs. Viewed December 15, 2005.

[5] Evcik D, Kizilay B, Gokcen E. "The effects of balneotherapy on fibromyalgia patients." *Rheumatol Int* 2002;22(2):56-59.

[6] Blunt KL, Rajwani MH, Guerriero RC. "The effectiveness of chiropractic management of fibromyalgia patients: a pilot study." *J Manipulative Physiol Ther* 1997;20(6):389-399.

[7] Hains G, Hains F. "A combined ischemic compression and spinal manipulation in the treatment of fibromyalgia: a preliminary estimate of dose and efficacy." *J Manipulative Physiol Ther* 2000;23(4):225-230.

[8] Gamber RG, Shores JH, Russo DP, et al. "Osteopathic manipulative treatment in conjunction with medication relieves pain associated with fibromyalgia syndrome: Results of a randomized clinical pilot project." *JAOA* 2002;102(6):321-325.

Chapter 13: High Blood Pressure

[1] Jorde R, Bønaa KH. "Calcium from dairy products, vitamin D intake, and blood pressure: the Tromsø study." *Am J Clin Nutr* 2000;71:1530-1535.

[2] Dwyer JH, Dwyer KM, Scribner RA, et al. "Dietary calcium, calcium supplementation, and blood pressure in African American adolescents." *Am J Clin Nutr* 1998;68:648-655.

[3] Pan Z, Zhao L, Guo D, et al. "Effects of oral calcium supplementation on blood pressure in population." *Zhonghua Yu Fang Yi Xue Za Zhi* 2000;34(2):109-112.

[4] Griffith LE, Guyatt GH, Cook RJ, et al. "The influence of dietary and nondietary calcium supplementation on blood pressure: an updated meta-analysis of randomized controlled trials." *Am J Hypertens* 1999;12 (1 Pt 1):84-92.

[5] Burke BE, Neuenschwander R, Olson RD. "Randomized, double-blind, placebo-controlled trial of coenzyme Q_{10} in isolated systolic hypertension." *South Med J* 2001;94(11):1112-1117.

[6] Singh RB, Niaz MA, Rastogi SS, et al. "Effect of hydrosoluble coenzyme Q_{10} on blood pressures and insulin resistance in hypertensive patients with coronary artery disease." *J Human Hyperten* 1999;13:203-208.

[7] Hodgson JM, Watts GF, Playford DA, et al. "Coenzyme Q_{10} improves blood pressure and glycaemic control: a controlled trial in subjects with type 2 diabetes." *Eur J Clin Nutr* 2002;56(11):1137-1142.

[8] Rosenfeldt F, Hilton D, Pepe S, et al. "Systematic review of effect of coenzyme Q_{10} in physical exercise, hypertension and heart failure." *Biofactors* 2003;18(1-4):91-100.

[9] Auer W, Eiber A, Hertkorn E, et al. "Hypertension and hyperlipidaemia: garlic helps in mild cases." *Br J Clin Pract* 1990; Suppl 69:3-6.

[10] Steiner M, Khan AH, Holbert D, et al. "A double-blind crossover study in moderately hypercholesterolemic men that compared the effect of aged garlic extract and placebo administration on blood lipids." *Am J Clin Nutr* 1996;64(6):866-870.

[11] Widman L, Wester PO, Stegmayr BK, et al. "The dose-dependent reduction in blood pressure through administration of magnesium. A double blind placebo controlled cross-over study." *Am J Hypertens* 1993;6(1):41-45.

[12] Sanjuliani AF, de Abreu Fagundes VG, Francischetti EA. "Effects of magnesium on blood pressure and intracellular ion levels of Brazilian hypertensive patients." *Int J Cardiol* 1996;56(2):177-183.

[13] Harris, WS. "N-3 fatty acids and serum lipoproteins: human studies." *American Journal of Clinical Nutrition* 1997:65(5 Suppl):1645S-1654S.

[14] Peacock JM, Folsom AR, Arnett DK, et al. "Relationship of serum and dietary magnesium to incident hypertension: The Atherosclerosis Risk in Communities (ARIC) Study." *Ann Epidemiol* 1999;9(3):159-165.

[15] Jee SH, Miller ER, Guallar E, et al. "The effect of magnesium supplementation on blood pressure: a meta-analysis of randomized clinical trials." *Am J Hypertens* 2002;15(8):691-696.

[16] Bonaa KH, Bjerve KS, Straume B, et al. "Effect of eicosapentaenoic and docosahexaenoic acids on blood pressure in hypertension. A population-based intervention trial from the Tromso study." *NEJM* 1990;322(12):795-801.

[17] Bao DQ, Mori TA, Burke V, et al. "Effects of dietary fish and weight reduction on ambulatory blood pressure in overweight hypertensives." *Hypertension* 1998;32:710-717.

[18] Toft I, Bonaa KH, Ingebretsen OC, et al. "Effects of n-3 polyunsaturated fatty acids on glucose homeostasis and blood pressure in essential hypertension. A randomized, controlled trial." *Ann Intern Med* 1995;123(12):911-918.

[19] Balk E, Chung M, Lichtenstein A, et al. "Effects of omega-3 fatty acids on cardiovascular risk factors and intermediate markers of cardiovascular disease: Summary." Evidence Report/Technology Assessment: No. 93. AHRQ Publication No. 04-E0101-1. March 2004. Agency for Healthcare Research and Quality, Rockville, MD.

[20] Morris MC, Sacks F, Rosner B. "Does fish oil lower blood pressure? A meta-analysis of controlled trials." *Circulation* 1993;88:523-533.

[21] Tam KC, Yiu HH. "The effect of acupuncture on essential hypertension." *Am J Chin Med* 1975;3(4):369-375.

[22] Guo W, Ni G. "The effects of acupuncture on blood pressure in different patients." *J Tradit Chin Med* 2003;23(1):49-50.

[23] Chiu YJ, Chi A, Reid IA. "Cardiovascular and endocrine effects of acupuncture in hypertensive patients." *Clin Exp Hypertens* 1997;19(7):1047-1063.

[24] Ferrara LA, Raimondi AS, d'Episcopo L, et al. "Olive oil and reduced need for antihypertensive medications." *Arch Intern Med* 2000;160(6):837-842.

[25] Perona JS, Canizares J, Montero E, et al. "Virgin olive oil reduces blood pressure in hypertensive elderly subjects." *Clin Nutr* 2004;23(5):1113-1121.

[26] Alonso A, Martinez-Gonzalez MA. "Olive oil consumption and reduced incidence of hypertension: the SUN study." *Lipids* 2004;39(12):1233-1238.

[27] Psaltopoulou T, Naska A, Orfanos P, et al. "Olive oil, the Mediterranean diet, and arterial blood pressure: the Greek European Prospective Investigation into Cancer and Nutrition (EPIC) study." *Am J Clin Nutr* 2004;80:1012-1018.

Chapter 14: High Cholesterol

[1] Davidson MH, Maki KC, Kong JC, et al. "Long-term effects of consuming foods containing psyllium seed husk on serum lipids in subjects with hypercholesterolemia." *Am J Clin Nutr* 1998;67:367-376.

[2] Anderson JW, Davidson MH, Blonde L, et al. "Long-term cholesterol-lowering effects of psyllium as an adjunct to diet therapy in the treatment of hypercholesterolemia." *Am J Clin Nutr* 2000;71:1433-1438.

[3] Moreyra AE, Wilson AC, Koraym A. "Effect of combining psyllium fiber with simvastatin in lowering cholesterol." *Arch Intern Med* 2005;165(10):1161-1166.

[4] Olson BH, Anderson SM, Becker MP, et al. "Psyllium-enriched cereals lower blood total cholesterol and LDL cholesterol, but not HDL cholesterol, in hypercholesterolemia adults: results of a meta-analysis." *J Nutr* 1997;127:1973-1980.

[5] Anderson JW, Allgood LD, Lawrence AL, et al. "Cholesterol-lowering effects of psyllium intake adjunctive to diet therapy in men and women with hypercholesterolemia: meta-analysis of 8 controlled trials." *Am J Clin Nutr* 2000;71:472-479.

[6] Anderson JW, Gilinsky NH, Deakins DA, et al. "Lipid responses of hyper-cholesterolemic men to oat-bran and wheat-bran intake." *Am J Clin Nutr* 1991;54(4):678-683.

[7] Romero AL, Romero JE, Galaviz S, et al. "Cookies enriched with psyllium or oat bran lower plasma LDL cholesterol in normal and hypercholesterol-emic men from Northern Mexico." *Am J Clin Nutr* 1998;17(6):601-608.

[8] Van Horn L, Liu K, Gerber J, et al. "Oats and soy in lipid-lowering diets for women with hypercholesterolemia: is there synergy?" *J Am Diet Assoc* 2001;101(11):1319-1325.

[9] Ripsin CM, Keenan JM, Jacobs DR, et al. "Oat products and lipid lower-ing." A meta-analysis. *JAMA* 1992;267(24):3317-3325.

[10] Chan DC, Watts GF, Mori TA, et al. "Randomized controlled trial of the effect of n-3 fatty acid supplementation on the metabolism of apolipoprotein B-100 and chylomicron remnants in men with visceral obesity." *Am J Clin Nutr* 2003;77:300-307.

[11] Miki KC, Van Elswyk ME, McCarthy D, et al. "Lipid responses to a dietary docosahexaenoic acid supplement in men and women with below average levels of high density lipoprotein cholesterol." *J Am Coll Nutr* 2005;24(3):189-199.

[12] Kris-Etherton PM, Harris WS, Appel J. "Fish consumption, fish oil, omega-3 fatty acids, and cardiovascular disease." *Circulation* 2002;106:2747-2757.

[13] Balk E, Chung M, Lichtenstein A, et al. "Effects of omega-3 fatty acids on cardiovascular risk factors and intermediate markers of cardiovascular diseases." Summary, Evidence Report/Technology Assessment No. 93. AHQ Publication No. 04-E010-1. Rockville, MD: Agency for Healthcare Research and Quality. March 2004.

[14] Neil HA, Miejer GW, Roe LS. "Randomised controlled trial of use by hypercholesterolaemic patients of a vegetable oil-sterol-enriched fat spread." *Atherosclerosis* 2001;156(2):329-327.

[15] Nguyen TT, Dale LC, von Bergmann K, et al. "Cholesterol-lowering effect of a stanol ester in a US population of mildly hypercholesterolemic men and women: a randomized controlled trial." *Mayo Clin Proc* 1999;74(12):1198-1206.

[16] Vanstone CA, Raeini-Sarjaz M, Parsons WE, et al. "Unesterified plant sterols and stanols lower LDL-cholesterol concentrations equivalently in hypercholesterolemic persons." *Am J Clin Nutr* 2002;76:1272-1278.

[17] De Graff J, Nolting PR, van Dam, MV, et al. "Consumption of tall oil-derived phytosterols in a chocolate matrix significantly decreases plasma total and low-density lipoprotein-cholesterol levels." *Br J Nutr* 2002;88:479-488.

[18] Adapted from De Graff J, Nolting PR, van Dam, MV, et al. "Consumption of tall oil-derived phytosterols in a chocolate matrix significantly decreases plasma total and low-density lipoprotein-cholesterol levels." *Br J Nutr* 2002;88:479-488.

[19] Chen JT, Wesley R, Shamburek RD, et al. "Meta-analysis of natural therapies for hyperlipidemia: plant sterols and stanols versus policosanol." *Pharmacotherapy* 2005;25(2):171-183.

[20] Kerckhoffs KA, Brouns F, Hornstra G, et al. "Effects on the human serum lipoprotein profile of b-glucan, soy protein and isoflavones, plant sterols and stanols, garlic and tocotrienols." *J Nutr* 2002;132:2494-2005.

[21] Washburn S, Burke GL, Morgan T, et al. "Effect of soy protein supplementation on serum lipoproteins, blood pressure, and menopausal symptoms in perimenopausal women." *Menopause* 1999;6(1):7-13.

[22] Adapted from Washburn S, Burke GL, Morgan T, et al. "Effect of soy protein supplementation on serum lipoproteins, blood pressure, and menopausal symptoms in perimenopausal women." *Menopause* 1999;6(1):7-13.

[23] Sirtori CR, Pazzucconi F, Colombo L, et al. "Double-blind study of the addition of high-protein soya milk v. cows' milk to the diet of patients with severe hypercholesterolaemia and resistance to or intolerance of statins." *Br J Nutr* 1999;82(2):91-96.

[24] Potter SM, Baum JA, Teng H, et al. "Soy protein and isoflavones: their effects on blood lipids and bone density in postmenopausal women." *Am J Clin Nutr* 1998;68(Suppl):1375S-1379S.

[25] Anderson JW, Johnstone BM, Cook-Newell ME. "Meta-analysis of the effects of soy protein intake on serum lipids." *N Engl J Med* 1995;333(5):276-282.

[26] Adapted from Anderson JW, Johnstone BM, Cook-Newell ME. "Meta-analysis of the effects of soy protein intake on serum lipids." *N Engl J Med* 1995;333(5):276-282.

[27] Zhan S, Ho Sc. "Meta-analysis of the effects of soy protein containing isoflavones on the lipid profile." *Am J Clin Nutr* 2005;81(2):397-408.

[28] Balk E, Chung M, Chew P, et al. "Effects of soy on health outcomes." Summary, Evidence Report/Technology Assessment No. 126. AHRQ Publication No. 05-E024-1. Rockville, MD: Agency for Healthcare Research and Quality. July 2005.

[29] Sabate J, Fraser GE, Burke K, et al. "Effects of walnuts on serum lipid levels and blood pressure in normal men." *N Engl J Med* 1993;328(9):603-607.

[30] Jenkins DJ, Kenall CW, Marchie A, et al. "Dose response of almonds on coronary heart disease risk factors: blood lipids, oxidized low-density lipoproteins, lipoprotein(a), homocysteine, and pulmonary nitric oxide. A randomized, controlled, crossover trial." *Circulation* 2002;106(11):1327-1332.

[31] Ros E, Nunez I, Perez-Heras A, et al. "A walnut diet improves endothelial function in hypercholesterolemic subjects: a randomized crossover trial." *Circulation* 2004;109:1609-1614.

[32] Mukuddem-Petersen J, Oosthuizen W, Jerling JC. "A systematic review of the effects of nuts on blood lipid profiles in humans." *J Nutr* 2005;135(9): 2082-2089.

[33] Feldman EB. "LSRO Report: The scientific evidence for a beneficial health relationship between walnuts and coronary heart disease." *J Nutr* 2002;132: 1062S-1101S.

[34] Hu FB, Stampfer MJ. "Nut consumption and risk of coronary heart disease: a review of epidemiologic evidence." *Curr Atheroscler Rep* 1999;1(3):204-209.

[35] Castano G, Mas R, Gamez R, et al. "Concomitant use of policosanol and beta-blockers in older patients." *Int J Clin Pharmacol Res* 2004;24(2-3): 65-77.

[36] Castano G, Menendez R, Mas R, et al. "Effects of policosanol and lovastatin on lipid profile and lipid peroxidation in patients with dyslipidemia associated with type 2 diabetes mellitus." *Int J Clin Pharmacol Res* 2002;22(3-4):89-99.

[37] Adapted from Castano G, Menendez R, Mas R, et al. "Effects of policosanol and lovastatin on lipid profile and lipid peroxidation in patients with dyslipidemia associated with type 2 diabetes mellitus." *Int J Clin Pharmacol Res* 2002;22(3-4):89-99.

[38] Castano G, Mas R, Fernandez JC, et al. "Effects of policosanol on older patients with hypertension and type II hypercholesterolaemia." *Drugs R D* 2002;3(3):159-172.

[39] Chen JT, Wesley R, Shamburek RD, et al. "Meta-analysis of natural therapies for hyperlipidemia: plant sterols and stanols versus policosanol." *Pharmacotherapy* 2005;25(2):171-183.

[40] Adapted from Chen JT, Wesley R, Shamburek RD, et al. "Meta-analysis of natural therapies for hyperlipidemia: plant sterols and stanols versus policosanol." *Pharmacotherapy* 2005;25(2):171-183.

Chapter 15: Insomnia

[1] National Center on Sleep Disorders Research, National Institutes of Health www.nhlbi.nih.gov/health/prof/sleep/sleep.txt (Viewed 8-9-06)

[2] Spence DW, Kayumov L, Chen A, et al. "Acupuncture increases nocturnal melatonin secretion and reduces insomnia and anxiety: a preliminary report." *J Neuropsychiatry Clin Neurosci* 2004;16(1):19-28.

[3] da Silva JB, Nakamura MU, Cordeiro JA, et al. "Acupuncture for insomnia in pregnancy – a prospective, quasi-randomized, controlled study." *Acupunct Med* 2005;23(2):47-51.

[4] "Traditional Medicine." World Health Organization, Media Centre. Revised May, 2003. Accessible at http://www.who.int/mediacentre/factsheets/fs134/en/. Viewed August 9, 2006.

[5] Zhdanova IV, Wurtman RJ, Regan MM, et al. "Melatonin treatment for age-related insomnia." *J Clin Endocrinol Metab* 2001;86(10):4727-4730.

[6] Haimov I, Lavie P, Laudon M, et al. "Melatonin replacement therapy of elderly insomniacs." *Sleep* 1995;18(7):598-603.

[7] Garfinkel D, Laudon M, Nof D, et al. "Improvement of sleep quality in elderly people by controlled-release melatonin." *Lancet* 1995;346(8974):541-544.

[8] Leatherwood PD, Chauffard F, Heck E, et al. "Aqueous extract of valerian root (*Valeriana officinalis L.*) improves sleep quality in man." *Pharmacol Biochem Behav* 1982;17(1):65-71.

[9] Ziegler G, Ploch M, Miettinen-Baumann A, et al. "Efficacy and tolerability of valerian extract LI 156 compared with oxazepam in the treatment of non-organic insomnia—a randomized, double-blind, comparative clinical study." *Eur J Med Res* 2002;7(11):480-486.

[10] Donath F, Quispe S, Diefenbach K, et al. "Critical evaluation of the effect of valerian extract on sleep structure and sleep quality." *Pharmacopsychiatry* 2000;33(2):47-53.

[11] Khalsa SBS. "Treatment of chronic insomnia with yoga: a preliminary study with sleep-wake diaries." *Biofeedback* 2004;29(4):269-278.

[12] Manjunath NK, Telles S. "Influence of Yoga & Ayurveda on self-rated sleep in a geriatric population." *Indian J Med Res* 2005;121(5):683-690.

Chapter 16: Menopause Hot Flashes

[1] Schwingl PJ, Hulka BS, Harlow SD. "Risk factors for menopausal hot flashes." *Obstetrics and Gynecology* 1994;84(1):29-34.

[2] Berkow R, Beers MH, Fletcher AJ, eds. *The Merck Manual of Medical Information.* (NJ: Whitehouse Station, Merck Research Laboratories, 1997), 1078.

[3] Berkow R, Beers MH, Fletcher AJ, eds. *The Merck Manual of Medical Information.* (NJ: Whitehouse Station, Merck Research Laboratories, 1997), 1078.

[4] Osmers R, Friede M, Liske E, et al. "Efficacy and safety of isopropanolic black cohosh extract for climacteric symptoms." *Obstet Gynecol* 2005; 105:1074-1083.

[5] Nappi RE, Malavasi B, Brundu B, et al. "Efficacy of *Cimicifuga racemosa* on climacteric complaints: A randomized, study versus low-dose transdermal estradiol." *Gynecological Endocrinology* 2005:20(1):30-35.

[6] Vermes G, Banhidy F, Acs N, et al. "The effects of Remifemin on subjective symptoms of menopause." *Advances in Therapy* 2005;22(2):148-154.

[7] Lock, M. *Encounters with Aging: Mythologies of Menopause in Japan and North America.* (Berkeley and Los Angeles: University of California Press, 1993.)

[8] Upmalis DH, Lobo R, Bradley L, et al. "Vasomotor symptom relief by soy isoflavone extract tablets in postmenopausal women: a multicenter, double-blind, randomized, placebo-controlled study." *Menopause* 2000;7(4):236-242.

[9] Albertazzi P, Pansini F, Bonaccorsi G, et al. "The effect of dietary soy supplementation on hot flushes." *Obstet Gynecol* 1998;91(1):6-11.

[10] Faure ED, Chantre P, Mares P. "Effects of a standardized soy extract on hot flushes: a multicenter, double-blind, randomized, placebo-controlled study." *Menopause* 2002;9(5):329-334.

[11] Fugate SE, Church CO. "Nonestrogen treatment modalities for vasomotor symptoms associated with menopause." *Ann Pharmacother* 2004;38(9): 1482-1499.

Chapter 17: Migraines

[1] Mauskop A, Fox B. *What Your Doctor May Not Tell You About Migraines.* (New York, NY: Warner Books) 2.

[2] Vickers AJ, Rees RW, Zollman CE, et al. "Acupuncture for chronic headache disorders in primary care: randomised controlled trial and economic analysis." *Health Technol Assess* 2004;8(48):1-35.

[3] Liguori A, Petti F, Bangrazi A, et al. "Comparison of pharmacological treatment versus acupuncture treatment for migraine without aura—analysis of socio-medical parameters." *J Tradit Chin Med* 2000;20(3):231-240.

[4] Melchart D, Thormaehlen J, Hager S, et al. "Acupuncture versus placebo versus sumatriptan for early treatment of migraine attacks: a randomized controlled trial." *J Intern Med* 2003;253(2):181-188.

[5] Allais G, DeLorenzo C, Quirico PE, et al. "Acupuncture in the prophylactic treatment of migraine without aura: a comparison with flunarizine." *Headache* 2002;42(9):855-861.

[6] Manias P, Tagaris G, Karageorgiou K. "Acupuncture in headache: A critical review." *Clin J Pain* 2000;16:334-339.

[7] Mauskop A, Altura BT, Cracco RQ, et al. "Intravenous magnesium sulphate relieves migraine attacks in patients with low serum ionized magnesium levels: a pilot study." *Clinical Science* 1995;89:633-636.

[8] Peikert A, Wilimzig C, Kohne-Volland R. "Prophylaxis of migraine with oral magnesium: results from a prospective, multi-center, placebo-controlled and double-blind randomized study." *Cephalalgia* 1996;16(4):257-63.

[9] Demirkaya S, Dora B, Topcuoglu MA, et al. "A comparative study of magnesium, flunarizine and amitriptyline in the prophylaxis of migraine." *J Headache Pain* 2000;1:179-186.

[10] Adapted from Demirkaya S, Dora B, Topcuoglu MA, et al. "A comparative study of magnesium, flunarizine and amitriptyline in the prophylaxis of migraine." *J Headache Pain* 2000;1:179-186.

[11] Facchinetti F, Sances G, Borella P, et al. "Magnesium prophylaxis of menstrual migraine: effects on intracellular magnesium." *Headache* 1991; 1(5):298-301.

[12] Tuchin PJ, Pollard H, Bonello R. "A randomized controlled trial of chiropractic spinal manipulative therapy for migraine." *J Manipulative Physiol Ther* 2000;23(2):91-95.

[13] Nelson CF, Bronfort G, Evans R, et al. "The efficacy of spinal manipulation, amitriptyline and the combination of both therapies for the prophylaxis of migraine headache." *J Manipulative Physiol Ther* 1998;21(8):511-519.

[14] Bronfort G, Nilsson N, Haas M, et al. "Non-invasive physical treatments for chronic/recurrent headache." *The Cochrane Database of Systematic Reviews* 2004, Issue 3. Art. No.:CD001878.pub2.

[15] Pothmann R, Danesch U. "Migraine prevention in children and adolescents: results of an open study with a special butterbur root extract." *Headache* 2005;45(3):196-203.

[16] Diener HC, Rahlfs VW, Danesch U. "The first placebo-controlled trial of a special butterbur root extract for the prevention of migraine: reanalysis of efficacy criteria." *Eur Neurol* 2004;51(2):89-97.

[17] Lipton RB, Gobel H, Einhaupl KM, et al. "Petasites hybridus root (butterbur) is an effective preventive treatment for migraine." *Neurology* 2004; 63(12):2240-2244.

[18] Grossman M, Schmidramsl H. "An extract of Petasites hybridus is effective in the prophylaxis of migraine." *Int J Clin Pharmacology Therapeutics* 2000;38(10):430-435.

[19] Johnson ES, Kadam NP, Hylands DM, et al. "Efficacy of feverfew as prophylactic treatment of migraine." *Br Med J* 1985;291:569-573.

[20] Murphy JJ, Heptinstall S, Mitchell JR. "Randomised, double-blind, placebo-controlled trial of feverfew in migraine prevention." *Lancet* 1988;2(8604): 189-192.

[21] Prusinski A, Durko A, Niczyporuk-Turek A. "Feverfew as a prophylactic treatment of migraine." *Neurol Neurochir Pol* 999;33(Suppl 5):89-95.

[22] Palevitch D, Earon G, Carasso R. "Feverfew (*Tanacetum parthenium*) as a prophylactic treatment for migraine: a double-blind placebo-controlled study." *Phytotherapy Res* 1997;11:508-511.

[23] Ernst E, Pittler MH. "The efficacy and safety of feverfew (*Tanacetum parthenium L.*): an update of a systematic review." *Public Health Nutr* 2000; 3(4A):509-514.

[24] Schoenen J, Lenaerts M, Bastings E. "High-dose riboflavin as a prophylactic treatment of migraine: results of an open pilot study." *Cephalalgia* 1994; 14(5):328-329.

[25] Boehnke C, Reuter U, Flach U, et al. "High-dose riboflavin treatment is efficacious in migraine prophylaxis: an open study in a tertiary care centre." *Eur J Neurol* 2004;11(7):475-477.

[26] Schoenen J, Jacquy J, Lenaerts M. "Effectiveness of high-dose riboflavin in migraine prophylaxis. A randomized controlled trial." *Neurology* 1998; 50(2):466-470.

[27] Sandor PS, Afra J, Ambrosini A, et al. "Prophylactic treatment of migraine with beta-blockers and riboflavin: differential effects on the intensity dependence of auditory evoked cortical potentials." *Headache* 2000;40(1):30-35.

[28] Rozen TD, Oshinsky ML, Gebeline CA, et al. "Open label trial of coenzyme Q_{10} as a migraine preventive." *Cephalalgia* 2002;22(2):137-141.

[29] Sandor PS, DiClemente L, Coppola G, et al. "Efficacy of coenzyme Q_{10} in migraine prophylaxis: a randomized controlled trial." *Neurology* 2005;64(4):713-715.

Chapter 18: Osteoarthritis

[1] Berman BM, Lao L, Langenberg P, et al. "Effectiveness of acupuncture as adjunctive therapy in osteoarthritis of the knee." *Ann Intern Med* 2004;141:901-910.

[2] Adapted from Berman BM, Lao L, Langenberg P, et al. "Effectiveness of acupuncture as adjunctive therapy in osteoarthritis of the knee." *Ann Intern Med* 2004;141:901-910.

[3] Vas J, Mendez C, Perea-Milla E, et al. "Acupuncture as a complementary therapy to the pharmacological treatment of osteoarthritis of the knee: randomised controlled trial." *Brit Med J* 2004;329(7476):1216.

[4] Adapted from Vas J, Mendez C, Perea-Milla E, et al. "Acupuncture as a complementary therapy to the pharmacological treatment of osteoarthritis of the knee: randomised controlled trial." *Brit Med J* 2004;329(7476):1216.

[5] Witt C, Brinkhaus B, Jena S, et al. "Acupuncture in patients with osteoarthritis of the knee: a randomised trial." *Lancet* 2005;366(9480):136-143.

[6] Acupuncture. National Institutes of Health Consensus Development Conference Statement. November 3-5, 1997. NIH Consensus Development Program. Accessible at http://consensus.nih.gov/1997/1997Acupuncture107html.htm. Viewed December 30, 2005.

[7] Michel BA, Stucki G, Frey D, et al. "Chondroitins 4 and 6 sulfate in osteoarthritis of the knee: a randomized, controlled trial." *Arthritis Rheum* 2005; 52(3):779-786.

[8] Uebelhart D, Malaise M, Marcolongo R, et al. "Intermittent treatment of knee osteoarthritis with oral chondroitin sulfate: a one-year, randomized, double-blind, multicenter study versus placebo." *Osteoarthritis Cartilage* 2004;12(4):269-276.

[9] Rovetta G, Monteforte P, Molfetta G, et al. "A two-year study of chondroitin sulfate in erosive osteoarthritis of the hands: behavior of erosions, osteophytes, pain and hand dysfunction." *Drugs Exptl Clin Res* 2004;30(1):11-16.

[10] McAlindon TE, LaValley MP, Gulin JP, et al. "Glucosamine and chondroi-tin for treatment of osteoarthritis: a systematic quality assessment and meta-analysis." *JAMA* 2000;283(11):1469-1475.

[11] Leeb BF, Schweitzer H, Montag K, et al. "A metaanalysis of chondroitin sulfate in the treatment of osteoarthritis." *J Rheumatol* 2000;27(1):205-211.

[12] Richy F, Bruyere O, Ethgen O, et al. "Structural and symptomatic efficacy of glucosamine and chondroitin in knee osteoarthritis: a comprehensive meta-analysis." *Arch Intern Med* 2003;163(13):1514-1522.

[13] Pavelka K, Gatterova J, Olejarova M, et al. "Glucosamine sulfate use and delay of progression of knee osteoarthritis: a 3-year, randomized, placebo-controlled, double-blind study." *Arch Intern Med* 2002;162(18):2113-2123.

[14] Bruyere O, Pavelka K, Rovati LC, et al. "Glucosamine sulfate reduces osteoarthritis progression in postmenopausal women with knee osteoarthri-tis: evidence from two 3-year studies." *Menopause* 2004;11(2):138-143.

[15] Muller-Fassbender H, Bach GL, Haase W, et al. "Glucosamine sulfate compared to ibuprofen in osteoarthritis of the knee." *Osteoarthritis Carti-lage* 1994;2(1):61-69.

[16] Herrero-Beaumont G, Roman JA, Trabado MC, et al. "Effects of glucos-amine sulfate on 6-month control of knee osteoarthritis symptoms vs. placebo and acetaminophen: results from the Glucosamine Unum in Die Efficacy (GUIDE) trial." Abstract accessible at http://www.abstractsonline. com/viewer/viewAbstractPrintFriendly.asp?CKey={2E7D5EAF-DE49-41FD-8067-626E44C2CA88}&SKey={58CE22F2-ABD7-467F-8B77-CA16B3EFE 39E}&MKey={F5B9F43A-15A0-467D-8458-5DF32518B4E3}&AKey={AA4 5DD66-F113-4CDD-8E62-01A05F613C0D}. Viewed January 9, 2006.

[17] Matheson AJ, Perry CM. "Glucosamine: a review of its use in the manage-ment of osteoarthritis." *Drugs Aging* 2003;20(14):1041-1060.

[18] McAlindon TE, LaValley MP, Gulin JP, et al. "Glucosamine and chondroi-tin for treatment of osteoarthritis: a systematic quality assessment and meta-analysis." *JAMA* 2000;283(11):1469-1475.

[19] Richy F, Bruyere O, Ethgen O, et al. "Structural and symptomatic efficacy of glucosamine and chondroitin in knee osteoarthritis: a comprehensive meta-analysis." *Arch Intern Med* 2003;163(13):1514-1522.

[20] Hesslink R, Armstrong D, Nagendran MV, et al. "Cetylated fatty acids improve knee function in patients with osteoarthritis." *J Rheumatol* 2002;29(8):1708-1712.

[21] Kraemer WJ, Ratamess NA, Anderson JM, et al. "Effect of a cetylated fatty acid topical cream on functional mobility and quality of life of patients with osteoarthritis." *J Rheumatology* 2004;31:767-774.

[22] Chrubasik S, Thanner J, Kunzel O, et al. "Comparison of outcome measures during treatment with the proprietary *Harpagophytum* extract Doloteffin in patients with pain in the lower back, knee or hip." *Phytomedicine* 2002; 9(3):181-194.

[23] Chantre P, Cappelaere A, Leblan D, et al. "Efficacy and tolerance of Harpagophytum procumbens versus diacerhein in treatment of osteoarthritis." *Phytomedicine* 2000;7(3):177-183.

[24] Gagnier JJ, Chrubasik S, Manheimer E. "*Harpagophytum procumbens* for osteoarthritis and low back pain: A systematic review." *BMC Complementary and Alternative Medicine* 2004;4:13. Accessible at http://www.biomedcentral.com/1472-6882/4/13. Viewed January 11, 2006.

[25] Adapted from Gagnier JJ, Chrubasik S, Manheimer E. "*Harpgophytum procumbens* for osteoarthritis and low back pain: A systematic review." BMC Complementary and Alternative Medicine 2004;4:13 doi:10.1186/1472-6882-4-13. Accessible at http://www.biomedcentral.com/1472-6882/4/13. Viewed January 11, 2006.

[26] Schruffler H. "Salus teufelskralle-tabletten." *Die Medizinische* 1980:22-25.

[27] Lecomte A, Costa JP. "Harpagophytum dans l'arthrose: Etudes en double insu contre placebo." *37°2 Le Magazine* 1992;15:27-30.

[28] Biller A. "Ergebnisse zweier randomisieter kontrollierter." *Phyto-pharmaka* 2002;7:86-88.

[29] Chantre P, Cappelaere A, Leblan D, et al. "Efficacy and tolerance of *Harpagophytum procumbens* versus diacerhein in treatment of osteoarthritis." *Phytomedicine* 2000;7(3):177-183.

[30] Frerick H, Biller A, Schmidt U. "Stufenschema bei coxarthrose." *Der Kassenarzt* 2001;5:34-41.

[31] Maccagno A, DiGiorgio EE, Caston OL, et al. "Double-blind controlled clinical trial of oral S-adenosylmethionine versus piroxicam in knee osteoarthritis." *Am J Med* 1987;83(Suppl 5A):72-77.

[32] Vetter G. "Double-blind comparative clinical trial with S-adenosylmethionine and indomethacin in the treatment of osteoarthritis." *Am J Med* 1987;83(Suppl 5A):78-80.

[33] Najm WI, Reinsch S, Hoehler F, et al. "S-adenosylmethionine (SAMe) versus celecoxib for the treatment of osteoarthritis symptoms: A double-blind cross-over trial." *BMC Musculoskeletal Disorders* 2004;5:6.

[34] Adapted from Najm WI, Reinsch S, Hoehler F, et al. "S-adenosyl methionine (SAMe) versus celecoxib for the treatment of osteoarthritis symptoms: A double-blind cross-over trial." *BMC Musculoskeletal Disorders* 2004;5:6.

[35] Soeken KL, Lee WL, Bausell RB, et al. "Safety and efficacy of S-adenosyl-methionine (SAMe) for osteoarthritis." *J Fam Pract* 2002;51(5):425-430.

[36] Hardy M, Coulter I, Morton SC, et al. "S-adenosyl-L-methionine for treatment of depression, osteoarthritis, and liver disease." Evidence Report/Technology Assessment No. 64. AHRP Publication No. 02-E034. Rockville: MD: Agency for Healthcare Research and Quality. October, 2002.

[37] Harlow T, Greaves C, White A, et al. "Randomised controlled trial of magnetic bracelets for relieving pain in osteoarthritis of the hip and knee." *BMJ* 2004;329:1450-1454.

[38] Adapted from Harlow T, Greaves C. White A, et al. "Randomised controlled trial of magnetic bracelets for relieving pain in osteoarthritis of the hip and knee." *BMJ* 2004;329:1450-1454.

[39] Pipitone N, Scott DL. "Magnetic pulse treatment for knee osteoarthritis: a randomised, double-blind, placebo-controlled study." *Curr Med Res Opin* 2001;17(3):190-196.

[40] Hartman CA, Manos TM, Winter C, et al. "Effects of T'ai Chi training on function and quality of life indicators in older adults with osteoarthritis." *J Am Geriatr Soc* 2000;48(12):1553-1559.

[41] Song R, Lee EO, Lam P, et al. "Effects of tai chi exercise on pain, balance, muscle strength, and perceived difficulties in physical functioning in older women with osteoarthritis: a randomized clinical trial." *J Rheumatol* 2003;30(9):2039-2044.

Chapter 19: Osteoporosis

[1] Passeri M, Biondi M, Costi D, et al. "Effect of ipriflavone on bone mass in elderly osteoporotic women." *Bone Miner* 1992;19(Suppl):S57-S62.

[2] Agnusdei D, Crepaldi G, Isaia G, et al. "A double-blind, placebo-controlled trial of ipriflavone for prevention of postmenopausal spinal bone loss." *Calcif Tissue Int* 1997;61(2):142-147.

[3] Ohta H, Komukai S, Makita K, et al. "Effects of 1-year ipriflavone treatment on lumbar bone mineral density and bone metabolic markers in postmenopausal women with low bone mass." *Horm Res* 1999;51(4):178-183.

[4] Alexandersen P, Toussaint A, Christiansen C, et al. Ipriflavone in the treatment of postmenopausal osteoporosis: a randomized controlled trial. *JAMA* 2001;285(11):1482-1488.

[5] Zhang X, Shu XO, Li H, et al. "Prospective cohort study of soy food consumption and risk of bone fracture among postmenopausal women." *Arch Intern Med* 2005;165(16):1890-1895.

[6] Alekel DL, St. Germain A, Peterson CT, et al. "Isoflavone-rich soy protein isolate attenuates bone loss in the lumbar spine of perimenopausal women." *Am J Clin Nutr* 2000;72:844-852.

[7] Chen YM, Ho SC, Lam SSH, et al. "Soy isoflavones have a favorable effect on bone loss in Chinese postmenopausal women with lower bone mass: A double-blind, randomized, controlled trial." *J Clin Endocrin Metab* 2003; 88(10):4740-4747.

[8] Lydeking-Olsen E, Beck-Jensen JE, Setchell KDR, et al. "Soymilk or progesterone for prevention of bone loss – a 2-year randomized, placebo-controlled trial." *Eur J Nutr* 2004;43(4):246-257.

[9] Shiraki M, Shiraki Y, Aoki C, et al. "Vitamin K2 (menatetrenone) effectively prevents fractures and sustains lumbar bone mineral density in osteoporosis." *J Bone Min Res* 2000;15(3):515-521.

[10] Iwamoto J, Takeda T, Ichimura S. "Effect of menatetrenone on bone mineral density and incidence of vertebral fractures in postmenopausal women with osteoporosis: a comparison with the effect of etidronate." *J Orthop Sci* 2001;6(6)487-492.

[11] Ushiroyama T, Ikeda A, Ueki M. "Effect of continuous combined therapy with vitamin K(2) and vitamin D(3) on bone mineral density and coagulofibrinolysis function in postmenopausal women." *Maturitas* 2002;41(3):211-221.

[12] Jellin JM, Gregory PJ, Batz F, et al. Pharmacist's Letter/Prescriber's Letter Natural Medicines Comprehensive Database. 7th ed. Stockton, CA: Therapeutic Research Faculty; 2005. pg 1300.

[13] Qin L, Au S, Choy W, et al. "Regular Tai Chi Chuan exercise may retard bone loss in postmenopausal women: A case-control study." *Arch Phys Med Rehabil* 2002;83(10):1355-1359.

[14] Chan K, Qin L, Lau M, et al. "A randomized, prospective study of the effects of Tai Chi Chun exercise on bone mineral density in postmenopausal women." *Arch Phys Med Rehabil* 2004;85(5):717-722.

Chapter 20: Pimples

[1] Yihou, X. "Treatment of facial skin diseases with acupuncture. A report of 129 cases." *J Traditional Chinese Med* 1990;10(1):22-25.

[2] Jin L. "Treatment of adolescent acne with acupuncture." *J Traditional Chinese Med* 1993;13(3):187-188.

[3] Thappa DM, Dogra J. "Nodulocystic acne: oral gugulipid versus tetracycline." *J Dermatol* 1994;21(10):729-731.

[4] Adapted from Thappa DM, Dorga J. "Nodulocystic acne: oral gugulipid versus tetracycline." *J Dermatol* 1994;21(10):729-731.

[5] Bassett IB, Pannowitz DL, Barnetson, RS. "A comparative study of tea-tree oil versus benzoyl peroxide in the treatment of acne." *Med J Aust* 1990; 153(8):455-458.

[6] See, for example, Michaelsson G, Ljunghall K. "Patients with dermatitis herpetiformis, acne, psoriasis and Darier's disease have low epidermal zinc concentrations." *Acta Derm Venereol* 1990;70(4):304-308.

[7] Hillstrom L, Pettersson L, Hellbe L, et al. "Comparison of oral treatment with zinc sulphate and placebo in acne vulgaris." *Br J Dermatol* 1977; 97(6):681-684.

[8] Michaëlsson G, Juhlin L, Vahlquist A. "Effects of oral zinc and vitamin A in acne." *Arch Dermatol* 1977;113(1):31-36.

[9] Michaëlsson G, Juhlin L, Ljunghall K. "A double-blind study of the effect of zinc and oxytetracycline in acne vulgaris." *Br J Dermatol* 1977;97(5): 561-566.

Chapter 21: PMS

[1] Habek D, Habek JC, Barbir A. "Using acupuncture to treat premenstrual syndrome." *Arch Gynecol Obstet* 2002;267(1):23-26.

[2] Xu TZ. "Clinical therapeutic effect of point-injection combined with body acupuncture on premenstrual tension syndrome." *Zhongguo Zhen Jiu* 2005;25(4):253-254.

[3] Yu JN, Liu BY, Liu ZS, et al. "Evaluation of clinical therapeutic effects and safety of acupuncture treatment for premenstrual syndrome." *Zhongguo Zhen Jiu* 2005;25(6):377-382.

[4] Acupuncture: Review and Analysis of Controlled Clinical Trials. World Health Organization. 2002. p16. Accessible at http://www.chiro.org/acupuncture/FULL/Acupuncture_WHO_2003. Pdf viewed Sept. 15, 2006.

[5] Schellenberg R, Kunze G, Pfaff ER, et al. "Treatment for the premenstrual syndrome with agnus castus fruit extract: prospective, randomised, placebo-controlled study." *BMJ* 2001;322:134-137.

[6] Adapted from Schellenberg R, et al. "Treatment for the premenstrual syndrome with agnus castus fruit extract: prospective, randomized, placebo-controlled study." *BMJ* 2001;322:134-7.

[7] Loch EG, Selle H, Boblitz N. "Treatment of premenstrual syndrome with a phytopharmaceutical formulation containing *Vitex agnus castus*." *J Womens Health Gend Based Med* 2000;9(3):315-320.

[8] Bendich A. "The potential for dietary supplements to reduce premenstrual syndrome (PMS) symptoms." *J Am Coll Nutr* 2000;19(1):3-12.

[9] Bertone-Johnson ER, Hankinson SE, Bendich A, et al. "Calcium and vitamin D intake and risk of incident premenstrual syndrome." *Arch Intern Med* 2005;165(11):1246-1252.

[10] Thys-Jacobs S, Ceccarelli S, Bierman A, et al. "Calcium supplementation in premenstrual syndrome: a randomized crossover trial." *J Gen Intern Med* 1989;4(3):183-189.

[11] Thys-Jacobs S, Starkey P, Bernstein D, et al. "Calcium carbonate and the premenstrual syndrome: effects on premenstrual and menstrual symptoms." *Am J Obstet Gynecol* 1998;179(2):444-452.

[12] Yakir M, Kreitler S, Brzezinski A, et al. "Effects of homeopathic treatment in women with premenstrual syndrome: a pilot study." *Br Homeopath J* 2001;90(3):148-153.

[13] Jang HS, Lee MS, Kim MJ, et al. "Effects of qi-therapy on premenstrual syndrome." *Int J Neurosci* 2004;114(8):909-921.

[14] Jang HS, Lee MS. "Effects of qi therapy (external qigong) on premenstrual syndrome: a randomized placebo-controlled study." *J Altern Complement Med* 2004;10(3):456-462.

Chapter 22: Prostate Enlargement

[1] Berges RR, Windeler J, Trampisch HF, et al. "Randomized, placebo-controlled, double-blind clinical trial of beta-sitosterol in patients with benign prostatic hyperplasia." Beta-sitosterol Study Group. *Lancet* 1995;345(8964):1529-1232.

[2] Adapted from Berges RR, Windeler J, Trampisch HF, et al. "Randomized, placebo-controlled, double-blind clinical trial of beta-sitosterol in patients with benign prostatic hyperplasia." Beta-sitosterol Study Group. *Lancet* 1995;345(8964):1529-1232.

[3] Klippel KF, Hiltl DM, Schipp B. "A multicentric, placebo-controlled, double-blind clinical trial of beta-sitosterol (phytosterol) for the treatment of benign prostatic hyperplasia." German BPH-Phyto Study group. *Br J Urol* 1997;80(3):427-432.

[4] Wilt TJ, MacDonald R, Ishani A. "Beta-sitosterol for the treatment of benign prostatic hyperplasia: a systematic review." *BJU Int* 1999;83(9): 976-983.

[5] Barlet A, Albrecht J, Aubert A, et al. "Efficacy of *Pygeum africanum* extract in the medical therapy of urination disorders due to benign prostatic hyperplasia: evaluation of objective and subjective parameters. A placebo-controlled double-blind study." *Wien Klin Wochenschr* 1990; 102(22):667-673.

[6] Chatelain C, Autet W, Brackman F. "Comparison of once and twice daily dosage forms of Pygeum africanum extract in patients with benign prostatic hyperplasia: a randomized, double-blind study, with long-term open label extension." *Urology* 1999;54(3):473-478.

[7] Ishani A, MacDonald R, Nelson D, et al. "*Pygeum africanum* for the treatment of patients with benign prostatic hyperplasia: a systematic review and quantitative meta-analysis." *Am J Med* 2000;109(8):654-664.

[8] Andro MC, Riffaud JP. "*Pygeum Africanum* extract for the treatment of patients with benign prostatic hyperplasia: a review of 25 years of published experience." *Curr Therap Res* 1995;56(8):796-817.

[9] Debruyne F, Koch G, Boyle P, et al. "Comparison of a phytotherapeutic agent (Permixon) with an alpha-blocker (Tamsulosin) in the treatment of benign prostatic hyperplasia: a 1-year randomized international study." *Eur Urol* 2002;41(5):497-506.

[10] Carraro JC, Raynaud JP, Koch G, et al. "Comparison of phytotherapy (Permixon) with finasteride in the treatment of benign prostate hyperplasia: a randomized international study of 1,098 patients." *Prostate* 1996;29(4): 231-240.

[11] Champault G, Patel JC, Bonnard AM. "A double-blind trial of an extract of the plant *Serenoa repens* in benign prostatic hyperplasia." *Br J Clin Pharmac* 1984;18:461-462. Letter to the Editor.

[12] Adapted from Champault G, Patel JC, Bonnard AM. "A double-blind trial of an extract of the plant *Serenoa repens* in benign prostatic hyperplasia." *Br J Clin Pharmac* 1984;18:461-462. Letter to the Editor.

[13] Wilt TJ, Ishani A, Stark G, et al. "Saw palmetto extracts for treatment of benign prostatic hyperplasia: a systematic review." *JAMA* 1998;280(18):1604-1609.

[14] Gerber GS. "Saw palmetto for the treatment of men with lower urinary tract symptoms." *J Urol* 2000;163(5):1408-1412.

[15] Boyle P, Robertson C, Lowe F, et al. "Updated meta-analysis of clinical trials of *Serenoa repens* extract in the treatment of symptomatic benign prostatic hyperplasia." *BJU Int* 2004;93(6):751-756.

[16] Wilt T, Ishani A, MacDonald R. "*Serenoa repens* for benign prostatic hyperplasia." The Cochrane Database of Systematic Reviews 2002, Issue 3. Art. No.: CD001423.

[17] Yasumoto R, Kawanishi H, Tsujino T, et al. "Clinical evaluation of long-term treatment using Cernitin pollen extract in patients with benign prostatic hyperplasia." *Clin Ther* 1995;17(1):82-87.

[18] Adapted from Yasumoto R, Kawanishi H, Tsujino T, et al. "Clinical evaluation of long-term treatment using Cernitin pollen extract in patients with benign prostatic hyperplasia." *Clin Ther* 1995;17(1):82-87.

[19] Buck AC, Cox R, Rees RW, et al. "Treatment of outflow tract obstruction due to benign prostatic hyperplasia with the pollen extract, Cernilton. A double-blind, placebo-controlled study." *Br J Urol* 1990; 66(4):398-404.

[20] MacDonald R, Ishani A, Rutks I, et al. A systematic review of Cernilton for the treatment of benign prostatic hyperplasia. *BJU Int* 2000;85(7):836-841.

[21] Schulz V, Hänsel R, Tyler VE. "Rational Phytotherapy: A physicians' guide to herbal medicine." 3rd ed. Berlin: Springer-Verlag; 1998: 231.

Chapter 23: Rheumatoid Arthritis

[1] Ruchkin IN, Burdeinyi AP. "Auriculo-electropuncture in rheumatoid arthritis (a double-blind study)." *Ter Arkh* 1987;59(12):26-30.

[2] Man SC, Baragar FD. "Preliminary clinical study of acupuncture in rheumatoid arthritis." *J Rheumatol* 1974;1(1):126-129.

[3] Adapted from Man SC, Baragar FD. "Preliminary clinical study of acupuncture in rheumatoid arthritis." *J Rheumatol* 1974;1:126-129.

[4] Acupuncture: Review and Analysis on Controlled Clinical Trials. World Health Organization. 2002. p23. Accessible at http://search.who.int/search?ie=utf8& site=default_collection&client=WHO&proxystylesheet=WHO&output= xml_no_dtd&oe=utf8&q=acupuncture+rheumatoid. Viewed August 18, 2006.

[5] Kremer JM, Lawrence DA, Petrillo GF, et al. "Effects of high-dose fish oil on rheumatoid arthritis after stopping nonsteroidal anti-inflammatory drugs." Clinical and immune correlates. *Arthritis Rheum* 1995;38(8): 1107-1114.

[6] Volker D, Fitzgerald P, Major G, et al. "Efficacy of fish oil concentrate in the treatment of rheumatoid arthritis." *J Rheumatol* 2000;27(10):2343-2346.

[7] Berbert AA, Kondo CR, Almendra CL, et al. "Supplementation of fish oil and olive oil in patients with rheumatoid arthritis." *Nutrition* 2005;21(2): 131-136.

[8] Kremer JM. "N-3 fatty acid supplements in rheumatoid arthritis." *Am J Clin Nutr* 2000;71(Suppl):349S-351S.

[9] Oh R. "Practical application of fish oil (n-3 fatty acids) in primary care." *J Am Board Fam Pract* 2005;18:28-36.

[10] MacLean CH, Mojica WA, Morton SC, et al. "Effects of omega-3 fatty acids on lipids and glycemic control in type II diabetes and the metabolic syndrome and on inflammatory bowel disease, rheumatoid arthritis, renal disease, systemic lupus erythematosus, and osteoporosis." Summary. Evidence Report/Technology Assessment No. 89. AHRQ Pub. No. 04-E012-1. Rockville, MD: Agency for Healthcare Research and Quality. March 2004.

[11] Fortin PR, Lew RA, Liang MH, et al. "Validation of a meta-analysis: the effects of fish oil in rheumatoid arthritis." *J Clin Epidemiol* 1995;48(11):1379-1390.

[12] Leventhal LJ, Boyce EG, Zurier RB. "Treatment of rheumatoid arthritis with gamma-linolenic acid." *Ann Intern Med* 1993;119(9):867-873.

[13] Zurier RB, Rossetti RG, Jacobson EW, et al. "Gamma-linolenic acid treatment of rheumatoid arthritis. A randomized, placebo-controlled trial." *Arthritis Rheum* 1996;39(11):1808-1817.

[14] Adapted from Zurier RB, Rossetti RG, Jacobson EW, et al. "Gamma-linolenic acid treatment of rheumatoid arthritis. A randomized, placebo-controlled trial." *Arthritis Rheum* 1996;39(11):1808-1817.

[15] Little C, Parsons T. "Herbal therapy for treating rheumatoid arthritis." Cochrane Database Syst Rev. 2001;(1):CD002948.

[16] Tao X, Younger J, Fan FZ, et al. "Benefit of an extract of *Tripterygium Wilfordii* Hook F in patients with rheumatoid arthritis: a double-blind, placebo-controlled study." *Arthritis Rheum* 2002;46(7):1735-1743.

[17] Cibere J, Deng Z, Lin Y, et al. "A randomized double blind, placebo controlled trial of topical *Tripterygium Wilfordii* in rheumatoid arthritis: reanalysis using logistic regression analysis." *J Rheumatol* 2003;30(3):465-467.

INDEX

Underscored page references indicate tables.

Boldface references indicate illustrations.